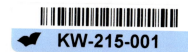
SZYCHER'S DICTIONARY

of

BIOMATERIALS

and

MEDICAL DEVICES

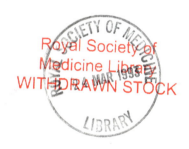
Michael Szycher, Ph.D.

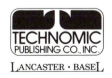
TECHNOMIC
PUBLISHING CO., INC.
LANCASTER · BASEL

1992

Szycher's Dictionary of Biomaterials and Medical Devices

a **TECHNOMIC**® publication

Published in the Western Hemisphere by
Technomic Publishing Company, Inc.
851 New Holland Avenue
Box 3535
Lancaster, Pennsylvania 17604 U.S.A.

Distributed in the Rest of the World by
Technomic Publishing AG

Printed in the United States of America
10 9 8 7 6 5 4 3 2 1

Main entry under title:
   Szycher's Dictionary of Biomaterials and Medical Devices

A Technomic Publishing Company book
Bibliography: p.

Library of Congress Card No. 91-67901
ISBN No. 87762-882-3

HOW TO ORDER THIS BOOK

BY PHONE: 800-233-9936 or 717-291-5609, 8AM-5PM Eastern Time
BY FAX: 717-295-4538
BY MAIL: Order Department
Technomic Publishing Company, Inc.
851 New Holland Avenue, Box 3535
Lancaster, PA 17604, U.S.A.
BY CREDIT CARD: American Express, VISA, MasterCard

CONTENTS

PREFACE

The field of Biomaterials and Medical Devices is not a monolithic field of science.

Biomaterials, by necessity, are an extension of several independent but nonetheless interdependent disciplines, such as polymer chemistry, biochemistry, metallurgy, and organic chemistry.

Since biomaterials are most frequently fabricated into medical devices, other disciplines are interfaced, such as medicine, pharmacology, and physiology. The biomaterials scientist is thus faced with an array of terminology from many fields, which must be understood and assimilated, to better understand and contribute to this new field.

This Dictionary contains many definitions from related disciplines; these definitions are frequently sought by biomaterials scientists in the usual pursuit of research, development, or manufacture of medical devices. Words in small capital letters indicate that further relevant or comparative information is provided in a separate entry. It is our hope to provide a comprehensive reference from related sources, and thus minimize the need for several dictionaries.

SZYCHER'S
DICTIONARY
OF
BIOMATERIALS
AND
MEDICAL DEVICES

A   Symbol for absorbance, activity, ampere, Ångstrom, area, MASS NUMBER.

AAMI   Abbreviation for the *Association for the Advancement of Medical Instrumentation.* An organization with a membership of about 5000 technology developers, users, and managers, who share their knowledge to "improve the development, management, and use of medical technology," by providing standards on equipment safety, performance, development, and use. AAMI sponsors certification programs for health care engineers and technicians.

Abbreviated New Drug Application (ANDA)   A simplified submission permitted for a duplicate of an already approved drug. Intended for products with the same or closely related ingredients, dosage forms, strength, administration route, use, and labeling as a product that has already been shown safe and effective. The ANDA includes information on chemistry and manufacturing controls, but does not have to include data from studies in animals or humans.

Abdomen   The portion of the body lying between the thorax and the pelvis.

Abherent   (1) Any coating or additive that prevents adhesion of a material to itself or to another material. Additives used for this purpose are often called anti-blocking agents or release agents. Fluorocarbons and silicones are widely used to reduce surface friction. (2) A membrane, film, or coating applied to a substrate to prevent or reduce its adhesion to another substrate brought into intimate contact.

Abietic Acid   A major active ingredient of rosin, where it is found in conjunction with other acids. Frequently used as a plasticizer in its many ester derivatives.

Ablation   The layer-by-layer decomposition of resins when heated suddenly to very high temperatures. Ablative materials are used to coat surfaces of rockets and missiles to prevent burnout upon reentry.

1

Ablative Polymers   Polymers that isolate underlying structures by decomposing layer by layer. "Teflon" is able to dissipate heat while decomposing to gases and a porous char.

Abrasion   Gradual erosion of surfaces by physical forces.

Abrasion Cycle   The number of repetitive abrasion motions that a specimen is subjected during an abrasion test.

Abrasion Resistance   The fundamental ability of a material to withstand surface rubbing, erosion, or scraping.

Abrasive   A finely divided, hard substance, capable of smoothing, cleaning, or polishing surfaces of other substrates.

Abrasive Finishing   A method of removing undesired rough edges, flash, gate marks, etc., from molded parts.

ABS   Abbreviation for the terpolymer *Acrylonitrile-Butadiene-Styrene*.

Abscess   Localized collection of pus, usually due to infection.

Absolute   Free from admixtures of other substances, or impurities.

Absolute Specific Gravity   The ratio of the weight of a standard volume of a substance to that of an equal volume of water at the same temperature.

Absolute Temperature   The fundamental temperature scale used in theoretical physics and chemistry, expressed in either degrees Kelvin or Rankine.

Absolute Viscosity   The tangential force per unit area necessary to move one parallel plate a unit distance, when the planes are filled with a specified fluid.

Absorbent   A material capable of incorporating other substances.

Absorption   The penetration of one substance into the bulk of another, by molecular or chemical means.

Absorption Peak   The wavelength of maximal electromagnetic absorption by a substance. Used to identify compounds, elements, or radicals.

ABS Resins   Thermoplastic materials consisting of terpolymers of acrylonitrile, butadiene, and styrene monomers in different proportions. The resins are hard and stiff and not brittle. Used in medical devices where impact resistance, heat resistance, and chemical resistance are important properties being sought.

Accelerated Test   Any test procedure where specified conditions are intensified to theoretically reduce the time required to obtain a given deterioration.

Accelerator   A substance that hastens a chemical reaction, usually in conjunction with a catalyst, or curing agent. Most widely used in curing thermosets and rubbers. Also called *promoters* and *cocatalysts*.

Acetaldehyde CH_3CHO. (ethanal, ethyl aldehyde, acetic aldehyde). A flammable, colorless fluid that reacts with cresol or phenol to form a family of thermosetting resins, or with polyvinyl alcohol to form polyvinyl acetal resins.

Acetal Resins   Acetal resins are polymers, generally referred to as polyoxymethylenes or polyacetals, produced by the addition polymerization of aldehydes through the carbonyl groups. The commercial products are stabilized by the esterification, or transesterification, of the hydroxyl end groups. The acetal resins, trade named "Delrin," "Celcon," etc., are highly crystalline polymers, among the strongest, and stiffest available thermoplastics, and are thus classified as engineering plastics. Acetal resins are not recommended for use in strongly acidic or basic environments.

Acetate   Compounds derived from acetic acid by replacing the acid hydrogen with a metal or radical, so the resultant product contains the acetate radical.

Acetates   Generic name for cellulose acetate resins. Commercially important acetates are cellulose acetate, "acetate rayon," vinyl acetate, and ethyl acetate, used as a solvent.

Acetic Aldehyde   See ACETALDEHYDE.

Acetic Ether   See ETHYL ACETATE.

Acetone CH_3COCH_3. (dimethyl ketone, 2-propanone). The first member in the ketone homologous series of solvents. Cellulosics, PVC, PVAC, PMMA, PVP, epoxy resins, and certain thermosetting resins are all soluble in this important solvent.

Acetone Extraction   A test for phenolic resins, in which the molded or laminated product is immersed in boiling acetone for a specified period of time, to extract acetone-soluble matter.

Acetone Resin   A synthetic resin derived from the reaction of acetone with materials such as phenol or formaldehyde.

N-Acetyl Ethanolamine $CH_3CONHC_2CH_4OH$. (hydroxyethylacetamide). A brown viscous liquid, soluble in alcohol and water. Plasticizer for polyvinyl alcohol and cellulosics; humectant; textile conditioner.

Acetyl Peroxide $(CH_3CO)O_2$. One of a series of peroxide catalysts, widely used to cross-link polymers and silicone rubbers, by the formation of free radicals upon heating.

4-Acetyl Resorcinol $C_6H_3(OH)_2COCH_3$. (2,4 dihydroxyacetophenone). One of a series of acetophenone light stabilizers for polymers. These light stabilizers work by absorbing most of the radiation in the ultraviolet range.

Acetyl Ricinolates   A generic name covering a variety of plasticizers used in many plastic substances.

Acetyl Triallyl Citrate   An important cross-linking agent, used in the peroxide-catalyzed curing of polyester resins to form clear and tough thermosetting resins.

Acetyl Triethyl Citrate   An FDA-approved plasticizer for food contact. Widely used as a plasticizer for cellulosics, particularly ethyl cellulose and polyvinyl acetate resins.

Acetyl Tri-2-Ethylhexyl Citrate   A low-efficiency vinyl plasticizer. Also finds use as a low-compatibility plasticizer for cellulosic resins.

3

Acetyl Value   Defined as the number of milligrams of potassium hydroxide required to neutralize the acetic value liberated by hydrolysis of one gram of an acetylated fat or oil.

Acetylation   Introduction of an acetyl radical (CH_3CO-) into the molecule of an organic compound having OH or NH_2 reactive groups.

Acetylcholine   A derivative of choline important because it acts as the chemical neurotransmitter of nerve impulses in the autonomic nervous system.

Acetylene   A colorless gas with a molecular weight of 26.04. It is a chemical intermediate in the production of vinyl chloride, acrylonitrile, vinyl acetate, and acrylic esters widely used in the manufacture of medical devices.

Acetylene Black   The powdery substance obtained from the incomplete combustion of acetylene. It is used as a colorant in plastics, a reinforcing agent in rubbers, and to impart electrical conductivity to resins.

Acetylene Polymers   See POLYACETYLENES.

Achlorydia   Pathological absence of hydrochloric acid secretion in the stomach.

Acid Acceptor   A compound that acts as a resin stabilizer by chemically combining with protons, which may be initially present in small amounts in the resin or which may be generated by the decomposition of the resin.

Acid Anhydride   An oxide of a nonmetallic element of an organic radical which is capable of forming an acid when united with water, or which can be formed by the abstraction of water from the acid molecule, or which can unite with basic oxides to form salts.

Acid Number   Acid number or acid value is a general term designed to express the degree of acidity of a given substance. See also ACID VALUE.

Acid Value   A general measure of the free acid content of a substance. It is expressed as the number of milligrams of a standard solution of potassium hydroxide neutralized by the free acid present in the sample. This value is frequently used in connection with polyesters and plasticizers, in which the acid value should be as low as possible.

Acid-Base Balance   In medicine, the mechanisms by which acids and alkalies are kept in normal equilibrium. Disturbance of this balance results in ACIDOSIS or alkalosis.

Acidimetry   The determination of the concentration of acid solutions by titration with a standard base solution of known strength.

Acidolysis   The process of reacting an acid with an ester. Also called *ester exchange*, and *trans-esterification*.

Acidosis   A condition in which the acid/base balance of body fluids is disturbed, thereby decreasing the alkaline contents.

Acids   A group of organic or inorganic compounds with a sour taste, which liberate hydrogen when reacted with metals, are capable of neutralizing alkaline compounds, and have pH values less than 7. Inorganic acids such as hydrochloric, nitric, and sulfuric are high-tonnage industrial chemicals. There are several classes of organic acids, including: (1) carboxylic acids (i.e., fatty acids, acetic acid); (2) aromatic acids (i.e., benzoic acid); (3) heterocyclic acids (i.e., pyromucic or furoic acid); (4) amino acids; (5) nucleic acids.

Aciduria   Acid condition of the urine.

Acquired   Any disease or abnormality not present at birth, but developed later in life. The opposite of CONGENITAL.

Acraldehyde   See ACROLEIN.

Acrolein CH_2CHCHO. (acrylic aldehyde, propenal, allyl aldehyde, acraldehyde). A reactive liquid obtained from the oxidation of allyl alcohol or propylene, and frequently used as an intermediate in the production of polyester resins and polyurethanes.

Acrylamide $CH_2CHCONH_2$. A crystalline solid at ambient temperature, capable of rapid polymerization, copolymerization, or cross-linking with other reactants that contain vinyl ligands. Used extensively as a cross-linking agent in hydrogels, adhesives, and coatings.

Acrylate   (1) Any of several monomers used in the manufacture of thermosetting acrylic resins, i.e., 2-hydroxyethyl acrylate (HEA), and hydroxypropyl acrylate (HPA). (2) Polymer of acrylic acid or its esters, used in surface coatings and the synthesis of hydrogels.

Acrylate Resins   See ACRYLIC RESINS.

Acrylic Acid $CH_2CHCOOH$. (acroleic acid, ethylenecarboxylic acid, vinylformic acid, propenoic acid). A colorless, unsaturated acid that polymerizes readily, used in the synthesis of acrylic resins.

Acrylic Aldehyde   See ACROLEIN.

Acrylic Ester   (Acryl Ester). An ester of acrylic acid, or any structural derivative of acrylic acid. These esters are readily polymerizable into high molecular weight acrylic resins.

Acrylic Fiber   Generic name for any manufactured fiber in which the monofilament is composed of at least 85% by weight of acrylonitrile units $-CH_2CH(CN)-$, according to the Federal Trade Commission.

Acrylic Resins   The term "acrylic" is used to designate products obtained from the polymerization of esters of acrylic acid ($H_2C:CHCOOH$), or methacrylic acid [$H_2C:C(CH_3)COOH$]. These acids, their nitriles and esters are all included in this group. The acrylates may be methyl, ethyl, butyl, or 2-ethylhexyl. The methacrylates may be methyl, ethyl, butyl, lauryl, and stearyl. Polymethyl methacrylate is used in those medical devices requiring good transmission of light, low water absorption, dimensional stability, and tensile strengths in the 7000–11,000 psi range.

Acrylonitrile $H_2C:CHCN$. (propenenitrile, vinyl cyanide). An intermediate in the manufacture of acrylic resins, fibers, acrylonitrile-based polymers, nitrile rubbers, and insecticides. This monomer is toxic by inhalation and skin absorption. Medical grade polymers should be free of unreacted acrylonitrile, since it is a known carcinogen.

Acrylonitrile-Butadiene Rubbers (NBR)   An important family of co-polymers, ranging from about 18 to 50% by weight of acrylonitrile in the molecular structure. These rubbers sometimes include a small amount of a third monomer to enhance some property. Originally known by their German names of *Perbunan*, and *Buna-N*.

Acrylonitrile-Butadiene-Styrene Resins   See ABS RESINS.

Acrylonitrile-Styrene Resins   Thermoplastic resins, consisting of copolymers of acrylonitrile and styrene monomers, having the transparency of styrene, but with improved impact and solvent resistance. The polymers are suitable for use in medical devices and food contact.

Activation   The process of rendering a thermoplastic surface more receptive to adhesives, or wetting by aqueous media, by means of chemical treatments, corona discharge, or flame treatment. Generally, increasing the hydrophilicity of a surface increases biocompatibility.

Activator   (1) An agent added to the primary catalyst, or accelerator, to enhance the action of the catalyst in the polymerization process. (2) A metallic oxide that promotes cross-linking in rubber vulcanization, such as ZnO.

Acupuncture   An ancient Chinese system of medicine in which needles are inserted into the body at some three hundred specific points for therapy and anesthesia. Acupuncture needles are usually made of stainless steel, and lately, titanium alloys.

Acute   The quick, sharp onset of a condition such as pain, usually of limited duration.

Addition Polymers   A large family of polymers formed by the simple combination of monomer units, without evolution of low molecular weight by-products, such as water or carbon dioxide. Polyethylene, polystyrene, vinyl, and acrylics are examples of addition polymers.

Additive   Any substance added to polymers to alter certain properties. In the medical device field, these materials are added to biomaterials in small amounts to improve processing characteristics, enhance heat stability, provide antioxidant protection, stabilize polymers against gamma radiation, etc.

Adenosine   An organic compound found in most cells, which unites readily with phosphate ions to form adenosine diphosphate (ADP), and adenosine triphosphate (ATP).

Adhere   To cause two surfaces to be permanently held together by physical or chemical forces.

Adherend   A substrate that is held to another body by an adhesive agent.

Adherometer   An instrument designed to measure the strength of an adhesive bond.

Adhesion   (1) The physicochemical state by which two surfaces are permanently held together by interfacial forces, which may consist of covalent forces, mechanical interlocking, or a combination of both. See also ADHESION, MECHANICAL; ADHESION, SPECIFIC. (2) In medicine, tissues growing together abnormally, following inflammation, injury, or surgery. Medical devices typically "adhere" to the surrounding tissue.

Adhesion, Mechanical   Adhesion between two surfaces in which the adhesive holds the parts together by an interlocking action.

Adhesion, Specific   Adhesion between two surfaces in which the adhesive holds the parts together by covalent or ionic forces.

Adhesive, Cold-Setting   An adhesive capable of hardening (setting) at temperatures below 20°C.

Adhesive, Contact   An adhesive apparently dry to the touch, which is capable of adhering to itself upon the application of minor mechanical pressure.

Adhesive, Dispersion   A two-phase system, in which the adhesive is suspended as small droplets in a liquid.

Adhesive, Foamed   An adhesive whose apparent density has been decreased by the presence of uniformly distributed gaseous cells.

Adhesive, Heat-Activated   An adhesive, dry at room temperature, that is rendered tacky or fluid upon application of heat.

Adhesive, Hot Melt   An adhesive that is applied in a molten state, and is capable of forming a bond upon cooling to a solid state.

Adhesive, Hot-Setting   An adhesive that sets at temperatures at or above 100°C.

Adhesive, Intermediate Temperature-Setting   An adhesive that sets at temperatures between 31°C, and 99°C.

Adhesive, Medical   Below is a listing of medical adhesive applications by polymer type:

TYPE	APPLICATIONS
Rubber-based	Laminations, ostomy devices, drug delivery.
Acrylics	ECG mounts, surgical tape, wound management, IV holddowns, external catheter holders, bone cements, mucoadhesives.
Silicones	Transdermal delivery systems, diagnostic devices, biocompatible systems.
Polyvinyl ether	Moisture-permeable skin patches.
PVP	Ostomy bags, mucoadhesives.
Epoxy	Medical device assemblies.
Urethanes	Sustained release wound dressings, medical device assemblies.

Adhesive, Pressure-Sensitive   A viscoelastic material, which remains permanently tacky, and that is capable of adhering to most solid surfaces, upon the application of minor pressure.

Adhesive, Solvent   An adhesive containing a volatile organic vehicle or rheological agent.

Adhesive, Solvent-Activated   An adhesive, dry at room temperature, that is rendered tacky upon contact with an organic solvent.

Adhesive Tape

Adhesive Tape   A Class I device consisting of a strip of cloth or plastic, coated on one side with an adhesive, and which may include a pad of surgical adhesive dressing without a disinfectant. The device is used to cover and protect wounds, to hold skin edges, to support an injured part, or to secure objects to the skin.

Adhesives   Materials capable of permanently joining one surface to another. Adhesives are widely used in the medical device industry to join a plastic device to another of the same polymer, a different polymer, or a nonplastic material. Adhesives used in these applications can be further classified into five types. (1) A Monomeric adhesive contains a monomer, and a catalyst, so that a bond is produced by polymerization at the adhesive/substrate interface. (2) A Solvent adhesive is one that mutually dissolves the polymers being joined, forming strong intermolecular bonds, prior to solvent vaporization. (3) Bonded adhesives are solvent solutions of polymers, sometimes containing tackifiers and plasticizers, which dry at room temperature. (4) Elastomeric adhesives contain elastomeric polymers dissolved in solvents, or suspended in water (latexes), and are intended to bond at, or near room temperature. (5) Reactive adhesives are those containing partially polymerized resins, and cure with the aid of catalysts or heat, to form a permanent bond.

Adipate Plasticizers   A family of adipate esters widely used to soften vinyl resins. In medical devices, the use of plasticizers should be carefully reviewed, since these additives are known to migrate.

Adiponitrile   NC(CH₂)₄CN. An intermediate used in the synthesis of nylon 66 polymers.

Adrenaline   (epinephrine). A hormone synthesized in the adrenal gland, with a pronounced effect on body metabolism, causing an increase in blood pressure and heart rate.

Adsorbent   A substance that has the ability to hold molecules on its surface. Activated charcoal is used in hemophoresis to cleanse the blood of certain toxins.

Adsorption   Adhesion of an extremely thin layer of molecules to the surface of solids or liquids with which they contact. Adsorption of plasma proteins is believed to be the first event in the coagulation of blood on the surface of biomaterials.

Aerator Cabinet   A Class II device consisting of a cabinet equipped with a ventilator system designed to circulate and exchange the air contained in the cabinet to remove residual ethylene oxide gas following sterilization.

Aerogel   Dispersion of a gas in a solid or a liquid.

Aerosol   Dispersion of a gas in a solid or a liquid, the particles often being in the colloidal size range. Fog and smoke are common examples of natural aerosols. In medicine, a spray used for sterilizing the air, or an atomized solution for inhalation purposes

Affinity   With respect to an adhesive, affinity is an attraction or surface polar similarity between the adhesive and an adherend, resulting in a stronger bond.

Agar   A phycocolloid derived from red algae; it is a polysaccharide mixture of agarose and agaropectin. Used in microbiology (culture medium), pharmaceuticals, and dental impressions.

Agglomeration   Combination or aggregation of colloidal particles suspended in a liquid into clusters of approximately spherical shape. Many diagnostic procedures depend on agglomeration or flocculation of particles as the primary response.

Agglutination   The combination or aggregation of particles of matter under the influence of a specific protein. The term is restricted to antigen-antibody reactions characterized by a clumping together of visible cells, such as bacteria or erythrocytes.

Agglutinin   An antibody directed toward surface antigens and capable of causing agglutination.

Agglutinin Adsorption   The removal of some antibodies in an antiserum by reaction with the cellular antigen.

Aggregation   A general term describing the tendency of large molecules or colloidal particles to combine into large clusters, especially in aqueous solution. Included in this term are the more specific terms such as AGGLUTINATION, COAGULATION, FLOCCULATION, AGGLOMERATION, and coalescence.

Agitator   Any rotating device that induces motion in fluid mixtures over a range of viscosities, thereby causing uniform dispersion of mixed components.

AIDS   (Acquired Immune Deficiency Syndrome). An autoimmune disease where the Human Immunodeficiency Virus (HIV) attacks the T-4 lymphocytes, thus severely limiting the host's ability to combat infections. In the U.S., AIDS was first described on June 5, 1981 by the Centers for Disease Control's Morbidity and Mortality Weekly Report describing a mysterious and deadly disease in otherwise healthy homosexual men. In the U.S., the number of AIDS cases has increased from 372 in 1981 to about 172,000 in 1991, and is projected to soar to 435,000 by 1993. Once a disease of whites, barely half of the 1991 caseload nationwide is white; 37 percent is black and 17 percent is hispanic. About 12 percent of AIDS cases are women. In 1990 nearly 1000 children were infected with the virus from birth.

Albumin   A protein normally found in circulating blood; when found in urine, it is usually indicative of a number of diseases.

Alcohol, Absolute   Ethyl alcohol that has been rendered anhydrous by distillation, and containing in excess of 99.9% pure alcohol.

Alcohol, Denatured   Ethyl alcohol to which certain denaturants have been added to adapt it to industrial uses and at the same time render it unfit for human consumption.

Alcohols   Classes of organic compounds where one or more hydroxyl (OH) groups are present in a hydrocarbon molecule, with no more than one hydroxyl group attached to a single carbon atom.

Alcoholysis　(1) The chemical process of reacting an alcohol with an ester. (2) A chemical reaction between an alcohol and another organic compound, analogous to hydrolysis. See also ESTER EXCHANGE.

Aldehydes　Members of a class of organic compounds characterized by the carbonyl group ($-CO-$), which is attached to a terminal carbon atom. The name aldehyde is derived from the fact that members of this family can be obtained when primary ALcohols are DEHYDrogenatEd either by dehydrogenation or oxidation reactions.

Aldol　(acetaldol; beta-hydroxybutyraldehyde). A clear to yellow syrupy liquid, used in the synthesis of accelerators, drugs, and synthetic polymers.

Aldol Condensation　A reaction between two aldehyde or two ketone molecules in which the position of one of the hydrogen atoms is changed in such a way as to form a single molecule having one hydroxyl and one carbonyl group.

Aldosterone　An adrenal minerolocortical steroid hormone. Probably the chief regulator of sodium, potassium, and chlorine metabolism.

Algesimeter　A Class I device designed to determine a patient's sensitivity to pain after using an anesthetic agent.

Alginates　Derivatives of alginic acid (e.g., calcium, sodium, or potassium salts). Used as thickeners, emulsifying agents, and film-formers by the pharmaceutical industry, and as first-aid dressings.

Aliphatic　Organic compounds characterized by open-chain structures, whose molecules do not have their carbon atoms arranged in a ring structure; contrasted with these are aromatic compounds, such as benzene, which have ring structures. Aliphatic compounds are named from the Greek aleiphar, which means fat or oil.

Alkali Resistance　The important characteristic of many plastic materials to resist the corrosive effects of strong bases.

Alkyd　A generic term used in conjunction with polyester resins. See also POLYESTER, MOLDING COMPOUNDS.

Alkyd Resins　See POLYESTER.

Alkyl　A general term for monovalent aliphatic hydrocarbon radicals, which have been derived from an alkane by removing one hydrogen from the formula. Contrast with corresponding aromatic radicals, which are known as ARYL.

Alkylene Oxide Polymers　See EPOXIDES.

Allergic　Subject to exaggerated or pathological reaction to substances that are without comparable effect on the average individual.

Allobar　Different forms of an element having different atomic weights, and therefore isotopic compositions.

Allomerism　A similarity in crystalline form between polymers with different chemical compositions. See also POLYALLOMERS.

Alloy　Synergistic polymer combinations with property advantages derived from a high level of thermodynamic compatibility between components. Alloys exhibit strong intermolecular forces and form single-phase systems with unique glass transition temperatures. The most significant commercial alloys are the styrene-modified polyphenylene oxides. Polymer blends, by comparison, have less intense thermodynamic compatibility than alloys, and thus result in less advantageous physical properties.

Allyl Alcohol CH_2CHCH_2OH. A transparent liquid widely used in the manufacture of plasticizers.

Allyl Diglycol Carbonate Resins   Thermosetting resins with outstanding optical clarity; frequently used in the manufacture of lenses. The resins are made by reacting the monomer of the same name with catalysts, such as diisopropyl peroxy carbonate, to yield materials with good abrasion resistance and good mechanical properties.

Allyl Resins   Polymers formed by the addition polymerization of compounds containing the group $(-CH_2:CHCH_2-)$. Allyl resins and monomers, of which diallyl phthalate is the best known, are premium materials noted for their unusual chemical and water-resistant characteristics, and their ability to maintain these properties under severe environmental conditions. The monomers and partial polymers are cured with peroxide catalysts to thermosetting resins; molding compounds are frequently reinforced with glass fibers.

Alpha   A prefix, denoting the location of a substituting group of atoms in the main group of a compound.

Alpha Olefins   A sub-group within the olefin family of unsaturated hydrocarbons of the general formula C_nH_{2n}, in which the number of carbons ranges from 5 to 20.

Alternating Copolymer   A copolymer in which the two monomeric units that comprise the chain alternate in a repeating, predictable fashion, such as $-A-B-A-B$.

Amalgam   A mixture or alloy of mercury with any of a number of metals or alloys, including tin, zinc, gold, and silver. Dental amalgams are mixtures of mercury with a silver-tin alloy, used in dental fillings.

Ambient   Completely surrounding a specimen. Indicative of the surrounding environmental conditions around a specimen, such as temperature, pressure, etc.

Ambient Temperature   The temperature of the environment surrounding a specimen. Frequently used to denote normal, prevailing room temperature of 23°C.

Amide   Organic compounds containing a $-CONH_2$ group. Closely associated to the organic acids with the $-COOH$ group. Examples of amides are acetamide and urea.

Amino   (amido). A prefix denoting the presence of an $-NH_2$ or $-NH$ group.

Amino Acids   (1) Naturally occurring organic acids characterized by the presence of a carboxyl and an amino group linked to the same carbon atom. (2) A substance formed during the digestive breakdown of proteins. (3) May be considered as the monomers that form the carbon skeleton of proteins. (4) Of the more than 80 amino acids known, only about 25 have been clearly established as protein constituents.

Amino Acids, Essential   The 10 essential amino acids that cannot be synthesized at all or in sufficient quantity in the body are: Arginine, Histidine, Isoleucine, Leucine, Lysine, Methionine, Phenylalanine, Threonine, Tryptophan, and Valine.

Amino Resins   (polyalkylene amides). A generic term identifying a heterogenous family of amino-rich polymers. The amino-bearing material is prereacted with formaldehyde to form a reactive monomer, which is subsequently polymerized by a polycondensation reaction, to produce cross-linked structures.

Aminoplasts   A term denoting thermosetting resins obtained from the condensation reaction of formaldehyde with amino groups in compounds such as urea and melamine. The best known aminoplasts are urea-formaldehyde and melamine-formaldehyde, used for their ability to form cross-linked, thermosetting structures.

Amorphous   Devoid of molecular crystallinity, stratification, or interchain orientation. Many polymers are amorphous at processing temperatures, some retaining this state at room temperature, such as ABS, Polycarbonate, Polysulfone, and Polyarylate. Amorphous polymers are generally clear, as opposed to crystalline polymers, which are generally opaque.

Ampholyte   Substance that can ionize to form either anions or cations, and thus may act as an acid or a base. Water is an ampholyte.

Amphoteric   Substances having the capacity to behave either as acids or bases. Amino acids are proteins that are amphoteric, i.e., their molecules contain both an acid group (COOH) and a basic group (NH$_2$).

Amyl Esters   Esters derived from amyl alcohol, OHC$_5$H$_{11}$, used as solvents and plasticizers for cellulosics, vinyls, acrylics, etc. Included are: amyl acetate, amyl formate, amyl oleate.

Anaerobic   Descriptive of (1) a chemical reaction, or (2) a microorganism that does not require the presence of air or oxygen. It also applies to certain polymers that solidify when kept out of contact with air.

Analgesic   A pharmacoactive substance capable of reducing or eliminating pain.

Anaphylatoxins   Low molecular weight, biologically active peptides defined by their activity on small blood vessels, smooth muscle, mast cells, and peripheral leukocytes.

Anaphylaxis   A severe form of allergic (hypersensitive) reaction to a substance. It can be fatal if not treated immediately.

Anastomosis   A communication between blood vessels and a synthetic vascular prosthesis by surgical means, i.e., abdominal aorta and femoral artery.

Anesthesia, Methods   To induce unconsciousness by general anesthesia, the agent may be administered so it reaches the brain via the blood stream. This can be performed in different ways. In inhalation anesthesia, gaseous anesthetic agents are introduced via the lungs. Examples: diethyl ether, chloroform, cyclopropane, halothane, methoxyflurane, and nitrous oxide. In intravenous anesthesia, the agent is injected directly into the blood, with the most commonly used agents being the barbiturates, often combined with some form of inhalation anesthesia. Rectal anesthesia is the third way, accomplished by placing the agent in the rectum where it is absorbed by the mucous membranes.

Anesthetics   Agents that cause a general or localized loss of feeling or sensation.

Angina   A sensation of choking or extreme pressure, caused by insufficient oxygen reaching the heart muscle.

Angioscope   A modified microscope for studying the capillary vessels.

Angiostomy   An artificial opening into an artery in the operation prior to an implantation.

Angstrom Unit   A unit of length. An Angstrom is one hundred millionth of a centimeter. Molecular distances are frequently expressed in Angstroms.

Anhydride   A chemical compound derived from an acid by elimination of a molecule of water.

Anhydrous   Descriptive of an inorganic compound that does not contain water, either adsorbed on its surface, or combined as water of crystallization. Not to be confused with ANHYDRIDE.

Aniline Formaldehyde Resins   Members of the aminoplasts family, made by the polycondensation of formaldehyde and aniline in an acid solution. See also AMINOPLASTS.

Aniline Resins   See ANILINE FORMALDEHYDE RESINS; AMINO RESINS.

Anion   An atom, molecule, or radical that has become electronegative by accepting an electron.

Anion Exchange Resins   See ION EXCHANGE RESINS.

Anisotropy   The tendency of a material to react differently to stresses applied in different directions. Medical devices are sometimes manufactured to match the natural anisotropy of skin or blood vessels.

Annealing   The physical process of relieving internal stresses in a polymer by heating below softening temperatures, and maintaining this temperature for a predetermined period of time. Annealing can be summarized as slow crystallization by heat treatment without large-scale melting. Annealing improves those properties of a given thermoplastic material that would normally be associated with high crystallinity.

Anti-Foaming Agents   Additives that reduce the surface tension of an aqueous solution or emulsion, thereby inhibiting or preventing the formation of foam. Silicone anti-foams are used during hemodialysis to reduce frothing and foaming of blood.

Anti-Gelling Agent   An additive that prevents a solution from forming a gel.

Antibacterial   A drug that counteracts, inhibits, or destroys bacteria. See also BIOCIDES.

Antiblocking Agents   Additives incorporated into polymers to reduce their tendency to stick during processing, storage, or use. Synthetic waxes and silicone oils are examples of antiblocking agents used in medical polymers.

Antibodies   Any one of the globulins that combine specifically with antigens and neutralize toxins. Globulins are complex substances produced by the body for defense against disease-causing microorganisms and antigens that have gained entry into the body.

Anticoagulant   A complex organic compound, often a carbohydrate, that has the property of retarding the clotting or coagulation of blood. Surfaces of vascular catheters are sometimes coated with anticoagulants to improve hemocompatibility.

Antifungal   A substance that counteracts the effects of fungal organisms that cause infections of the skin, mucous membranes, etc.

Antigen   Any substance that is capable of inducing the formation of antibodies.

Antimicrobial   See ANTIBACTERIAL.

Antioxidant   A substance capable of inhibiting the tendency of polymers to undergo oxidation when exposed to oxygen at normal or elevated temperatures. Antioxidants are most frequently used in conjunction with oxidation-susceptible polymers such as polyolefins, ABS, acetals, and polyurethanes.

Antiozonant   A substance added to polymers to retard or prevent deterioration caused by continuous exposure to an atmosphere containing ozone gas.

Antiseptic   A germicide that is used on skin or living tissue for the purpose of inhibiting or destroying microorganisms. This term is frequently confused with disinfectant, which is a germicide used solely to destroy microorganisms on inanimate objects. An antiseptic germicide is used on or in living tissue.

Apparent Density   The weight per unit volume of a material, including all voids inherent in the material as tested. Used in connection with powders, granules, pellets, etc. See also BULK FACTOR.

Aromatic Compound   An important class of organic compounds characterized by an unsaturated ring of carbon atoms. Most of the ring compounds are related to benzene (C_6H_6), or its derivatives. The name is associated with the penetrating odor of the first few compounds isolated; this odor was described as "aromatic." This classification, however, is no longer limited to an odor or type of odor.

Aromatic Hydrocarbon   A hydrocarbon containing one or more six-carbon rings, and having properties similar to benzene. This large family of compounds includes many plastics solvents.

Arrhenius Principle   This principle is concerned with chemical reaction rates, stating that in general for every 10°C (18°F) rise in temperature, the first-order chemical reaction doubles, and vice versa. The Arrhenius equation has the form:

$$k = Ae^{-E/RT} \text{ where}$$

A = proportionality constant
e = base for natural logarithms
E = activation energy
T = absolute temperature

Examples of procedures that utilize the Arrhenius aging techniques are: ASTM D-3045 heat aging of plastics without load; and ASTM D-2990 tensile, compressive, flexural creep, and creep rupture of plastics.

Arrythmia Detector   A Class III device, it is a system that monitors the electrocardiogram, and is designed to produce a visible or audible signal when an arrythmia is encountered.

Arterial Blood Sampler   A Class II device used to obtain arterial blood and determine the concentration of dissolved gases. The kit usually includes a syringe, needle, cork, and heparin.

Arteriography   Radiographic study of part of the arterial system to diagnose disturbances of blood supply. Modern arteriography depends on polymer-based blood-compatible catheters.

Artificial Embolization Device   A Class III device that is placed in blood vessels to permanently obstruct blood flow to an aneurysm or other vascular malformation.

Aryl   A compound whose molecules have the ring structure characteristic of benzene, naphthalene, phenanthrene, etc. An aryl group may be phenyl (C_6H5-), or naphthyl ($C_{10}H9-$).

Asepsis   The continued exclusion of harmful or undesirable microorganisms. Thus, the culturing of cells in vitro is carried out aseptically. The medium is sterilized to remove all living organisms, and then inoculated with the required cell structure. The system is no longer sterile, but aseptic, as no unwanted organisms are present. See also ANTISEPTIC, DISINFECTION.

Aseptic   A substance that kills microorganisms and sterilizes the area to which it is applied, rendering it sterile.

Assay   In modern terminology, an analysis for only a certain constituent or constituents of a mixture, while all others are intentionally neglected.

A-Stage Resin   An early phase in the reaction of certain thermosetting resins in which the material is still soluble in solvents, and fusible. See also B-STAGE RESIN and C-STAGE RESIN.

ASTM   Abbreviation for *American Society for Testing and Materials*, a nonprofit corporation organized in 1898, that is one of the world's leaders in the development of voluntary standards for materials, products, systems, and services. ASTM publishes over 8500 standards in diverse fields such as medical devices, plastics, biotechnology, etc. ASTM's membership of 32,000, of which 4000 are international members, is organized into 134 different technical committees that do the actual work of writing standards. Committee members voluntarily contribute their time and effort.

ASTM Consensus Standards   ASTM defines a standard as "a rule for an orderly approach to a specific activity, formulated and applied for the benefit and with the cooperation of all concerned." ASTM Consensus Standards are accepted rules of behavior developed by democratic procedures. ASTM has developed five different types of full consensus standards. They are:

(1) *Standard Test Method*—a definitive procedure for the identification, measurement, and evaluation of qualities, characteristics, or properties of a material, product, system, or service that produces a test result.

(2) *Standard Specification*—a precise statement of a set of requirements to be satisfied by a material, product, system, or service that also indicates the procedures for determining whether each of the requirements is satisfied.

(3) *Standard Practice*—a definitive procedure for performing one or more specific operations or functions that does not produce a test result.

(4) *Standard Guide*—offers a series of options or instructions, but does not recommend a specific course of action.

(5) *Standard Classification*—a systematic arrangement or division of materials, products, systems, or services into groups based on similar characteristics such as origin, composition, properties, or use.

Asymmetry   A molecular arrangement in which a particular carbon atom is covalently joined to four different groups.

Atactic   Pertaining to an arrangement that is more or less random.

Atactic Polymers   Polymers with molecular backbones in which pendant groups are arranged randomly, above and below the main carbon chain, when the latter are arranged so as to be coplanar. The opposite of stereospecific polymers.

Ataxiagraph   A Class I device used to determine the extent of ataxia (failure of muscular coordination) by measuring the swaying of the body when the patient is standing erect and with closed eyes.

Atom   The smallest possible unit of an element, comprised of a nucleus containing one or more protons and (except hydrogen) two or more neutrons, and one or more electrons that revolve around it.

Atomic Absorption Spectroscopy   An analytical method for the determination of certain elements in a sample. The sample is first converted into an atomic vapor so that elements exist mostly as neutral atoms in the ground state. In this state, each specific element in the atomic vapor absorbs a characteristic monochromatic resonance radiation, leading to a fingerprint indicative of the presence and quantity of each element in the sample.

ATR-FTIR (Attenuated Total Reflectance – FTIR Spectroscopy). ATR-FTIR is a variation of Fourier Transform Infrared Spectroscopy used to obtain infrared spectra of surfaces and to perform depth profiling. Surface characterization in the range of 0.3 to 4.0 microns may be performed on flat samples. See also FTIR.

Audit (Regulatory). A documented activity performed in accordance with written procedures on a periodic basis to verify, by examination and evaluation of objective evidence, compliance with those elements of the quality assurance program under review.

Autoclave (1) A pressure vessel with a door, widely used to sterilize medical devices, surgical instruments, etc. (2) An apparatus in which devices may be sterilized by air-free saturated steam at temperatures in excess of 100°C. Water is heated in a closed system to generate steam temperatures suitable for sterilization at about 121°C.

Autoimmune Diseases An abnormal state where a confused immune system attacks the ''self'' of the body instead of the ''nonself'' of invading microorganisms. The most common autoimmune diseases are: Graves' Disease (antibodies attack thyroid gland); Insulin-Dependent Diabetes Mellitus (T cells attack insulin-producing pancreatic cells); Multiple Sclerosis (T cells attack sheaths around nerve cells); Myasthenia Gravis (antibodies attack neuromuscular junctions); Psoriasis (T cells attack skin); Reiter's Syndrome (T cells attack tissues in eyes, joints, and genital tract); Rheumatic Fever (antibodies attack heart muscle); Rheumatoid Arthritis (T cells attack joints); Systemic Lupus Erythematosus (widespread antibody attack affects joints, skin, kidneys, and other organs).

Autooxidation A spontaneous, self-catalyzed oxidation occurring in the presence of air; it usually involves a free-radical mechanism. Seen in the degradation of high polymers exposed to gamma radiation, UV exposure for prolonged periods, etc.

Average Molecular Weight The average molecular weight of the chains of a polymer, independent of the specific chain length. The value falls between weight average and number average molecular weight.

Azeotrope See AZEOTROPIC MIXTURE.

Azeotropic Distillation A type of distillation in which a substance is added to the mixture to be separated in order to form an azeotropic mixture. The azeotrope thus formed will have boiling points different from the boiling points of the original mixture and will permit greater ease of separation.

Azeotropic Mixture A liquid mixture of two or more substances that behaves like a single substance by forming constant boiling mixtures.

Azobisformamide An aliphatic azo compound widely used as a blowing agent in PVC, polystyrene, and many other polymers.

B

B   Chemical symbol for the element barium. Abbreviation for *Base*.

Bacillus   A rod-shaped bacteria.

Back Pressure   The resistance of heated plastic material to forced flow.

Bacteremia   The presence of viable bacteria in blood. Contaminated medical devices implanted in blood may cause bacteremia.

Bacteria, Saprophytic   (Necrobacteria). A heterogenous class of bacteria that live by ingesting dead organic matter. Saprophytic bacteria may be found around heavily infected medical devices, where they live on any necrotic tissue surrounding the implant.

Bactericide   A chemical agent capable of destroying bacteria, especially those causing disease.

Bacteriostat   A chemical agent that when incorporated into a plastics compound prevents or retards the growth of bacteria on the surfaces of formed products. Ex: quaternary ammonium salts and hexachlorophene.

Bacterium   A procaryotic microorganism. Responsible for many human diseases. Found in the form of rods (bacilli), spheres (cocci) or, spiral structures.

Ball Rebound Test   A method for determining the elastic response of polymeric materials by measuring the energy absorbed when a steel ball impacts the material. The ball is dropped from a fixed height, and the rebound height measured; the difference between the two heights indicates the energy absorbed. The more elastic the polymer, the greater the rebound height.

Ball Viscometer   A viscometer that employs solid spheres of specified weight and diameter as the shearing mechanism.

Ballistocardiograph   A Class II device, including a supporting structure on which a patient is placed, that moves in response to blood ejected from the heart. The device usually includes a visual display.

Banbury Mixers   A mixing machine consisting of two counter-rotating spiral blades encased in segments of cylindrical housings, intersecting so as to leave a ridge between the blades. Banbury mixers are frequently used for compounding solid radiopacifiers into biomaterials.

Bandage, Elastic   A Class I device consisting of either a long flat strip or a tube of elasticized material used to support or compress a part of the body.

Bandage, Liquid   A Class I device composed of a sterile liquid used to cover an opening in the skin, or as a dressing for burns.

Barrel   The tubular portion of an extruder, where mixing, heating, and plastication of the polymer takes place.

Barrier Resin   A crystalline resin used to prevent moisture or gas diffusion. The chief factors involved are polarity, crystallinity, and degree of cross-linking.

Base   A compound with one or more of the following: bitter taste, slippery feeling in solution, ability to turn litmus blue, and ability to react (neutralize) acids to form salts.

Basement Membrane   A thin, amorphous, sheetlike structure found underneath epithelial cells in skin and other organs. The basement membrane varies widely in thickness depending on site, and contains several distinct layers. Closest to the cells is the lamina lucida, a layer of sparse 10-nm fibrils running perpendicular to the cell surface. Closest to the connective tissue is the lamina fibroreticularis, consisting of loose and thin fibrils. Sandwiched between these two layers is the lamina densa, mostly amorphous in appearance, but occasionally composed of thin microfibrils running parallel to the cell surface. Together the lamina densa and the lamina lucida are referred to as the basal lamina. See also COLLAGENS, BASEMENT MEMBRANES.

Basement Membrane Components   The following is a list of all known basement membrane components, including those of the epidermal-dermal junction.

MACROMOLECULE	CHAIN STRUCTURE	ROLE IN BASEMENT MEMBRANE
Bullous pemphigoid	An	Unknown
Laminin	AB_1B_2	Cell-substrate attachment
Type IV collagens	Heteropolymer	Tissue support
Heparain sulfate	Sulfated GAG	Permeability barrier
Fibronectin	Dimers	Cell attachment
Entactin	Unknown	Unknown

Batch   A manufactured unit, or a blend of multiple units of the same formulation and processing.

Benzaldehyde   (benzoic aldehyde, Oil of Bitter Almonds). A solvent used in conjunction with polyester and cellulosics.

Benzalkonium Chloride   A mixture of alkyl dimethylbenzylammonium chlorides. Used as an antiseptic, fungicide, and cationic detergent.

Benzene   (benzol). C_6H_6. A solvent and intermediate in the production of phenolics, epoxies, styrene, and nylon. Hydrogenation of benzene produces cyclohexane, a solvent and raw material for preparing adipic acid, which is in turn, a reactant in the synthesis of nylon. In medical devices benzene is rarely used since it is a carcinogen.

Benzene Ring   The six carbon atoms forming a closed hexagon in the benzene molecule.

Benzofuran Resins   See COUMARONE-INDENE RESINS.

Benzoic Acid C_6H_5COOH. (carboxybenzene, benzenecarboxylic acid, phenylformic acid). A crystalline substance found in benzoin gum, used in the manufacture of benzoate plasticizers, polyethylene glycol, and benzophenone UV absorbers.

Benzophenone   (diphenyl ketone). A UV absorber and plasticizer for cellulosic esters.

Benzoyl Peroxide   A catalyst used in the polymerization of styrene, vinyl, and acrylic resins. A free radical cross-linking agent frequently used in the cure of medical-grade silicone elastomers.

Beta   (1) A prefix, usually abbreviated as the Greek letter β, denoting the location of a substituting group of atoms in the main group of a compound. (2) A type of radiation.

Beta Gauge   Device used for continuously measuring the thickness of plastic films, sheets, or shapes without making physical contact. The apparatus consists of a source of beta rays, and a detecting element.

Beta Particle   A particle created at the instant of emission from a radioactive atomic nucleus. A negatively charged beta particle is identical to an ordinary electron.

Bi   Prefix meaning two; exceptions are bicarbonate, bisulfate, and bitartrate, in which it indicates the presence of hydrogen in the molecule.

Bile acid   Steroids found in bile, having a hydroxyl group, and a five-carbon atom side chain terminating in a carboxyl group. Cholic acid is the most important bile acid in human bile.

Bilirubin   Red coloring matter of bile. Also occurs in blood serum as a decomposition product of hemoglobin. Some devices implanted in blood are stained green/yellow by bilirubin absorption.

Binary   Descriptive of a system containing two, and only two components.

Binder   (1) An adhesive material used for holding particles of dry substances together. (2) The important component of an adhesive formulation that is primarily responsible for the adhesive forces that hold two surfaces together.

Bio   The Greek suffix meaning life.

Bioactive Material   A material that has been specifically designed to elicit a desired biological activity.

Bioadhesion   The temporary or permanent bonding of cells and/or tissue to the surface of a material.

Bioadsorbable/Soluble Polymers   Biomedical polymers that are bioadsorbable or water-soluble include:

- Poly(lactic acid/glycolic acid)
- Poly(amino acids)
- Poly(hydroxybutyrate)
- Poly(caprolactones)
- Poly(oxyethylene glycolate)
- Poly(alkylene oxalates)
- Poly(ethylene oxide)
- Albumin (cross-linked)
- Collagen (cross-linked)
- Poly(anhydrides)
- Poly(orthoesters)

Bioassay   The determination of the potency or concentration of a compound by its effect upon animals, isolated tissue, cultured cells, or microorganisms, compared to a standard (control) preparation.

Bioattachment   The temporary or permanent bonding of cells and/or tissue to the surface of a material due to mechanical interlocking.

Bioavailability   Rate and extent to which a drug is absorbed or is otherwise available to the treatment site in the body.

Biocatalyst   See ENZYME.

Biocides   Agents incorporated into, or coated onto, the surfaces of plastics to kill or inhibit the growth of microorganisms such as bacteria, molds, and fungi. Some plastics, i.e., acetals, acrylics, epoxies, phenoxies, ABS, nylons, polycarbonate, polyesters, fluorocarbons, and polystyrene are naturally resistant to attack by microorganisms. Many other plastics, under some circumstances, are affected by the growth of these organisms on their surfaces. Biocidal agents include chlorinated hydrocarbons, organometallics, halogen-releasing compounds, quaternary ammonium compounds, etc.

Biocompatibility   The inherent ability of a material to appropriately interact with the host in a specific application. Biocompatibility may be further subdivided into: (1) Hemocompatibility, (2) Histocompatibility, and (3) Osteocompatibility.

Biocompatibility Testing   There are three reasons for biocompatibility testing: (1) To identify any adverse reactions that may lead to failure, or which may contribute to unacceptable clinical outcome; (2) To determine if devices constructed of new materials or processes function as intended under simulated use conditions; (3) To advance new technology.

Biocompatible Carbons   Pyrolytic carbon, glassy carbon, carbon fibers, and carbon composites used to enhance the biocompatibility of prostheses.

Biocompatible Ceramics/Glass/Glass Ceramics   High-density alumina, calcium phosphates, aluminum calcium phosphorous oxide ceramics, bioactive glasses, and bioactive glass ceramics.

Biocompatible Surface Modifiers   Coatings and surface derivatizations to control tissue adhesion, reduce drag, improve hemocompatibility, and increase bacterial resistance. They can act as immobilizing agents for chemotherapy. Examples: silicones, hydrogels, glow-discharged PTFE, long-chain alkyl groups, PEO groups, anticoagulants, thrombolytic agents, anti-platelet agents, antibiotics, and various enzymes.

Biodegradability   In general, the susceptibility of a substance to decomposition by a living body or microorganism.

Biodegradation   In the context of medical devices, (1) the rate at which certain polymers are depolymerized and absorbed within the human body, i.e., the biodegradation of resorbable sutures made of poly(lactic/glycolic) acid; (2) the undesirable degradation of polymers by enzymatic action following surgical implantation.

Biodeterioration   The degradation of polymers, which results from the

21

action on the material by all living forms, e.g., bacteria, fungi, insects, and rodents.

Bioengineering   See BIOMEDICAL ENGINEERING.

Bioequivalence   Scientific basis on which generic and brand-name drugs are compared. To be considered bioequivalent, the bioavailability of two products must not differ significantly when given in studies at the same dosage, under similar conditions.

Bioequivalence Requirement   A requirement imposed by the FDA for in vitro and/or in vivo testing of specified drug products, which must be satisfied prior to marketing.

Bioequivalent Drug Products   Pharmaceutic equivalents or alternatives that are *not* significantly different with respect to rate and extent of absorption when administered at the same molar dose under similar experimental conditions. Some drugs may be considered pharmaceutic equivalents that are equal in extent of absorption but not in rate; this is possible when differences in absorption rate are considered clinically insignificant. Example: aspirin and acetaminophen are well-absorbed drugs, and small differences in the rate of absorption are of very little clinical consequence.

Bioethics   An interdisciplinary science established in 1971, encompassing the ethical and social issues resulting from advances in medicine and the biomedical sciences.

Bioimplant   Term denoting a prosthesis made of biosynthetic material.

Bioinstrument   A sensor or device attached to or implanted in the human body to record and transmit physiological data to a receiving and monitoring station.

Biokinetics   The science that studies the movements of tissue and related phenomena that occur during the development of organisms.

Biological   (1) Pertaining to biology. (2) A medicinal preparation made from living organisms and their products; these include sera, vaccines, etc.

Biologically Derived Materials   Processed biologic tissue (porcine heart valves, bovine carotid arteries, human umbilical veins), reconstituted collagen and/or elastin, hyaluronic acid, chondroitin sulfate, and chitosans used in cardiovascular, soft-tissue augmentation and ophthalmologic applications.

Biologics   Refers to such pharmaceutical products as vaccines, toxins, toxoids, antitoxins, immune serums, blood derivatives, immunologic diagnostic aids, and related preparations. The usual intent of the term is to describe materials of biologic origin having *immunologic* effect. There is some interest in abandoning the older term ''biologics'' for the more encompassing ''immunobiologics.''

Biolysis   The disintegration of organic matter through the chemical (enzymatic) action of living organisms.

Biomaterials   A systemic, pharmacologically inert substance designed for implantation or incorporation within the human body. Biomaterials can be polymers, metals, ceramics, and composites. They must be compatible with the body, and nontoxic; they must closely duplicate the properties of the tissues they replace.

Biomaterials, Surface Roughness   The relative surface roughness of biomaterials is described as:

(1) *Very Smooth* — pyrolitic carbons, polished metals
(2) *Smooth* — silicone rubbers, polyurethanes, PVC
(3) *Microrough* — grafted polyethylene; PTFE
(4) *Medium Rough* — woven dacron; teflon fabrics
(5) *Very Rough* — knitted, velour fabrics, macroporous film, sand-blasted materials

Biomaterials Industry   Organizations that design, fabricate, and/or manufacture materials used in the health and allied fields. The industry may be classified as follows:

(1) Artificial Organs
   — *Artificial pancreas*
   — *Artificial kidney*
   — *Artificial heart*
(2) Biosensors
   — *In vivo/in vitro blood chemistries*
(3) Biotechnology
   — *Process/purification membranes*
   — *Surface immobilization of enzymes/cells*
   — *Cell culture systems*
   — *Fermentation polymers*
(4) Cardiovascular
   — *Vascular grafts*
   — *Heart valves*
(5) Commodities/Disposables
   — *Diagnostic catheters*
   — *Syringes*
(6) Drug Delivery Systems
   — *Topical drug delivery*
   — *Transdermal drug delivery*
   — *Extracorporeal therapy*
(7) Maxillofacial; Dental; ENT; Cranial
   — *Soft tissue augmentation*
   — *Mandibular implants*
   — *Ossicular replacement/reconstruction*
   — *Intracochlear prosthesis*
(8) Ophthalmology
   — *Contact/intraocular lenses*

- *Artificial cornea*
- *Vitreous implants*
- *Bioadhesives*
(9) Orthopedics
- *Artificial hips, knees*
- *Bone replacements*
- *Fixation devices*
- *Fixation cements*
- *Tendon prostheses*
- *Ligament prosthesis*
(10) Packaging
- *Personal care/hygiene*
- *Sterilizable films, trays*
- *Parenterals*
(11) Wound Management
- *Artificial skin*
- *Bioadhesives*
- *Burn dressings*
- *Staples*
- *Wound dressings*

Biomaterials Market　In 1990 the total U.S. market for polymeric biomaterials was estimated at $3.2 billion a year, with $2.5 billion for medical disposables. It was further estimated that over 2 million prosthetic implants a year were performed in the U.S. and Europe. Silicone accounted for about 10%, polyurethanes 5%, and collagen-based products 2%.

Biomechanics　The science of action of forces, internal or external, upon living bodies.

Biomedical　The combined sciences of biology and medicine, dealing with those aspects of biology and engineering that relate to medicine.

Biomedical Polymers　The attributes of an ideal biomedical polymer are listed below. Biomedical polymers should not:
- Cause uncontrolled thrombosis
- Damage blood cellular elements
- Alter blood proteins
- Destroy or denature enzymes
- Deplete electrolytes
- Cause adverse immune response
- Damage adjacent tissue
- Be carcinogenic, mutagenic, or teratogenic

Biomedical Tissue Adhesives　Adhesives specifically designed to bond living tissue. Examples: cyanoacrylates; gelatin resorcinol; fibrin glue; and the subclass of hemostatic agents that includes collagen, gelatin foam, succinylated amylose, and oxidized regenerated cellulose.

24

Bionics   The science of biological structure and function as applied to electronic devices.

Biopharmaceutics   The area of study embracing the relationship between the physical, chemical, and biological sciences as they apply to drugs, dosage forms, and drug actions.

Biopsy   The removal of a small portion of tissue from the body for diagnostic purposes.

Bioresorption   The process of removal by cellular activity (through phagocytosis or enzymatic attack) and/or physical dissolution of a material in the biological environment.

Bioreversible   Capable of being changed back to the original biologically active chemical form by processes within the organism; usually applied to drugs.

Biosensor   An analytical device consisting of immobilized biological enzymes, antibodies, etc., in intimate contact with a transducer capable of converting a biochemical signal into a measurable electrical signal. A variety of biosensors exist based on the following principles: conductrimetry, redox reactions, field-effect transistor, thermistor, optoelectronic, photodiode, fiber optic, gas-sensing, piezoelectric crystals, and ion-selective electrodes.

Biospectrometry   The spectroscopic analysis of types and amounts of substances present in tissue, or fluids from a living body.

Biosynthesis   (1) The formation of chemical compounds by living organisms. (2) Practical application of the results of recombinant DNA research, especially in regards to hormones, interferon, insulin, anticlotting agents, etc.

Biotechnology   The application of scientific and engineering principles to the processing of materials by biological agents to provide goods and services.

Biotelemetry   The recording and measuring of vital phenomena occurring in living organisms that are at a distance from the measuring device.

Biotoxicology   Scientific study of poisons produced by living organisms, their causes, detection, effects, and treatment of conditions produced by them.

Biotransformation   The conversion of drugs and ingested substances to their metabolites within living organisms.

Biotransformation Reactions   For most biotransformation reactions, the metabolite of the drug is more polar than the parent compound, thus leading to quicker elimination. Phase I reactions include oxidation, reduction, and hydrolysis, whereas Phase II or synthetic reactions are more complicated. This is shown below.

PHASE I REACTIONS	*PHASE II REACTIONS*
OXIDATION	GLUCORONIDE CONJUGATION
Aromatic hydroxylation	Ether glucoronide
Side chain hydroxylation	Ester glucoronide
N, O, and S dealkylation	Amide glucoronide

Biotransformation Reactions

PHASE I REACTIONS	PHASE II REACTIONS
Deamination	
Sulfoxidation, N-oxidation	PEPTIDE CONJUGATION
N-hydroxylation	Glycine conjugation
REDUCTION	
Azoreduction	METHYLATION
Nitroreduction	N-methylation
Alcohol dehydrogenase	O-methylation
HYDROLYSIS	ACETYLATION
Ester hydrolysis	SULFATE CONJUGATION
Amine hydrolysis	MERCAPTURIC ACID SYNTHESIS

Birefringence   (Double Refraction). The difference between any two refractive indices. May be used to determine the degree of crystallinity of polymers.

Bis   Prefix meaning "twice" or "again." Used in chemical nomenclature to indicate that a chemical grouping or radical occurs twice in a molecule, e.g., bisphenol A, where two phenols appear, or ethylene bis stearamide, where two stearic acids reacted with ethylene amine to form the amide linkage.

Bisphenol A   An intermediate in the production of epoxy, polycarbonate and phenolic resins. The name was derived from the condensation reaction in which two (bis) molecules of phenol are reacted with one molecule of acetone.

Blend   A uniform combination of two or more materials, either of which could be used alone for the same purpose as the blend.

Block Copolymer   A copolymer with chains composed of shorter homopolymer chains that are covalently linked together. The blocks can be regular or randomly placed. Block copolymers usually display higher impact strengths than either homopolymer, or plain physical mixtures of the two homopolymers.

Blocked Curing Agent   A curing agent that can be activated by physical or chemical means. Activation usually results in molecular splitting, in which one of the products is capable of curing a resin.

Blocking   An undesirable adhesion between layers of plastic, which may develop during pressure of storage, heat, sterilization, etc. The tendency to block is reduced by chemicals added to the plastic called anti-blocking agents.

Blood   A complex, liquid tissue of pH 7.4, comprised of erythrocytes, leucocytes, platelets, plasma proteins, and serum. Experimental work has been reported on the effectiveness of fluorocarbons to carry oxygen, and the use of polyvinyl pyrrolidone as a plasma extender.

Blood, Functions   The most important functions of blood are: transport of oxygen and carbon dioxide; transport of hormones, cells, and immunological agents; elimination of toxic substances; and maintenance of appropriate body temperature.

Blood Carbon Dioxide Analyzer   A Class III device consisting of an in-dwelling catheter with a PCO_2 transducer tip, used to measure the partial pressure of carbon dioxide in blood, to aid in determining the patient's circulatory, ventilatory, and metabolic status.

Blood Factors   (Coagulation Factors). Proteins derived in the multistep process of blood clotting. Twelve blood factors are essential to normal blood clotting whose absence, diminution, or excess may lead to abnormalities of the clotting mechanism. For example, Factor VIII which is deficient in persons with hemophilia A causes affected individuals to be susceptible to abnormal bleeding. Lately, biotechnology-derived recombinant forms of Factor VIII open the promise of effective treatment to hemophiliacs.

Blood Flow to Human Tissue   Some organs are significantly more perfused with blood than others, as shown below:

TISSUE	% CARDIAC OUTPUT	BLOOD FLOW (ml/100 gr/min)	ml/min
Adrenals	1	550	60
Kidneys	24	450	1440
Thyroid	2	400	120
Liver			
Hepatic	5	20	300
Portal	20	75	1200
Heart	4	70	240
Brain	15	55	900
Skin	5	5	300
Muscle (basal)	15	3	900
Connective tissue	1	1	60
Fat	2	1	60

Blood Hydrogen Ion Analyzer   A Class III device consisting of an indwelling catheter with a pH electrode at the tip, used to measure the hydrogen ion concentration in blood as an aid in determining the patient's acid-base balance.

Blood Oxygen Analyzer   A Class III device consisting of an indwelling catheter with a PO_2 electrode tip, used to measure in vivo partial pressure of oxygen, as an aid in determining respiratory, ventilatory, and metabolic status.

Blood Oxyhemoglobin Analyzer   A Class III device consisting of an indwelling catheter designed to measure electrophotometrically the oxygen-carrying capability of blood to aid in determining a patient's physiological status.

Bloom   An undesirable cloudy effect on the surface of a plastic article due to the incompatibility and migration of a compounding ingredient such as a lubricant, antioxidant, plasticizer, etc.

Blowing Agent   Any substance that alone or in combination with other substances is capable of producing a cellular structure. In medical foams, the toxicity of the blowing agent, or the decomposition products of the foaming reaction is a matter of regulatory concern.

Body Fluid Compartments   The total amount of water in a 70 kg man is about 40 liters. About 25 liters are inside the 100 trillion cells of the body and are collectively called the intracellular fluid. An additional 15 liters are stored outside the cells and are called extracellular fluid. Finally, the BLOOD contains the remaining 5 liters, where 3000 ml of this is plasma and the remainder, 2000 ml, is red blood cells.

Body Water, Daily Loss   Normally, at 68°F, the body loses about 2400 ml of water daily, but this may climb to about 6700 ml during diaphoresis, as shown below:

	NORMAL TEMP.	HOT WEATHER	DIAPHORESIS
Insensible loss			
Skin	350	350	350
Lungs	350	250	650
Urine	1400	1200	500
Sweat	100	1400	5000
Feces	200	200	200
TOTAL	2400	3400	6700

Bond, Chemical   An attractive force between atoms strong enough to permit the combined aggregate to function as a unit. Covalent bonding results most commonly when electrons are shared by two atomic nuclei.

Bond Strength   (1) The unit load applied in tension, compression, flexure, peel, impact, cleavage, or shear, required to break an adhesive assembly, with failure occurring at the interfacial plane of the bond. (2) The degree of attraction existing between atoms within a molecule.

Boyer-Beamen Rule   The relationship between the glass transition temperature T_g and the melting temperature T_m of a polymer. The ratio (when the temperature is expressed in degrees Kelvin) usually lies between 0.5 and 0.7; symmetrical polymers, such as linear polyethylene, exhibit a ratio closer to 0.5, while unsymmetrical polymers, such as polystyrene, exhibit ratios closer to 0.7.

BR   Abbreviation for *Butadiene Rubber.*

Brabender Plastograph   (Brabender Plasti-Corder). An instrument capable of continuously measuring the torque exerted in shearing a polymer specimen over a range of shear rates and temperatures, including anticipated running conditions. The instrument records torque, time, and temperature on a graph, from which processing information can be gleaned. Useful in predicting effects of additives, fillers, plasticity, cure, heat stability, and polymer consistency.

Brain Death   In the U.K., brain death is diagnosed under the following circumstances:

- There is a score of three on the Glasgow coma scale, i.e., no utterance, no eye opening, and no pain response.
- Brain-stem reflexes are absent, including pupil, caloric responses, corneal, gag and cough reflexes.

— There is no respiratory effort in response to hypercapnia.

— There is a structural cause for the observed state, and no reversible factors such as drugs that depress neuroligical functions.

Brain death is now the accepted definition for medical death, which allows decisions about the withdrawal of intensive care treatment and organ donation. Thus, brain-stem criteria are used to certify as medically dead a potential donor for, say, a kidney or heart transplantation.

Brain Death Causes   The most common causes of brain death are: (1) diffuse primary cranial injury; (2) subarachnoid hemorrhage; (3) raised intracranial pressure with irreversible brain-stem damage; (4) cerebral ischemia/anoxia; and (5) severe encephalitis.

Branched Polymer   A polymer in which the molecules have side chains or branching. The opposite of a linear polymer.

Branching   The growth of a new polymer chain from an active site on an established chain, in a direction different from the original chain, similar to the branching of a tree. Branching occurs as a result of chain transfer processes, or from the polymerization of difunctional monomers, and has important effects on the physical properties of the finished polymer.

Breathable   The special ability of some polymers to allow the passage of air or water vapor; polyurethanes, silicones, and other amorphous polymers are considered breathable.

Breathable Films   A film that is permeable to gases, due to diffusion, or due to the presence of molecular pores throughout its mass.

Breathing   The ability of a plastic film to allow passage of air or water moisture as a result of diffusion, or due to a degree of porosity.

Breathing Frequency Monitor   A Class II device used to measure respiratory rate. The device provides an audible or visible alarm when the respiration rate falls outside predetermined limits.

Brittleness Temperature   The temperature at which polymers rupture by sudden impact under specified conditions. This temperature is related to the glass transition temperature T_g.

Bronchial Tube   A Class II device used to differentially intubate a bronchus in order to isolate a portion of the lung distal to the tube.

Bronchoscopy   Visualization of the windpipe (trachea) and the bronchial structures via an endoscope, a lighted instrument passed into these passages, for examination purposes.

B-Stage Resin   An intermediate stage in the reaction of certain thermosetting resins in which the material swells when in contact with certain solvents and softens when heated, but is not entirely soluble or fusible.

Bulk Density   The density of a molding compound in powder form, expressed as the ratio of weight to volume (g/cm^3 or lb/ft^2).

Bulk Factor   The ratio of the volume of a given mass of powder molding material to the volume of the same mass of the material after molding or forming. The bulk factor is also equal to the ratio of the density after molding to the apparent density of the powder.

Bulk Modulus   See MODULUS OF ELASTICITY.

Bulk Polymerization   (Mass Polymerization). The polymerization of a monomer in the absence of any medium other than a catalyst or accelerator. Polystyrene, polymethyl methacrylate, polyhydroxy ethyl methacrylate, polyethylene, and styrene-acrylonitrile are prototype polymers produced by bulk polymerization. Most of the medical hydrogels are formed by this process.

Buna-N   See ACRYLONITRILE-BUTADIENE RUBBERS.

Buna-S   See STYRENE-BUTADIENE RUBBERS.

Butadiene $CH_2:CHCHCH:CH_2$. A gas obtained from petroleum cracking widely used in the formation of copolymers with styrene, acrylonitrile, vinyl chloride, etc., to impart flexibility to the finished product.

Butadiene-Acrylonitrile Copolymers (NBR)   See ACRYLONITRILE-BUTA-DIENE RUBBERS.

Butadiene Rubber (BR)   See POLYBUTADIENE.

Butadiene-Styrene   See BUTADIENE-STYRENE THERMOPLASTICS.

Butyl   The radical C_4H_9, occurring only in combination.

1,4-Butylene Glycol   (1,4 butane diol). An important intermediate in the production of poly vinyl pyrrolidone, polyesters, and polyurethane elastomers.

Butylenes   A class of hydrocarbons frequently utilized to copolymerize with styrene, acrylics, olefins, and vinyl resins.

Butyl Methacrylate   A polymerizable monomer used in the production of acrylic resins.

***p*-tert-Butylphenyl Salicylate**   An FDA approved plasticizer for food contact, which can also be used as a light stabilizer.

Butyl Rubber   A synthetic elastomer produced by the copolymerization of isobutylene with a small amount of either isoprene or butadiene. Butyl rubber is extensively used in the production of rubber stoppers for drug vials.

Butyl Stearate   A nontoxic lubricant and secondary plasticizer for vinyls.

Butyraldehyde   A monomer used with polyvinyl alcohol to form polyvinyl butyrate.

Butyrate   (1) The salt or ester of butyric acid, (2) the common name for *Cellulose Acetate Butyrate* (CAB) terpolymers.

C   Symbol for CARBON.

Ca   Symbol for calcium, a mineral essential to life; an important body electrolyte. Has a positive inotropic effect on the heart, intimately involved in the selectively permeable transport of substances through cell membranes. Vital element to the composition of bone.

CA   Abbreviation for *Cellulose Acetate.*

CAB   Abbreviation for *Cellulose Acetate Butyrate.*

Cadmium   Soft, blue white element, of atomic weight 48. Highly toxic, especially by inhalation of dust or fume. A known carcinogen. Soluble compounds are highly toxic.

Calcium Ricinolate   A white powder derived from castor oil, used as a nontoxic stabilizer for PVC resins.

Calcium Stearate   A nontoxic stabilizer and lubricant, used in combination with zinc and magnesium salts in the production of stabilizers.

Calcium-Zinc Stabilizers   A family of stabilizers containing mixtures of calcium and zinc compounds, approved by the FDA for food contact.

Calender   A large machine performing the operation of calendering onto thermoplastic resins. See also CALENDERING.

Calender Coating   The process of coating substrates with thermoplastic resins by forcing both the substrate and the thermoplastic resin through calender rolls.

Calendering   The process of forming sheets or coatings by passing thermoplastic resins through a series of heated rolls. The gap between the last pair of heated rolls determines the final thickness of the sheet, which is subsequently cooled by chilled rolls. The plastic is usually premixed and plasticated on separate equipment (such as a Banbury Mixer), then continuously fed into the nip of the first pair of heated calender rolls.

Calorie   The amount of heat necessary to raise one gram of water one degree centigrade at one atmosphere.

Calorimeter   A device for measuring the amount of heat liberated during thermal reactions.

Cancer   A general term that includes the various types of malignant neoplasm (carcinoma or sarcoma) which invade surrounding tissue, metastasize, are likely to recur after surgery, and cause death unless adequately treated. According to the American Cancer Society an estimated 1.1 million people will be diagnosed with cancer in the U.S. in 1991, as shown below:

TYPE	MEN	WOMEN
Bladder	37,000	13,200
Breast	–	175,000
Colon/rectum	78,500	79,000
Lung	101,000	60,000
Uterus	–	46,000
Lymphoma	23,800	20,800
Ovary	–	20,700
Skin melanoma	17,000	15,000

Cancer

TYPE	MEN	WOMEN
Pancreas	13,700	14,500
Prostate	122,000	–
Leukemia	15,800	12,200
Oral	120,600	10,200
Kidney	15,800	9,500
All types	545,000	555,000

The odds of men developing prostate cancer is 1 in 11. The odds of women developing breast cancer is 1 in 9.

Candida   A common type of yeast-like fungus found on skin, throat, vagina, and feces. May contaminate the surface of implanted devices.

CAP   Abbreviation for *Cellulose Acetate Propionate*.

Capillarity   The attraction between molecules, similar to surface tension, which results in the rise of a liquid in small tubes or fibers, or in the wetting of a solid by a liquid.

Capillary   Relates to tiny blood or lymph vessel.

Capillary Rheometer   An instrument used for measuring the flow properties of molten polymers, consisting of a capillary tube, a pressure device, means of maintaining a desired temperature, and means of measuring differential flow rates and pressures.

Capillary Viscometer   The two types of instruments described under Capillary Rheometer—one for concentrated solutions and polymer melts, and the other for dilute solutions.

Caprolactone   Reaction product of peracetic acid and cyclohexanone; an intermediate in the manufacture of caprolactam. Used in adhesives, urethanes, and elastomers. Synthesis of bioerodible devices.

Carbamide Phosphoric Acid   (urea phosphoric acid). A catalyst used in the polymerization of acid-setting resins.

Carbanion   A negatively charged organic ion, such as H_3C-, having at least one electron more than the corresponding free radical. Important intermediates in base-catalyzed polymerization and alkylation reactions.

Carbohydrate   A compound of carbon, hydrogen, and oxygen that contains the saccharose grouping or its first reaction product, and in which the ratio of hydrogen to oxygen is the same as in water.

Carbon   One of the most abundant elements in nature, found in all living tissue without exception. Forms the structural basis of virtually all carbohydrate, protein, and lipid molecules.

Carbon Black   A generic name for the entire family of colloidal carbons, produced by the incomplete combustion of gas, oil, or another hydrocarbon. Carbon black is used to impart electrical conductivity to biomaterials.

Carbon Fibers   A group of fibrous materials consisting primarily of elemental carbon, prepared by (1) pyrolysis of organic fibers, (2) crystal growth under high pressure, and (3) growth from a vapor state by thermal decomposition. Used in the manufacture of reinforced orthopedic composites.

Carbon Tetrachloride   A powerful solvent for many resins. Not used extensively with biomaterials because of toxicity concerns.

Carbonate   A compound resulting from the reaction of either a metal or an organic compound with carbonic acid.

Carbonyl Group   The divalent group $C = O$, which occurs in a wide range of chemical compounds. It is present in aldehydes, ketones, organic acids and sugars.

Carboxylic   Term for the COOH group, the radical found in organic acids.

Carboxylic Acid   Any organic acid comprised chiefly of alkyl (hydrocarbon) groups, usually in a straight chain, terminating in a carboxylic acid group. Exceptions are formic and oxalic acids.

Carboxymethyl Cellulose   (CMC, CM cellulose). A semisynthetic, water-soluble polymer, in which CH_2COOH groups are substituted on the glucose units of the cellulose through an ether linkage. Since the reaction occurs in an alkaline medium, the product is the sodium salt of the carboxylic acid. Extensively used in pharmaceuticals and controlled delivery tablets.

Carcinogen   Any substance that causes the development of cancerous growths in living tissue. Such substances are classified as (1) confirmed carcinogens, those that are known to induce cancer in man, and (2) experimental carcinogens, those found to cause cancer in animals under experimental conditions. *Among known carcinogens*: Acrylonitrile, chloroaniline, epichlorohydrin, ethylene dibromide, toluene bis chloroaniline, methylene bis chloroaniline, 2-nitropropane.

Cardiac   Pertaining or referring to the heart.

Cardiac Angiography   The visualization, under fluoroscopy, of the interior of the heart, or heart blood vessels, performed by inserting a catheter into an artery, and injecting contrast media.

Cardiac Arrest   Any condition in which the heart fails to depolarize, leading to cessation of ventricular activity.

Cardiac Catheterization   The surgical insertion of a fine tube into the chambers of the heart for diagnostic purposes.

Cardiac Output   The amount of blood pumped by the heart per minute. Measured with a cardiac output catheter.

Cardiopulmonary Bypass (CPB)   A Class III multicomponent device designed to perform the dual function of the heart and lungs during open heart surgery.

Cardiopulmonary Bypass Blood Pump   A Class II device that uses a revolving roller mechanism to pump blood through the circuit during open heart surgery.

Cardiopulmonary Bypass Catheter   A Class II device comprising catheters, cannulas, and tubing used in cardiopulmonary bypass surgery to cannulate vessels, perfuse the coronary arteries, and interconnect with an oxygenator/perfusion pump apparatus.

Cardiopulmonary Bypass Defoamer   A Class III device used in conjunction with an oxygenator during open heart surgery to remove gas bubbles from the pumped blood.

Cardiopulmonary Bypass Heat Exchanger   A Class II device consisting of a heat exchange system, to warm or cool the blood or perfusion fluid flowing through the device.

Cardiopulmonary Bypass Oxygenator   A Class III device used to exchange gases between blood and a gaseous environment to satisfy the metabolic requirements of a patient during open heart surgery.

Cardiopulmonary Bypass Tubing   A Class II device consisting of polymeric tubing that is used in the pump head, where it is cyclically compressed by the rotors to cause the blood to flow through the bypass circuit.

Cardiovascular Flow Meter   A Class II device which, when connected to a flow transducer, energizes the transducer, and displays the blood flow signal.

Cardioversion   Conversion, by electrical means, of a cardiac tachyarrhythmia to a more normal rhythm, that is more physiologically tolerable.

Casein Plastics   A family of resins derived from casein. Because of their poor water resistance and dimensional stability, these resins are not widely used.

Casing   (Cross-linking by Activated Species of Inert Gases). A process developed by Bell Telephone, where plastic surfaces are exposed to activated inert gases in a glow discharge tube, so that printing inks and adhesives will bond firmly to the articles.

Casting   The process of forming solid or hollow articles from fluid plastic mixtures in a mold with little or no pressure. Following solidification, the articles are removed by the process known as demolding.

Casting Resins   Liquid monomers, oligomers, or prepolymers, capable of hardening (polymerizing) in molds. Acrylics, styrenes, polyesters, epoxies, silicones, nylons, and polyurethanes are frequently used as casting compounds.

Castor Oil   A pale yellow oil derived from Ricinus communis beans. It is an important raw material for plasticizers, nylons, alkyd resins, and certain medical-grade polyurethane casting compounds.

Catabolism   The breakdown process of food during digestion into less complex substances.

Catalysis, Heterogenous   A catalytic reaction in which the reactants and the catalyst comprise two separate phases, e.g., liquids containing finely divided solids as a disperse phase.

Catalysis, Homogenous   A catalytic reaction in which the reactants and the catalyst comprise only one phase.

Catalyst   A substance that causes or greatly accelerates a chemical reaction, without being permanently affected by the reaction. In biology, catalysts that perform these functions are known as enzymes. In general, catalysts are thought to increase the rate of chemical reactions; negative catalysts (inhibitor, retarder) decrease the rate. Catalysts are categorized as: polymerization, organic synthesis, gas synthesis, oxidative, hydrogenating, and dehydrogenating.

Catalyst, Stereospecific   An organometallic catalyst that permits control of molecular geometry of polymeric molecules. Example: a Ziegler-Natta catalyst for the polymerization of polypropylene, polyethylene, and other polyolefins.

Catenane   A compound with interlocking rings, which are not chemically bonded, but which cannot be separated without breaking at least one valence bond. The model resembles the links of a chain.

Catheter   A hollow cylinder, designed to be inserted into any body canal, such as veins, arteries, urethra, etc. Catheters are widely used to infuse or withdraw materials into or out of the body.

Catheterization   A surgical process in which a small hollow tube is introduced into an organ, to empty it, as in urinary catheterization, for diagnostic, or for therapeutic purposes.

Catheterization, Cardiac   The insertion of a catheter through peripheral vessels, which reaches all the heart chambers, for an exact diagnosis of an organic defect, e.g., a valvular defect or a congenital deformity. Three catheterization procedures are currently favored: right, retrograde, and transseptal catheterization.

Cation   An atom, molecule, or radical that has lost an electron and has thus become positively charged.

Cationic Reagent   A family of surfactants, characterized by the presence of positive ions in the active constituent.

CAT Scan   (Computerized Axial Tomography). A complex X-ray procedure, which produces a reconstructed image of a transverse section of the body. It allows in-depth visualization of body sections useful in the noninvasive diagnosis of disease or injury.

Cautery   An agent used for scarring tissues by means of heat or caustic chemicals.

Cell   (1) The fundamental structural and functional unit of all life. Composed of an outer membrane, which encloses the protoplasm and the nucleus. (2) Any completely enclosed hollow unit, as in a cellular plastic, foam, or honeycomb. In cellular plastics terminology, the single void produced by a blowing agent. (3) Any self-contained unit having a functional purpose, e.g., voltaic cell, electrolytic cell, fuel cell, or solar cell.

Cell Collapse   A defect in foamed plastics characterized by surface defects, created by the collapse of internal cells. Usually created during the foaming process by rapid gas permeation or weakening of cellular walls.

Cell Immobilization   The transformation of cells from a free mobile state to the fixed state, either by cellular attachment to a substrate or by entrapment in a biocompatible matrix. Three major methods are utilized: AGGREGATION (cross-linking with glutaraldehyde); ADSORPTION (carrier binding onto substrates); and entrapment (in biocompatible hydrogels such as polyacrylamide, alginates, and carrageenan).

Cellophane   Regenerated cellulose.

Cellular Plastic   A plastic composed of numerous microscopic cells evenly distributed throughout its mass. A cellular plastic may be created by (1) incorporation of a blowing agent that decomposes at elevated temperature to liberate a gas, (2) mechanical frothing of a gas, (3) incorporation of a soluble material that is subsequently leached, and (4) addition of a solvent-extractible material.

Cellulose   A family of carbohydrate polymers of high molecular weight, derived from cotton, plants, and tree stems.

Cellulose Acetate   The acetic acid ester of cellulose, which results in transparent thermoplastic material. Not frequently used in medical applications.

Cellulose Acetate Butyrate   A mixed ester of butyric and acetic acids with fibrous cellulose. Not frequently used in medical applications.

Cellulose Acetate Propionate   A thermoplastic resin formed by reacting fibrous cellulose with propionic and acetic acids.

Cellulose Esters   Cellulose derivatives based on the esterification of acetic, nitric, propionic, and butyric acids.

Cellulose Ethers   Cellulose derivatives based on the etherification of cellulose, including methyl, ethyl, and carboxymethyl resins. Widely used in such pharmaceutical applications as tablet coatings, controlled drug delivery orals, etc.

Cellulosic Plastics   A large family of thermoplastics, made by substituting various chemical groups for the hydroxyl groups contained in the cellulose molecule.

Cementing   The process of permanently joining plastics to themselves, or to other substances, by means of solvents, dopes, or chemical cements. Solvent cements comprise a mutual solvent for the cement and substrate; dope cements contain a solvent solution of a plastic similar to the plastic substrate; chemical cements are based on reactive species that polymerize to form strong bonds.

Centigrade   A measurement of heat based on a scale divided into 100 degrees, where water freezes at $0°$ and boils at $100°$. Normal body temperature on this scale is $37°$.

Centipoise   A unit of viscosity, comprised of one hundredth of a POISE. Water at room temperature has a viscosity of about one centipoise.

Centistoke   A unit of viscosity, comprised of one hundredth of a STOKE. A stoke is equal to the viscosity in poises of a liquid, times the density of the liquid in grams per cc.

Centrifugation   A separation technique based on the application of centrifugal force to a mixture or suspension of materials of similar densities.

This technique is widely used in pharmaceutical, biological, and diagnostic procedures.

Cephalosporin   Any member of a family of antibiotics, containing a fused beta-lactam-dihydrothiazine ring system with an N-acyl side chain and an acetoxy group attached to the ring. These antibiotics are thought to be free from allergic reactions common to penicillin.

Ceramic Fibers   The use of reinforcing fibers made of refractory oxides such as aluminum, magnesium, and zirconium. The fibers add high strength and modulus to certain resins.

Cerebrospinal Fluid Systems   The entire cavity enclosing the brain and spinal cord has a volume of approximately 1650 ml and about 140 ml of this volume is occupied by cerebrospinal fluid (CSF). Cerebrospinal fluid is produced in the choroid plexus at a rate of 750 ml/day, which is about five times as much as the total volume of fluid in the cerebrospinal cavity. The CSF is found in the ventricles of the brain, and in the subarachnoid space around both the brain and the spinal cord. These spaces are interconnected, with the fluid pressure regulated at a constant level.

Cervical Cap   A Class II device, it is a cup-like receptacle that fits over the cervix to collect menstrual flow, or to aid in artificial insemination.

Cervical Dilator   A Class III device used to dilate the cervix, comprised of an instrument with two opposing blades manually operated.

Cervical Drain   A Class II device designed to provide an exit channel for draining discharge from the cervix after pelvic surgery.

CFR   Abbreviation for *Code of Federal Regulations*. A collection of regulations established by law. Copies may be obtained from the Superintendent of Documents, Government Printing Office, Washington D.C., 20402.

Chain   A series of atoms of a particular element directly connected by covalent bonds, which constitutes the structural configuration of a compound. These chains are usually composed of carbon atoms.

Channel Black   A specific type of carbon black, made by impingement of a flame against a metal plate. The carbon residue is scraped at predetermined interval.

Channel Depth Ratio   The ratio of the depth of the first flight at the feeding section of an extruder, to the depth of the last flight in the metering section.

Channel Volume Ratio   The volume ratio of the first flight at the feeding section to the volume of the last flight in the metering section. Generally, the term COMPRESSION RATIO is used instead of channel volume ratio.

Chelating Agent   Substance capable of sequestering and holding metallic ions in a "claw" composed of a ring structure of nitrogen, oxygen, and sulfur, each of which donates two electrons to form a coordinate bond with the chelated ion.

Chemical Change   Rearrangement of atoms, ions, or radicals resulting in the formation of new substances, often displaying entirely different properties. Such a change is called a CHEMICAL REACTION.

Chemical Nomenclature   The origin and use of the names of elements, compounds, and other chemical entities, individually and as a group, as well as the various accepted conventions for systematizing them. Present nomenclature follows the reforms adopted by the International Union of Pure and Applied Chemistry (IUPAC).

Chemical Reaction   A change that may occur by combination, replacement, decomposition, or some suitable combination of these. Common reactions are oxidation, reduction, ionization, combustion, polymerization, hydrolysis, condensation, enolization, saponification, rearrangement, etc. Chemical reactions involve only rupture of the bonds that hold the molecules together, and should not be confused with a NUCLEAR REACTION, in which the atomic nucleus is involved.

Chemical Resistance   The fundamental ability of a polymer to withstand chronic exposure to acids, alkalis, organic solvents, and other corrosive chemical environments.

Chemical Technology   A generic term covering the spectrum of physico-chemical knowledge of materials, processes, and operations used in the chemical industry. It includes (1) basic phenomena such as catalysis and polymerization; (2) properties, behavior, and handling of materials; and (3) the formulation, compounding, fabrication, and testing of chemicals.

Chemically Foamed Plastic   A cellular plastic in which the cells are formed by a chemical blowing agent, or by the chemical reaction of constituents.

Chemisorption   The formation of bonds between the surface molecules of a material of high surface energy and a gas or liquid in contact with it.

Chemosterilant   Materials or processes that sterilize male insects, thus preventing their reproduction.

Chemotaxis   The directed migration of cells in response to a concentration gradient of a soluble attractant. Chemotaxis is the most often reported mechanism of directed cell motility, and is thought to be regulated by diffusion of the attractant from its source into an attractant-poor environment.

Chemotherapy   The treatment of disease by the administration of chemicals (drugs).

CHEMTREC   Abbreviation for *Chemical Transportation Emergency Center*, established in Washington D.C. by the Chemical Manufacturers Association to provide emergency information on materials involved in transportation accidents.

Chill Roll   A temperature-controlled cold roll, which cools an extruded or cast polymer film prior to winding into rolls.

Chlorinated Hydrocarbons   A general term covering a wide variety of liquids and solids resulting from the addition of chlorine to hydrocarbons, such as methane, ethylene, and benzene. They are widely employed as nonflammable solvents and monomers for synthesis of plastics.

Chlorinated Polyether   Corrosion-resistant thermoplastics obtained by polymerization of the monomer chlorinated oxetane.

Chlorinated Polyethylenes   A family of polyethylene polymers modified by the chemical substitution of chlorine on the linear backbone. They range from amorphous rubbers at 25 to 40% of chlorine by weight, to hard elastoplastics at 65 to 75% chlorine.

Chlorofluorocarbon Resins   Resins made by the polymerization of monomers composed of chlorine, fluorine, and carbon only. These materials are very biocompatible, inert, and display low coefficients of friction, making them useful in many medical applications.

Chlorotrifluoroethylene   A colorless gas obtained by either dehalogenation or dehydrohalogenation of saturated chlorofluorocarbons or chlorohydrocarbons. Used as a monomer in the polymerization of polychlorotrifluoroethylene (PCTFE) resins.

Cholinergics   Drugs that act on the involuntary nervous system to increase activity of internal organs such as the heart and lungs, and to produce expansion of blood vessels.

Chromatography   The process of selective retardation of one or more components of a fluid solution as the fluid advances through a column packed with finely divided substances, the retardation resulting from the distribution of the components between one or more thin phases and the liquid. The process is used for analysis and separation of liquid mixtures.

Chromatophore   An atom or group of atoms that imparts a characteristic color to a substance.

Chromogenic Substrate   An enzyme substrate that is capable of being converted to a characteristic colored product as a direct result of enzyme action. Chromogenic substrates are extensively used to detect enzyme-linked antibodies with in vitro diagnostic techniques such as ELISA and immunoblotting.

Chromophore   A chemical grouping which when present in an aromatic compound (the chromogen) gives color to the substance, by causing a displacement or appearance of absorbent bands in the visible spectrum.

Chromosomes   The carriers of the genes that determine the sex and physical characteristics of each person.

Chronaximeter   A Class II device that measures neuromuscular excitability by means of a strength-duration curve that can be used for diagnosis of neurological dysfunctions.

Chronic   A state or disease condition, that lasts for a long period of time without any appreciable change.

Chronotropic   Substances having an effect on heart rate; drugs that speed up heart rate are said to have a positive effect, those that slow it down are said to be negatively chronotropic.

Circulation   The course of the blood from the heart, to the body, and back to the heart.

Circulation, Blood Quantities   By far the greatest amount of blood is contained in the systemic veins, as shown below:

```
Large veins and venous reservoirs . . . . . . . . . . .34%
Small veins, venules, and venous sinuses  . . . . . . .25%
Pulmonary vessels . . . . . . . . . . . . . . . . . . . 2%
Heart  . . . . . . . . . . . . . . . . . . . . . . . . 9%
Large arteries  . . . . . . . . . . . . . . . . . . . . 8%
Small arteries  . . . . . . . . . . . . . . . . . . . . 5%
Capillaries . . . . . . . . . . . . . . . . . . . . . . 5%
Arterioles  . . . . . . . . . . . . . . . . . . . . . . 2%
```

Circulation, Collateral   Parallel or secondary circulation from other vessels.

Circulation, Coronary   Flow of blood to the heart, via coronary arteries.

Circulation, Cross-Sectional Areas   If all vessels of each type were put side by side, their total cross-sectional areas would be:

```
Aorta  . . . . . . . . . . . . . . . . . . . . . . . 2.5 cm²
Small arteries  . . . . . . . . . . . . . . . . . .  20 cm²
Arterioles  . . . . . . . . . . . . . . . . . . . .  40 cm²
Capillaries . . . . . . . . . . . . . . . . . . . 2500 cm²
Venules  . . . . . . . . . . . . . . . . . . . . . 250 cm²
Small veins . . . . . . . . . . . . . . . . . . . .  80 cm²
Venae cavae  . . . . . . . . . . . . . . . . . . . .  8 cm²
```

Circulation, Extracorporeal and Assisted   During open heart surgery, e.g., installation of a valve prosthesis or correction of a congenital malformation, the heart cannot maintain circulation. In such a case it becomes necessary to provide extracorporeal circulation. Although it is technically possible to replace the function of only the right half of the heart (right bypass), the usual practice is to bypass the whole heart. At the same time, an artificial lung is used so that blood is oxygenated and carbon dioxide is removed, thus creating a heart-lung bypass. There is also a need for devices to provide circulatory assistance to support a failing heart, popularly known as artificial hearts. Several artificial hearts are presently under development for both temporary and permanent assistance.

Circulation, Functional Parts   The functional parts of the circulation are: arteries, arterioles, capillaries, venules, and veins. The function of the arteries is to transport blood under high pressure to the tissues. The arterioles act as control valves through which blood is released into the capillaries. The capillaries exchange fluid and nutrients between the blood and the interstitial spaces. The venules collect blood from the capillaries; they gradually coalesce into progressively larger veins. The veins function as conduits for transport of blood from the tissues back to the heart.

Circulation, Pulmonary   Flow of blood through the lungs.

Circulation, Systemic   Flow of blood through the major parts of the body.

Circumcision Instrument   A Class II device, which includes a plastic bell circumcision device, shield, and clamp.

Cirrhosis   A degenerative disease of the liver in which liver cells are destroyed and replaced by nonfunctioning fatty or fibrous tissue.

Cis   A chemical prefix, from the Latin "on this side," denoting an isomer in which certain atoms are on the same side of a plane. The opposite of TRANS.

Class I Devices, General Controls   Primarily intended for devices that pose no potential risk to health, and thus can be adequately regulated without imposing standards or the need for premarket review. This category provides a broad general control. It requires that manufacturers of these devices register with the FDA, provide a listing of products, maintain adequate reports, and comply with good manufacturing practices. Examples: stethoscopes, periodontic syringes, nebulizers, vaginal insufflators.

Class II Devices, Performance Standards   Applicable when general controls are not adequate to assure the safety and effectiveness of a device, based on the potential risk to health posed by the device. To classify a device in the Class II category, the FDA must find that enough data are available on which to base adequate performance standards that would control the safety and effectiveness of these devices. Examples: diagnostic catheters, electrocardiographs, wound dressings, percutaneous catheters, gastrointestinal irrigation systems.

Class III Devices, Premarket Approval   Applicable when a device is a "critical device," i.e., life-supporting and/or life-sustaining, unless adequate justification is given for classifying it in another category. Class III contains devices produced after 1976 that are not sufficiently similar to pre-1976 devices, and devices that were regulated as new drugs before 1976. Examples: bronchial tubes, ventilators, vascular grafts, pacemakers, cardiopulmonary bypass, surgical meshes. See Appendix for CRITICAL DEVICE LISTING.

Clean Air Act   This act addresses three broad types of air pollution problems: (1) The Ozone Protection Act forces manufacturing plants to attain norms deemed necessary to protect the earth's ozone layer. (2) The acid rain provisions force plants to cut emissions of acid gases. (3) The toxic air section specifies that any pollution source, that imposes a cancer risk greater than a certain probability be eliminated.

Clean Room   The cleanliness is rated according to the number of particles above certain sizes in a specific volume of air. For example, Class 100,000 rating means that a room contains no more than 100,000 particles/ft^3 of air if the particles are 0.5 μm, or 700 particles/ft^3 of air if the particles are 5 μm or larger. Clean Room Criteria include the following:

- Room is air conditioned
- Room uses high-efficiency filters

- Room is maintained under positive pressure
- Air locks are provided for entry and exit of personnel
- Curtain of ionized air is present at every entry
- Humidity is controlled at 20% to inhibit organism growth
- Personnel required to wear masks, hats, gloves, and gowns

Coacervation   An equilibrium state of colloidal or macromolecular systems. Defined as the partial miscibility of two or more optically isotropic liquids, at least one of which is in the colloidal state.

Coagulation   The process of changing from a liquid to a thickened or solid state, as in the formation of a clot of blood.

Cold Flow   See CREEP.

Cold Molding   A manufacturing process, similar to compression molding, except that no heat is applied during the molding/compression cycle. The molded part is subsequently hardened or cured by subsequent heating. Silicone-based medical prostheses may be fabricated from cold-molded shapes.

Cold Pressing   A bonding operation that relies solely on pressure, without the application of heat.

Collagen   An important connective tissue protein that functions to hold tissues together. Composed of an albumin-like protein, similar to gelatin. Found in soft tissue, most bone and cartilage.

Collagen Deposition During Wound Repair   The primary types deposited in the wound bed during fibroplasia and associated granulation tissue are types I and III collagen. Normal skin contains about 80–90% type I and 10–20% type III. During the course of wound healing, increased type III is seen for the first few days after wounding. Particularly important in the process of dermal wound healing is type IV collagen synthesis by epidermal cells and the regeneration of basement membranes, although the synthesis of type IV collagen and associated glycoproteins such as laminin is delayed until the wound is reepithelialized and epidermal cells are no longer in a migratory phase. See also COLLAGEN TYPES.

Collagen Types   Collagen is a generic term encompassing at least 11 types of molecules, many with two or more subtypes. All consist largely of the unique collagen triple helix, and in most cases they perform a structural function in aggregate form. These are listed below:

TYPE	TRIMER MW	AGGREGATE FORM	LOCALIZATION
I	300,000	67 nm bands	Dermis, tendon, bone, cornea
II	300,000	67 nm bands	Cartilage, sclera
III	300,000	67 nm bands	Cardiovascular, dermis
IV	550,000	Mat	Basement membrane
V	400,000	Fibril	Dermis
VI	550,000	Fibril	Dermis
VII	500,000	Dimer	Anchoring fibrils
VIII	500,000	Unknown	Unknown

TYPE	TRIMER MW	AGGREGATE FORM	LOCALIZATION
IX	210,000	Unknown	Cartilage
X	190,000	Unknown	Cartilage
$\alpha1\alpha2\alpha3$	300,000	Unknown	Cartilage

Collagens, Basement Membrane　　Several distinct types of collagens are found in all basement membranes. These collagens are organized into structures distinct from typical cross-striated collagen fibrils seen in connective tissue stroma. They cannot be defined ultrastructurally without using collagen type-specific antibodies as markers. The collagens found in basement membranes are:

COLLAGEN TYPE	FIBRIL LENGTH (nm)	LOCALIZATION
IV	425	All basement membranes and organs
V	300	Lamina reticularis in muscle; basal lamina in kidney, lung,etc.
VI	120	Lamina reticularis
VII	450	Skin anchoring fibrils
VIII	unknown	Endothelial cells

Collapse　　In foam terminology, the inadvertent and undesirable densification of a cellular plastic.

Colligative Property　　A property that is numerically equal for any group of substances, independent of their respective chemical structures.

Colloid　　Any substance capable of forming stable suspensions or emulsions with a liquid. Colloidal suspensions should not settle to any noticeable degree, and should not diffuse readily through vegetable or animal membranes. High molecular weight substances capable of forming colloidal suspensions are usually in the range of 10^{-7} to 10^{-5} cm in diameter.

Colloid Chemistry　　A subdivision of physical chemistry, comprising the phenomenological study of matter when one or more of its dimensions lie in the range between 1 millimicron (nanometer) and 1 micron (micrometer). Natural colloidal systems include blood, milk, and rubber latex.

Colloidal Mill　　A piece of equipment capable of manufacturing emulsions and colloidal suspensions, comprising a high-speed rotor and a fixed or counter-rotating element in close proximity to the rotor.

Collodion　　A solution of cellulose nitrate in a mixture of alcohol and ether.

Colony Counter　　A Class I device used to determine the number of bacterial colonies present on a bacteriological culture medium contained in a petri dish. This is a measure of the degree of bacterial infection.

Colony-Stimulating Factors (CSFs)　　Immune system growth factors that control the differentiation, growth, and activity of white blood cells. GM-CSF stimulates the production of both granulocytes and macrophages, helping to overcome immune deficiencies and fight infection. Other proteins having narrower responses include G-CSF and M-CSF.

Color Concentrate　　A plastics compound containing a high percentage of pigments or dyes, used for blending with another resin so the correct and desired amount of color is easily achieved. The concentrate provides a dustless and convenient method of obtaining reproducible colors in plastics compounds. The term *masterbatch* is sometimes used for color concentrates, as well as for concentrates of other important additives such as catalysts, radio-opacifiers, and lubricants.

Color Migration   The movement (diffusion) of dyes and pigments through the matrix of a material.

Color Stability   The maintenance of original color in a polymer. See also LIGHT RESISTANCE.

Colorants   Dyes or pigments that impart color to polymers. Dyes are synthetic or natural compounds of microscopic size, soluble in organic solvents, yielding transparent colors. Pigments are organic or inorganic substances, with larger particle size, insoluble in organic solvents. Organic pigments produce nearly transparent colors, whereas inorganic pigments produce opaque colors (with some exceptions).

Colorfastness   See LIGHT RESISTANCE.

Colorimeter   An instrument used for matching colors with results approximating those obtained by expert visual inspection. The sample is illuminated by light from three primary color filters, and qualitatively scanned by an electronic detection system. Colorimeters are frequently used in conjunction with spectrophotometers, for close color control in production operations.

Colorimetry   An analytical method based on the knowledge that polymers undergo characteristic color changes when exposed to certain chemicals.

Colostomy   A surgical opening into the colon, to relieve an intestinal obstruction, or other disease of the colon, allowing the discharge of feces through the opening instead of through the rectum. Colostomy devices were among the earliest uses of synthetic polymers in medicine.

Colostomy Rod   A Class II device used during the loop colostomy procedure. A loop of colon is surgically extracted through the abdominal wall and the stiff colostomy rod is placed through the loop to prevent slippage of the colon.

Colposcope   A Class II device designed to permit direct viewing of tissues of the vagina and cervix by means of a telescopic system located within the vagina.

Colposcopy   An examination of the vagina and cervix with a device called a colposcope, that permits visualization of the internal surfaces of these body parts.

Coma   A level of unconsciousness from which a person cannot be aroused, due to disease, drug abuse, poisoning, injury, etc.

Combustible Liquid   An organic liquid that evaporates flammable vapors at 150°F or below. Many organic solvents used in the fabrication of medical devices are combustible according to this definition. Exceptions are the chlorinated and fluorinated solvents.

Combustion   An exothermic oxidation reaction that may occur with any organic compound, as well as certain elements, e.g., hydrogen, sulfur, phosphorus, and magnesium. The heat evolved by combustion is due to rupture of chemical bonds and the formation of new compounds. Substances vary greatly in their combustibility, that is, in their ignition points (solids and gases) or their flash points (liquids).

Comminute   To pulverize or reduce solids to small sizes by mechanical methods, such as grinding.

Communicable Disease   A contagious disease that can be spread to uninfected persons in a variety of ways.

Comonomer   A monomer that is physically mixed with another monomer for a copolymerization reaction, the result of which is a copolymer, such as ethylene vinyl acetate, or butadiene styrene.

Compatibility   The ability of two or more substances to mix together without spontaneous separation. In device terminology the term may be applied to compatibility with the human body, referring to the ability of the device to interface with tissue without causing harm to the patient.

Complement   A system of nine serum proteins that interact with antigen and antibody to produce cytolytic, chemotactic and anaphylactic effects.

Complement, Bioactive Products   With respect to host defenses and inflammation (experienced after prosthetic implants), the most important products of complement are high molecular weight fragments of C3 with opsonic activity, and low molecular weight peptides of C3 and C5 that exhibit anaphylatoxin activity and directly stimulate leukocytes.

Complement Activation   The complement activation cascade may be initiated by microbial pathogens, endogenous immune complexes, or complement adsorption onto foreign surfaces. Activation results in the production of a series of activation peptides and anaphylatoxins, which increase vascular permeability. The most potent of these peptides, C5a, is also chemotactic for inflammatory cells and stimulates release of toxic oxygen products and lysosomal enzymes by neutrophils.

Complement Activation, Interactions   Complement system proteases interact directly with the coagulation, fibrinolytic, kinin-generating systems, and membrane attack complexes that promote platelet aggregation.

Complement Fixation   The binding of serum complement in a reaction with antigen and antibody. Complement fixation and activation on the surface of biomaterials is thought to induce mural thrombus.

Complexing Agents   See CHELATING AGENTS, SEQUESTERING AGENTS.

Compliance   In tensile testing, the reciprocal of Young's Modulus. In device terminology, the ability of an implant to closely match the physiological and mechanical properties of tissues at the implant site.

Component   (Regulatory). Any material, substance, piece, part, or assembly used during device manufacture that is intended to be included in the finished device.

Composite   An article or substance containing two or more different substances. In plastics, the term is frequently used in reference to structures containing reinforcing fibers or polymers (dispersed, discontinuous phase) incorporated into compatible polymeric matrixes (continuous phase). Reinforced composites are used in dental, orthodontic, and orthopedic devices.

Composite Material   A compound of two or more materials consisting of at least three structures; Materials A and B, plus a bound interface AB.

Compound   A mixture of polymer(s) and ingredient(s) necessary to modify the polymer to a form suitable for processing, fabrication, and stability in the intended implant site.

Compounding   The art of mixing polymers with additives such as lubricants, stabilizers, fillers, and pigments in a form suitable for production of finished products.

Compressibility   The change in volume per unit volume produced by a change in pressure. The reciprocal of bulk modulus.

Compression Mold   A precision-machined mold used in the process of compression molding.

Compression Molding   A method of molding in which the preheated polymer is forced into a cavity. The material is subjected to pressure and (usually) heat until cure has been effected. The process most often employs thermosetting resins, such as silicones, for the production of medical devices.

Compression Ratio   In extrusion terminology, the ratio of the volume of material held in the first flight at the feed zone to the volume held in the last flight in the metering section. This ratio provides an indication of the compaction performed on the material, and the amount of mechanical work done on the melt by the screw.

Compression Set   A permanent deformation of a material resulting from the application of compressive stress.

Compression Zone   The portion of an extruder barrel in which melting of the extrudate is completed.

Compressive Modulus   The ratio of compressive stress to compressive strain below the proportional limit. Theoretically equal to Young's Modulus determined from stress-strain curves.

Compressive Strength   The maximal load sustained by a test specimen in a compressive test divided by the original area of the specimen.

Compressive Stress   The compressive load per unit area of original cross section carried by the specimen during a compression test.

Condensation   (1) A chemical reaction in which two or more molecules combine, with the separation of water, alcohol, or other simple substance (condensate). If a polymer is formed by condensation, the process is referred to as polycondensation. (2) The change of state of a substance from the vapor to the liquid state.

Condensation Agent   A chemical substance that acts as a catalyst during a polycondensation reaction. It may also be a substance that provides a complement reactant necessary for a polycondensation reaction to occur.

Conditioning   The act of subjecting a test specimen to standard environmental and/or stress history conditions prior to testing. Typical conditions for medical devices are 40–50% relative humidity at room temperature.

Conductance   The electrical conductivity of a solution, defined as the reciprocal of resistance. Most commonly used in connection with electrolytic solutions.

Conductivity, Electrical   The reciprocal of volume resistivity; the conductance of a unit cube of material.

Configuration   In an organic molecule, the specific location or disposition of substituent atoms or groups around asymmetric carbon atoms.

Conformal Coatings   Thin surface coatings of polymers designed to protect substrates from environmental degradation, abrasion, etc.

Conformation   The shapes or arrangements in three-dimensional space that an organic molecule assumes by rotating carbon atoms or their substituents around single covalent bonds.

Congenital   A condition, deformity, or disease present at birth.

Conjugated   In chemistry, the regular alternation of single and double bonds between atoms and molecules, such as those seen in the benzene ring.

Conjugated Double Bonds   A chemical term signifying double bonds separated from each other by single bonds, such as 1,3 butadiene, $CH_2 = CH - CH = CH_2$.

Connective Tissue   The body's mechanical stability and strength are provided by the connective tissue: fibrous tissue, adipose tissue, cartilage, and bone. The intercellular substance contains collagen fibers, which display high tensile strength, and elastin, which displays great elasticity. The mechanical properties of the connective tissue depend on the relative number of these fibers. The least elastic are the tendons, which consist mainly of collagenous connective tissue fibers.

Consistency   The rheological property of a material by virtue of which it tends to resist deformation.

Contact Adhesive   A liquid adhesive that dries to a film that is tack-free to other materials but not to itself. A typical medical-grade contact adhesive can be made of a silicone elastomer dissolved in chlorinated solvents. The adhesive is applied to both surfaces to be joined, and partially dried. When pressured together for a few seconds a bond of high initial strength is obtained.

Contact Lens   A lens made of a variety of polymers worn directly on the eye in place of eye glasses. It may also be worn by a person after cataract surgery, in which case the device performs the functions of the diseased natural lens removed during surgery.

Contact Pressure Resins   Liquid resins that thicken on heating, and when used for bonding require little or no pressure to effect bonding.

Continuous Phase   In a suspension, the liquid medium in which the solid particles are dispersed. The solid particles are the discontinuous phase.

Continuous Polymerization   An economically advantageous type of polymerization in which the monomers are continuously fed to a reactor, and the polymer produced is continuously removed. Medical-grade Pellethane polyurethane is produced by a continuous extruder-reactor polymerization process disclosed in U.S. Patent 3,642,964.

Controlled-Release   Descriptive of devices capable of delivering drugs at a controlled, sustained rate for prolonged periods of time. It may involve (1) encapsulation of the drug, (2) incorporation into a neutral polymeric matrix, (3) coating the devices, and (4) absorbing the drug into various substrates.

Control Number   (Regulatory). Any distinctive combination of letters, numbers, or both, from which the complete manufacturing history, control, packaging, and distribution of a production run, lot, or batch of finished devices can de determined.

Contusion   A bruise. Swelling and discoloration of the skin following an injury.

Converting   A term descriptive of processes by which a multitude of packaging products are produced. Converting involves coating, impregnating, laminating, embossing, printing operations, etc., necessary to produce finished packaged products.

Coordination Catalysts   Catalysts comprising a mixture of (1) an organometallic compound, such as triethyl aluminum and (2) a transition-metal compound, i.e., titanium tetrachloride, used in the production of high molecular weight olefins and dienes. They are often called *Ziegler-Natta catalysts*, in honor of the inventors.

Coordination Compound   A complex compound comprising a central atom bonded to other atoms by coordinate covalent bonds based on a shared paired electron, both of which are of a single atom or ion. These compounds are frequently used as polymerization catalysts.

Copolycondensation   The copolymerization of two or more monomers by the condensation polymerization process.

Copolymer   A high molecular weight substance containing several types of repeating structures. A styrene-methyl methacrylate copolymer is obtained by polymerizing styrene and methyl methacrylate together. It is sometimes used for terpolymers (acrylonitrile, butadiene, styrene), quadripolymers, etc. Three common types of copolymers are block copolymers, graft copolymers, and random copolymers.

Cornea   The clear, transparent portion of the eye that permits the entry of light, refracts light rays, and helps focus the eyes. Contact lenses are placed directly over the cornea to correct ophthalmic deficiencies.

Corona Discharge   The flow of electrical energy from a conductor to the surrounding air or gas. The discharge is produced by high voltage, over 5000 volts, resulting in a characteristic pale violet glow.

Corona Discharge Treatment   An important surface treatment which renders normally inert polymers, such as olefins, and fluorocarbons, more receptive to coatings, adhesives, and inks. The corona discharge oxidizes the surface of the polymer by the formation of polar groups on reactive site.

Corrosion   (l) The degradation of polymers as a result of environmental forces. (2) The destruction of body tissues by strong acids and bases. (3) The electrochemical degradation of metals due to environmental factors.

Corrosion Resistance   The important ability of polymers to resist environmental degradation.

Corticosteroids   Natural or synthetic compounds from the adrenal cortex that act as anti-inflammatory and immunosuppressive agents. Some pacemaker lead tips are coated with steroids to avoid inflammation of the endocardium and thus provide better electrical conductivity after prolonged implantation.

Cosmeceutical   A coined word signifying the grey area between a cosmetic and a pharmaceutical. Some cosmetic preparations claim medicinal effects, e.g., wrinkle removal, skin rejuvenation, etc. Traditionally, only pharmaceuticals were allowed to claim medicinal effects.

Cosmetic   Any preparation in the form of a liquid, semi-liquid paste, or powder applied to the skin to improve its appearance, for cleaning, softening, or protection, but without specific medicinal or curative effects.

Coumarone-Indene Resins   Thermoplastic resins produced by polymerizing a coal tar naphtha containing coumarone and indene. Not used in medical devices.

Coupling Agent   A chemical substance capable of reacting with both the reinforcing agent and the resin matrix of a composite material to promote a stronger bond at the interphase. Silane coupling agent(s) are frequently used for this purpose.

CP   (l) Abbreviation for *Cellulose Propionate Resins*. (2) In chemistry, abbreviation for *Chemically Pure*.

Cps   Abbreviation for *Centipoise*, a unit of viscosity.

CPVC   Abbreviation for *Chlorinated Polyvinyl Chloride Resin*.

CR   Abbreviation for *Chloroprene Rubber*.

Crazing   Microscopic fine cracks that may extend in a network on, or under, the surface of a polymer. An undesirable effect in plastics articles characterized by a frosty appearance, due to (l) shrinkage, (2) flexing, (3) solvents, (4) temperature changes, and (5) environmental shocks.

Creep   The time-dependent dimensional change of a polymer under load. Creep at room temperature is also called *cold flow*.

Creep Rupture   A failure mechanism resulting in rupture of a polymer under continuously applied stress at a point below the normal tensile stress. This phenomenon is caused by the viscoelastic nature of many polymers.

Critical Component   (Regulatory). Any component of a critical device whose failure to perform can reasonably be expected to cause failure of a critical device, or to affect its safety or effectiveness.

Critical Device   (Regulatory). A device intended for surgical implant into the body or to support or sustain life, and whose failure to perform when properly used in accordance with instructions for use provided in the labelling can reasonably be expected to result in a significant injury to the user.

Critical Operation   (Regulatory). Any operation in the manufacture of a critical device which, if improperly performed, can reasonably be expected to cause the failure of a critical device or to affect its safety or effectiveness.

Critical Strain   The strain at yield point.

Critical Surface Tension   The value of surface tension of a liquid below which a liquid will wet the surface of a polymer. The critical surface tension is measured by contact angle studies and is measured in dynes/cm. Values of some medically important polymers are: acetal = 47, epoxy = 47, fluoroethylene propylene = 16, polyamide = 46, polycarbonate = 46, polyethylene = 46, polymethyl methacrylate = 49, polysulfone = 41, polytetrafluoroethylene = 18, silicone = 39. Surface tension of common liquids are: glycerol = 63, petroleum oil = 29, epoxy adhesive = 47, water = 73.

Critical Technologies   (Key Technologies). Those products, processes, systems, devices, and their applications that create geographically pervasive and significant effects on modes of conducting business, national behavior, production processes, recovery and utilization of resources, or the health and well-being of mankind. According to a 1991 report by the 13-member National Critical Technologies Panel, the 21 technologies listed as national priorities and critical to the future of the United States are (in alphabetical order):

1. Aeronautics	2. Applied molecular biology
3. Ceramics	4. Composites
5. Computer simulation	6. Data storage and peripherals
7. Electronics and phototonics	8. Energy technologies
9. Computer-aided manufacturing	10. High-definition imaging
11. High-performance metals/alloys	12. Intelligent processing systems
13. Materials synthesis	14. Medical technology
15. Micro/nanofabrication	16. Micro/optoelectronics
17. Pollution minimization	18. Sensors and signal processing
19. Software	20. Surface transportation
21. Systems management technology	

Cross-Linking   As applied in polymer chemistry, the formation of covalent bonds between adjacent molecular chains. When extensive, as in most thermosetting resins, cross-linking makes one infusible supermolecule of all molecular chains, also rendering the material insoluble in most organic liquids. Cross-linking may be achieved by chemical agents that produce free radicals, by using multifunctional monomers, or by irradiation with high-energy electron beams.

Cross-Linking Index   The average number of cross-linked units per primary polymer molecule in the system as a whole.

Cryogenic   Pertaining to very low temperatures, such as -150°F or below. Cryogenic temperatures are used to granulate elastomeric polymers.

Cryogenic Surgical Device   A Class II device used to destroy nervous tissue by the application of extreme cold to the target site.

Cryptometer   An instrument for measuring the opacifying power of surface coatings.

Crystal   A homogeneous solid displaying an orderly and repetitive steric arrangement of its atoms.

Crystal Lattice   The spatial arrangement of atoms or radicals in a crystal.

Crystalline Polymers   Polymers containing a portion of their atoms and molecules arranged in a perfect crystal lattice. These polymers exhibit excellent chemical resistance, sharp melting points, low melt viscosity, and significant tensile, flexural, and heat distortion improvements with reinforcement. Typical crystalline polymers are: polypropylene, polyacetal, nylon 6/6, and polybutylene terephthalate.

Crystallinity   A state of molecular structure in some polymers attributed to the existence of crystals with a definite geometric form.

Crystallization   The phenomenon of crystal formation by nucleation and accretion.

C-Stage Resin   The final, cured state of a thermosetting resin.

CTA   Abbreviation for *Cellulose Triacetate.*

Culture   A process in which microorganisms in a specimen such as blood, urine or throat swab are placed in a nutrient broth and allowed to grow, so that they can be identified, and appropriate treatment given.

Curative   Any substance or agent that effects a fundamental and desirable change in a material to make it more suitable for practical purposes.

Cure   To change the physicochemical properties of a material, by polymerization, cross-linking or vulcanization. Usually accomplished by the combined actions of heat, pressure, and a catalyst. The term is properly used when referring to thermosetting resins, although it is incorrectly used in conjunction with the polymerization of thermoplastic resins.

Curing Agents   (Hardeners, Curatives). Substances or mixtures of substances added to a compound to promote or control the curing reaction. Curing agents are reactive substances that become part of the molecular structure during cure.

Curing Temperature   The temperature at which a thermosetting or elastomeric material is subjected in order to attain final cure. The term is used primarily in conjunction with thermosetting resins and rubbers.

Curing Time   The time necessary to attain full cure in a thermosetting resin or rubber.

Cutaneous Oxygen Monitor   A Class II device used to monitor relative changes in the cutaneous oxygen tension by means of a noninvasive sensor placed on the patients skin.

Cyanoacrylate   (Adhesive). An adhesive based on alkyl-2-cyanoacrylates. These adhesives are characterized by rapid anaerobic polymerization and bonding properties, making them suitable as ''instant'' adhesives for hard and soft tissue implants. Lately, the cytotoxic properties of these adhesives have restricted their use.

Cycle   The sequential operations comprising a process, or part of a process.

Cyclic Compound   An organic compound whose structure is characterized by one or more closed rings. There are three major groups of cyclic compounds: (l) alicyclic, (2) aromatic, and (3) heterocyclic.

Cycloaliphatic Epoxy Resin   A polymer prepared by epoxidation of multicycloalkenyls with organic peracids. Used as adhesives and encapsulants in certain medical devices.

Cyclohexane   A colorless liquid derived from the catalytic hydrogenation of benzene.

Cyclohexanone $CH2_2(CH_2)_4CO$. A colorless liquid produced by the oxidation of cyclohexane or cyclohexanol. Used in the synthesis of nylon 6/6 and nylon 6. A powerful solvent for urethanes, acrylics and vinyl resins.

Cyclohexyl Methacrylate $H_2C{:}C(CH_3)COOC_6H_{11}$. A colorless monomer, with characteristic odor, used in the manufacture of optical lenses and certain dental composites.

Cystoscopy   Examination of the urinary bladder and the lower portion of the urinary tract with a lighted device called a cystoscope.

Cystourethroscope   A Class II device for examining the posterior urethra and bladder.

Cytapheresis   A procedure in which cells of one or more kinds (leukocytes, platelets, etc.) are separated from whole blood and retained, the plasma and other formed elements being retransfused into the donor; it includes LEUKAPHERESIS and thrombocytapheresis.

Cytochemistry   The branch of chemistry that studies the chemical composition of cells and cell membranes.

Cytokines   Important mediators of inflammatory responses by virtue of their ability to attract and activate macrophages and lymphocytes. Among the most important cytokines are: Interleukin-1, Tumor Necrosis Factor, Interferon, and Myeloid Growth Factors.

Cytokinins   A term coined in 1965 to describe a group of natural or synthetic growth substances derived from the purine adenine, characterized by their ability to promote cell division and differentiation in culture. Nearly all known cytokines are adenine derivatives with substituents in the N-6 position.

Cytology   The science that examines and studies cells.

Cytoplasm   The extra-nuclear components of the living cell, including mitochondria, spherosomes, etc. Comprised primarily of water and proteins.

Cytotechnologist   A medical laboratory technologist specializing in cytology. The cytotechnologist processes and stains specimens of exfoliated cells obtained from the female reproductive tract, the oral cavity, and other body cavities, and examines the specimens to detect minute abnormalities that may indicate malignant disease, hormonal changes, inflammation, or infection.

Cytotoxic   Any substance, drug, or other matter that is harmful to cells.

D

Damping   Hysteresis, or variations in properties resulting from dynamic loading conditions. Damping is a fundamental mechanism occurring in viscoelastic polymers, providing an important mechanism for dissipating energy, preventing brittle failure, and improving fatigue performance.

Deaerate   To remove air from a substance. Deaeration is an important step in the production of two-component, castable polyurethanes, to remove air that would cause objectionable bubbles.

Death   The cessation of all physical and chemical processes that invariably occurs in all living organisms. At present there is no standardized diagnosis of clinical death, no precise definition of human death. It has been recommended that the U.S. recognize the cessation of brain function as the definition of death, even in cases where life-support systems could maintain respiratory and circulatory functions by artificial means. See also BRAIN DEATH.

Debridement   Removal of diseased, dirty or foreign matter from a wound.

Defibrillator   A Class III device used to produce an electrical shock (for restoring normal heart rhythm), or to terminate cardiac arrhythmias. It releases a large burst of DC current (up to 400 watt-sec) sufficient to depolarize all the myocardium simultaneously, thus restoring normal cardiac rhythm.

Deflashing   The finishing process of removing of flash or rind produced by spaces between mold cavity edges.

Defoamer   An agent that, when added to a fluid containing entrained gas bubbles, causes the bubbles to coalesce into larger bubbles that rise to the surface and break.

Degradation   An undesirable change in chemical structure, physical properties, or appearance in a polymer caused by heat, light, chemical environment, or mechanical forces.

Degree of Cure　The extent to which cross-linking (curing) has progressed in a thermosetting resin or rubber.

Degree of Polymerization　The average number of monomer units per polymer molecule, a measure of molecular weight. The degree of polymerization is given in percentage terms, i.e., 95% conversion.

Dehydration　Removal of water from any substance, either by ordinary drying or heating, absorption, adsorption, chemical reaction, condensation of water vapor, centrifugal force, or hydraulic pressure.

Dehydrogenation　The removal of hydrogen from a compound by chemical means.

Dehydrohalogenation　The process of splitting hydrogen chloride from polymers containing chlorine atoms such as PVC, caused by excessive heat and/or light. This process may be slowed by addition of heat stabilizers and UV absorbers.

Delamination　The undesirable separation of one or more layers in a laminate caused by failure at the adhesive interphase.

Delustrants　Chemical agents used to produce dull surfaces on synthetic monofilaments to obtain a more natural silk-like appearance.

Denier　The weight in grams of 9000 meters of synthetic fiber in the form of a continuous monofilament.

Density　Mass per unit volume of a substance at room temperature, expressed in metric units such as grams per cubic centimeter, English units such as pounds per cubic foot, or pounds per gallon.

Dental Mercury　A Class II device composed of mercury used as a component in an amalgam alloy in the restoration of dental cavities or broken teeth.

Dentistry　The science and art dealing with the health and care of all oral tissues, with emphasis on (1) prevention, diagnosis, and treatment of teeth and gingivae; (2) replacement of missing teeth; (3) correction of malformations or irregularities of teeth and adjacent bones; and (4) the study and care of nondental diseases affecting the oral cavity.

Deoxy　A prefix denoting replacement of a hydroxyl group with hydrogen. An example is deoxyribonucleic acid (DNA).

Depolymerization　The reversion of a polymer into its constituent monomers, or by chain scission into a polymer of lower molecular weight. Reversion may occur as a result of physical, chemical, and mechanical factors.

Dermatology　The branch of medicine that studies the skin, its chemistry, physiology, histopathology, and the relationship of cutaneous lesions to systemic disease.

Deterioration　An undesirable permanent change in the physical or chemical properties of a polymer evidenced by an impairment of these properties.

Development　Those technical activities of a nonroutine nature concerned with translating research findings or other scientific knowledge into commercial products or processes.

Device   Any instrument, apparatus, implement, machine, contrivance, implant, in vitro reagent, or other similar or related article, including any component part or accessory that is:

(1) Recognized in the official National Formulary, the United States Pharmacopeia, or any supplement to these publications

(2) Intended for use in the diagnosis of disease or other condition, or in the cure, mitigation, treatment, or prevention of disease, in man or other animals

(3) Intended to affect the structure or any function of the body of man or other animals

(4) Does not achieve any of its principal intended purposes through chemical action within or on the body of man or other animals and that is not dependent on being metabolized for the achievement of any of its principal intended purposes

Device, Biofeedback   A Class II device that provides a signal corresponding to the status of the patient's physiological parameters (brain alpha waves, muscle activity, skin temperature, etc.) so that the patient can voluntarily control these parameters.

Device, Biopsy   A Class II device used to remove samples of tissue for diagnostic purposes.

Device, Bleeding Time   A Class II device usually employing two spring-loaded blades that produce two small incisions in the skin. The length of time required for the bleeding to stop is a measure of the effectiveness of the coagulation system, particularly the platelets.

Device, Blood Access   A Class II device intended to provide access to the blood for hemodialysis or equivalent uses.

Device History Record   (Regulatory). A compilation of records containing the complete production history of a finished device.

Device Master Record   (Regulatory). A compilation of records containing the design, formulation, specifications, complete manufacturing procedures, quality assurance requirements, and labelling of a finished device.

Di   A prefix indicating two, or twice. An example is a diisocyanate, meaning that the molecule contains two isocyanate groups. The terms BI and BIS are nearly equivalent.

Diagnosis Related Group   A system developed by the Health Care Financing Administration, the branch of the Department of Health and Human Services responsible for administering Medicare. The objective is to control health costs by establishing incentives to hospitals to limit length of stay and control consumption of resources. There are 468 clinical DRGs, organized into 23 Major Diagnostic Categories (MDCs), which are related to clinical specialties as follows:

Diseases and Disorders of:

(1) Nervous System	(2) Eye
(3) Ears, Nose & Throat	(4) Respiratory System
(5) Circulatory System	(6) Digestive System
(7) Hepatobiliary and Pancreas	(8) Skeletal & Conn. Tissue
(9) Skin, Breast	(10) Endocrine, Metabolic
(11) Kidney, Urin. Tract	(12) Male Repro. System
(13) Female Repro. System	(14) Pregnancy, Childbirth
(15) Newborns, Perinatal	(16) Blood, Immunity
(17) Malignancies, Neoplasms	(18) Parasitic Diseases
(19) Mental	(20) Substance-Induced
(21) Injury, Poisoning	(22) Burns

(23) Factors Influencing Health Status and Other Contacts with Health Services.

Dialysance   The small rate of net exchange of solute molecules passing through a membrane in dialysis.

Dialysate   Fluid flowing through a semipermeable membrane during the process of dialysis.

Dialysis   The process of separating molecules of one size from molecules of another size, in which solute molecules are transferred from one liquid to another through a membrane in response to concentration gradients. Dialysis is frequently utilized to cleanse the blood of patients with kidney failure.

Dialysis, Extracorporeal and Intracorporeal   In extracorporeal dialysis (hemodialysis) blood is purified by an artificial kidney (a hemodialyzer) where waste products diffuse through a semipermeable membrane that is continuously rinsed by a dialyzing solution (dialysate). In intracorporeal dialysis a membrane in the body is used for diffusion; in clinical application, the peritoneal cavity is employed. The method is known as PERITONEAL DIALYSIS. The two procedures are complementary. Hemodialysis is more effective but technically more complex and presents the risk of transmitting hepatitis to the technical staff. Peritoneal dialysis is simpler to perform but less effective, and prone to tunnel infection. Hemodialysis is completed within 3-6 hours; peritoneal dialysis requires almost three times as long. In dialysis, three physical processes can be used: DIFFUSION, OSMOSIS, and ULTRAFILTRATION.

Dialysis, Peritoneal   In peritoneal dialysis the patient's own peritoneal membrane is used as a dialysis membrane. A catheter is inserted into the abdomen; about 1.5-2 liters of sterile dialysate fluid is allowed to flow into the abdomen. Diffusion takes place in 10-30 minutes, and the liquid is then removed by aspiration, with the procedure repeated 20-30 times. Thus, in peritoneal dialysis the abdominal cavity is used as an "artificial kidney."

Dialyzable   A solute capable of being passively removed through a semiper-meable membrane.

Diamondizing   A coating technique (submicron to 5 microns in thickness) that imparts an extremely durable, abrasion-resistant, biocompatible, carbon-based coating to plastics and metal substrates. It provides glasslike abrasion resistance to clear plastics such as polycarbonate, acrylics, and polyarylate. Diamond-like coatings are amorphous solid matrices of carbon and hydrogen atoms covalently bonded in tetrahedral form, similar to crystalline, tetrahedral pure carbon (diamond). Diamond-like coatings provide the following combinations of properties for medical devices:

- Wear resistance
- Low friction
- Non-pyrogenicity
- Hardness
- Biocompatibility
- Prevention of ion migration

Diaphanography   Transillumination of the breasts, with photography of the transilluminated light on infrared-sensitive film.

Diaphoresis   Abnormal perspiration, especially profuse perspiration.

Diaphoretic   (1) Pertaining to, characterized by, or promoting diaphoresis. (2) An agent that promotes diaphoresis.

Diaphragm Contraceptive   A Class II device, a closely fitted membrane placed between the posterior aspect of the pubic bone, and the posterior vaginal fornix, to prevent pregnancy.

Diathermy   A Class II device used in applying therapeutic deep heat to specific areas of the body, as adjunctive therapy for the relief of pain in muscle spasms and joint contractures.

Diatomite   (Diatomaceous Earth). Naturally occurring deposits of skeleton remains of aquatic plants called diatoms. Used as a reinforcing agent in some medical grade silicone elastomers.

Dibasic   Pertaining to acids or salts that have two active hydrogen atoms per molecule. Substances having one active hydrogen are called MONOBASIC, those with three TRIBASIC.

Dibutyltin Di-2-Ethylhexoate   A waxy solid formed by reacting dibutyltin oxide with 2-ethylhexoic acid. Used as a catalyst for curing silicone resins and polyether-based urethane foams.

Dibutyltin Dilaurate $(C_4H_9)_2Sn(OOCC_{11}H_{23})_2$. An important catalyst for the production of urethane elastomers. Also used as a stabilizer for vinyl resins when optical clarity is desired.

Dichlorodifluoromethane CCl_2F_2. (Freon 12). A nonhazardous blowing agent for foamed polymers.

1,1-Dichloroethylene   See METHYLENE CHLORIDE.

Dichroism (l) A property of many refracting crystals exhibiting different colors when viewed from different directions. (2) The exhibition of different colors by some solutions with different degrees of concentration or dissolution.

Dicyclohexyl Phthalate (dioctyl phthalate, DCHP). An efficient plasticizer for PVC, widely used in medical tubing for its clarity and low cost. However, it can leach from the tubing and thus into the infusion liquid, creating a toxicity hazard.

Die A metal block containing a precision-machined orifice through which a molten plastic is extruded, shaping the extrudate to the desired profile.

Die Adaptor The portion of an extrusion die that holds the die block.

Die Block The part of an extrusion die that holds the forming bushing and core.

Die Cone (Torpedo). The tapered portion of an extrusion die that guides the extrudate to the webs of the spider.

Die Cutting The process of cutting shapes from sheets of plastic by applying hydraulic or mechanical pressure to a knife edge.

Die Land The final element of an extrusion die that imparts to the extrudate its final profile.

Die Lines (l) In blow molding, vertical defect lines caused by damaged die elements or compound contamination; (2) in extrusion, parallel defect lines caused by damaged dies or compound degradation.

Die Plates In injection molds, the members that are attached respectively to the fixed and moving heads of the compression press.

Die Spider In extrusion terminology, the membranes or wires supporting a mandrel within the head and die assembly.

Die Swell In extrusion terminology, the increase in diameter of the extrudate compared to the die opening through which it is extruded.

Die Swell Ratio In extrusion terminology, and particularly in blow-molding, the ratio of the outer parison to the outer diameter of the extrusion die.

Dielectric Polymers with very weak electrical conductivity so different parts of its surface display different electrical charge. These polymers typically exhibit conductivities in the order of one millionth of a reciprocal ohm per centimeter.

Dielectric Heating (Radio Frequency Heating, High Frequency Heating). Heating a polymer by internal molecular friction and stress induced by an alternating current of sufficient frequency and intensity. Most polymers have dielectric loss characteristics sufficiently high to be heated in this highly efficient fashion.

Dielectric Heat Sealing An important sealing method, widely used for sealing films made of thermoplastics with sufficient dielectric loss, in which the films are heated rapidly by dielectric heating, causing adhesion between the films. Medical packaging is frequently sealed by dielectric heat sealing.

Dielectric Loss   A loss of energy resulting in the temperature rise of a dielectric material placed in an alternating electrical field of sufficient frequency and intensity.

Dielectric Loss Angle   (Dielectric Phase Difference). The arithmetic difference between ninety degrees and the dielectric phase angle.

Dielectric Phase Angle   The angular difference in phase between the sinusoidal voltage applied to the dielectric material and the resulting current.

Dielectric Strength   A measure of the maximum voltage required to puncture a dielectric material, expressed in volts per mils of thickness. The voltage value is the average root-mean-square voltage gradient between two electrodes under which the electrical breakdown occurs under standard test conditions.

Diene Polymers   A large family of polymers characterized by the presence of unsaturated hydrocarbons or diolefins having double bonds. In conjugated dienes the double bonds are separated by only one single bond; in unconjugated dienes the double bonds are separated by at least two single bonds. Included in this family are: copolymers of ethylene, propylene, isoprene, butadiene, and cyclopentadiene.

Diethyl Adipate   (dioctyl adipate, DOA). A primary plasticizer for vinyls, polystyrene, and ethyl cellulose resins. Used in medical grade vinyls because it is FDA approved for food contact, and because it imparts resistance to extraction to tubings and catheters compounded with it.

Diethylene Glycol   bis (allyl carbonate). A thermosetting resin belonging to the family of allyl resins, used extensively in the manufacture of colorless, optically clear lenses, with outstanding chemical and abrasion resistance.

Di(2 Ethylhexyl) Phthalate   (dioctyl phthalate, DOP). An important primary plasticizer for PVC resins. Generally recognized as imparting the best over-all properties to vinyls. However, it can easily be extracted from vinyl tubings, creating a toxicity hazard to patients.

Differential Thermal Analysis (DTA)   An analytical method, similar in some respects to Thermogravimetric Analysis (TGA), except that the specimen is heated simultaneously with an inert control material, each having its own temperature sensing and recording apparatus. The curve plotting weight losses of both materials under the same heating rate is known as the DTA curve.

Diffusion   The spontaneous mixing of one substance with another resulting from the movement of molecules of each substance through the empty molecular spaces of the other substance. Diffusion occurs in and between gases, liquids and solids. The new technology of controlled drug release is based in large part on the diffusion of drugs through nonporous polymer films.

Diffusion Couple   An assembly of two materials in such intimate contact that each may diffuse into the other.

Diisobutyl Aluminum Chloride   A catalyst for the polymerization of olefins.

Diisobutyl Ketone (DIBK)   (2,6-dimethyl-4-heptanone). A slow evaporating solvent for vinyls, cellulosics and certain acrylic resins.

Diisocyanates   Organic compounds having two isocyanate groups (–NCO), used in the production of polyurethane elastomers, foams, adhesives, etc. Other uses include incorporation into adhesives to improve bonding to many substrates.

Diisooctyl Phthalate (DIOP)   A primary plasticizer for PVC, with performance similar to DOP. DIOP is FDA approved for medical applications involving contact with water.

Dilatancy   A rheological phenomenon characterized by an increase in viscosity with increasing rates of shear. It is the opposite of pseudoplasticity.

Dilatomer   See PYCNOMETER.

Dilator   A Class II device designed to augment (dilate) an intended body passage.

Dilator, Esophageal   A Class II device consisting of a cylindrical instrument and weighed with mercury or metal, used to dilate a stricture of the esophagus.

Dilator, Rectal   A Class II device designed to dilate the anal sphincter and canal when the anal opening may interfere with its function or the passage of an examining instrument.

Dilator, Ureteral   A Class II device consisting of a specially shaped catheter or bougie used to dilate at a place where a stone has become lodged, or where a stricture has occurred.

Diluent   A substance that lowers the concentration, viscosity, or cost of another more expensive material. In adhesives, diluents are used for thinning out liquids, increasing or decreasing rates of evaporation, lowering costs, etc. If it is an inert powder added to an elastomer merely to increase its volume (and thereby reduce cost) is called a filler.

Dilute Solution Viscosity   The viscosity of a dilute solution of a polymer, measured under standard conditions, as an indication of the molecular weight and degree of polymerization of a resin.

Dimensional Stability   The innate ability of a plastic part to retain the precise dimensions in which it was extruded, molded, cast, or fabricated.

Dimer   (1) A molecule formed by the union of two identical simpler molecules, (2) a substance composed of dimers. For instance, propane C_4H_8 is a dimer of ethane C_2H_4.

Dimeric Acid   A coined, generic term for high molecular weight dibasic acids that polymerize with diols and glycols to make plasticizers.

Dimethylformamide (DMF) $(CH_3)NCOH$. A colorless, strong solvent for polyurethanes, vinyls, nylons, and other resins. Its strong solvent action makes it suitable for adhesive and coating compositions.

Dimethyl Ketone   See ACETONE.

Dimethyl Polysiloxanes   (dimethyl silicone fluids). An important family of fluid silicones of the composition $[(CH_3)_2SiO]_n$, widely used as lubricating agents, antifoams, and gels in the medical industry. See also SILICONES.

1,4 Dioxane (diethylene ether). A powerful solvent for polyurethanes and vinyls, similar in action to THF, but at a lower cost.

Dip Coating A coating process wherein the object to be coated is immersed in a vessel containing a solution, dispersion, or heated fluid coating material, then withdrawn and subjected to heat or drying to solidify the film deposit. FLUIDIZED BED COATING is a typical example of this technique.

Dip Forming (Dip Coating). A process similar to dip coating, except that the cured or dried deposit is stripped from the dipping mandrel. Devices such as intraaortic balloons are manufactured in this fashion. Also many developmental prosthesis are fabricated this way, the most notable being diaphragms for artificial heart devices.

Discoloration (1) Any undesirable change from an initial coloration possessed by a polymer. (2) A lack of uniformity in color where color should be uniform over the whole surface of a plastic article, also known as mottling, segregation, two-toning.

Disinfection The removal or destruction of those living organisms that may otherwise cause specific damage or infection. In disinfection, it is not necessary to remove all microorganisms, but only those that can produce undesirable results. Thus, disinfection is a less lethal process than sterilization and lacks the margin of safety achieved by sterilization techniques. See also STERILIZATION.

Dispersant Any liquid component capable of solvating a resin, so as to aid in dispersing and suspending it.

Disperse Phase In a suspension, the disperse phase refers to the solid particles dispersed in the liquid medium, thus being the discontinuous phase. In contrast, the liquid is called the continuous phase.

Dispersing Agents Any substance added to a suspending medium to promote and maintain the separation of discrete fine particles of solids or liquids.

Dispersion A two-phase or multi-phase system comprising a finely divided material (the discontinuous phase) uniformly distributed in another material (the continuous phase). In the medical industry, the term dispersion usually denotes a finely divided solid dispersed in a liquid. Dispersions are classified as: (1) emulsions (liquids in liquids), (2) suspensions (solids in liquids), (3) foams (gases in liquids), and (4) aerosols (liquids in gases).

Dispersion Resins A special type of PVC resin with small spherical particles (one micron or less in diameter), suitable for compounding with liquid plasticizers by simple stirring techniques, forming plastisols and organosols.

Dissipation Factor, Electrical The ratio of conductance of a capacitor in which the material is the dielectric. Most polymers have a low dissipation factor, a desirable property because it minimizes the waste of electrical energy.

Dissipation Factor, Mechanical   The ratio of the loss modulus to the modulus of elasticity.

Dissolution   The process by which a chemical or drug becomes dissolved in a solvent. In biological systems, aqueous drug dissolution is a prerequisite of systemic absorption. The rate at which drugs with poor aqueous solubility dissolve from a solid dosage form often controls the rate of systemic absorption.

Di-tert-butyl Peroxide   A stable liquid used as a high temperature polymerization catalyst for a variety of olefin and vinyl monomers.

DMF   Abbreviation for *Dimethylformamide Solvent*.

Doctor   Any device used to spread a coating onto a substrate in a layer of controlled uniformity and thickness.

Doctor Bar   (Doctor Blade, Doctor Knife). A precision-machined flat bar used for regulating the amount of liquid material on the rollers of a coating machine, or to control the thickness of a coating after it has been applied to a substrate.

Doctor Roll   A roll operating at a different speed or in the opposite direction as compared to the primary roll of a coating machine, thus regulating and controlling the uniformity and thickness of coating material before it is applied to the substrate.

Donor   (1) An organism that supplies living tissue to be used in another body (recipient), as a person who furnishes blood for transfusion, or an organ for transplantation. (2) A substance or compound that contributes part of itself to another substance (acceptor).

Donor, Universal   A person with group O blood; such blood is sometimes used in emergency transfusion. Transfusion of blood cells rather than whole blood is preferred.

DOP   Abbreviation for *Dioctyl Phthalate* or *Di(2-ethylhexyl phthalate) Plasticizer*.

Dosage   The exact quantity of a drug that has been prescribed for a given time period.

Double Bond   A type of intermolecular structure in which a pair of valence bonds joins a pair of carbon or other atoms, or a covalent linkage in which atoms share two pairs of electrons. In general, double bonds are represented in chemical formulas by the symbols " $=$ " or " $:$ ", as in ethylene, $H_2C = CH_2$ or $H_2C:CH_2$.

Drawdown   In extrusion terminology, the process of stretching the hot extrudate away from the die at speeds higher than the merging melt, thus reducing the cross-sectional dimensions of the extrudate.

Drawdown Ratio   In extrusion terminology, the ratio of thickness of die opening to the final thickness of the product.

DRG   See DIAGNOSIS RELATED GROUP.

Drug   According to FDA, the term drug applies to the following products:

(1) Articles recognized in the official U.S. Pharmacopeia, the official Homeopathic Pharmacopeia of the United States, the official National Formulary, or any supplement to any of these publications.

(2) Articles intended for use in the diagnosis, cure, mitigation, treatment or prevention of disease in man or other animals.

(3) Articles (other than food) intended to affect the structure or any function of the body of man or other animals.

(4) Articles intended for use as a component of any articles specified in the three previous clauses, but not including devices or their components, parts or accessories.

Drug, Generic   According to the FDA, a generic drug is considered bioequivalent if the rate and extent of adsorption do not show a significant difference from the pioneer product, when administered at the same molar dose of the therapeutic ingredient under the same experimental conditions.

Drug, Generic; Approval   Under the 1984 act, to gain FDA approval a generic drug product must:

- Contain the same active ingredients as the pioneer drug
- Be identical in strength, dosage form, and route of administration
- Have the same indications and precautions for use and other labelling instructions
- Meet the same batch-to-batch requirements for identity, strength, purity, and quality
- Be manufactured under the same GMP regulations as required for pioneer products

Drug Categories   Each drug substance in use today is classified by one or more means as follows: (1) according to site of action; (2) according to therapeutic activity or application; (3) according to the pharmacological mechanism of action; and (4) according to the source or chemical origin and pharmacological properties of the drug. Under these categories, diphenhydramine could be classified as: (1) a drug acting upon histamine H_1 receptors; (2) an antihistamine; (3) a histamine H_1 receptor antagonist; and (4) a derivative of ethylamine.

Drug Delivery Systems   Due to the varying drug release characteristics of the drug products, various terms are utilized to describe available types. A prolonged action drug product is designed to provide a constant supply of drug at a constant rate. In contrast, a sustained release drug product is designed to deliver an initial therapeutic dose of drug that is followed by a slower and constant drug release. A repeat action drug product is designed to release one dose of drug initially and a second dose of drug at a later time.

Drug and Device Market   (European Market). The European drug and device market is estimated at nearly $76 billion in 1991 as follows: Austria: $1,153 million; Belgium: $2,387 million; Denmark: $690 million; Finland:

$817 million; France: $17,501 million; Germany: $20,778 million; Greece: $570 million; Iceland: $156 million; Ireland: $310 million; Italy: $11,355 million; Netherlands : $2,667 million; Norway: $548 million; Portugal: $751 million; Spain: $4,030 million; Sweden: $1,372 million; Switzerland: $1,574 million; and the U.K.: $9,074 million.

Drug Equivalents   The following terms may be used to define the type or level of "equivalency" between drug products:

(1) *Biological Equivalents* – pharmaceutical equivalents which, when administered to the same individuals in the same dosage regimen, will result in comparable bioavailability.

(2) *Pharmaceutical Equivalents* – drug products that contain the same amount of the same therapeutically active ingredient(s) in the same dosage form.

(3) *Therapeutic Equivalents* – pharmaceutical equivalents which, when administered to the same individuals in the same dosage regimen, will provide essentially the same therapeutic effect.

Drug-Related Devices   Of the approximately 1700 generic medical devices identified by the FDA, approximately 70 types are referred to as "drug-related." These devices can be divided into three categories, as follows:

(1) The primary intended use is for the delivery of a drug to the patient.

(2) The primary intended use is not drug delivery; however, the product can be functionally used for that purpose.

(3) A drug is essential to the safe and effective use of the device and may be delivered to the patient during the use of the device.

For purposes of the FD&C Act, intended use means that use intended by the person who placed the product in commercial distribution, as illustrated by labelling claims, advertising matter, oral or written statement. Functional use, on the other hand, is often determined by the end user. See Appendix II for DRUG-RELATED DEVICES CLASSIFICATION.

Drugs, Nonproprietary Names   Some of the recommendations of the United States Adopted Names (USAN) Council regarding prefixes and suffixes for the construction of nonproprietary drug names are listed below:

Anabolic steroids	bol-; -bol
Androgens	andr-; -stan; -ster
Anesthetics (local)	-caine
Anorexics	-orex
Antiadrenergenics (β receptor)	-olol
Antibiotics (cefazolin types)	cef-
Antibiotics (streptomyces strain)	-mycin
Antibiotics (tetracycline deriv.)	-cycline
Anticoagulants (coumarin types)	-arol

Antiinflammatory (ibuprofen type)	-profen
Antiinflammatory (indomethacin type)	-methacin
Antimicrobial sulfonamides	sulfa-
Bronchodilators (phenethylamine)	-terol
Cortisone derivatives	-cort-
Diuretics (thiazide derivatives)	-thiazide
Estrogens	-estr-
Tranquilizers	-azepam
Progestins	-gest-

Drugs, Phases of Clinical Testing   To be accepted for interstate commerce a drug must undergo clinical testing. The following is a summary of the required phases:

	NO. OF PATIENTS	LENGTH	PURPOSE
Phase 1	20–100	Several months	Safety
Phase 2	> 500	Months to years	Effectiveness
Phase 3	Thousands	1–4 years	Dosage

Drugs, Routes of Administration

TERM	SITE
Mouth	Mouth
Sublingual	Under the tongue
Parenteral	Injection
Intravenous	Vein
Intraarterial	Artery
Intracardiac	Heart
Intraspinal or intrathecal	Spinal
Intraosseous	Bone
Intraarticular	Joint
Intrasynovial	Joint-fluid area
Intracutaneous or intradermal	Skin
Subcutaneous	Beneath the skin
Intramuscular	Muscle
Epicutaneous (topical)	Skin surface
Transdermal	Through the skin
Conjunctival	Conjunctiva
Intraocular	Eye
Intranasal	Nose
Aural	Ear
Intrarespiratory	Lung
Rectal	Rectum
Vaginal	Vagina
Urethral	Urethra

Drugs, Schedules   The Comprehensive Drug Abuse and Control Act of 1970 established five ''Schedules'' for the classification and control of drug substances that are subject to public abuse. The schedules provide for decreasing levels of control from Schedule I to those classified as Schedule V drugs.

They are described as follows:

- *Schedule I*: Drugs with no accepted medical use, or other substances with a high potential for abuse. In this category are heroin, LSD, and similar substances.
- *Schedule II*: Drugs with accepted medical uses and a high potential for abuse, which if abused may lead to severe psychological or physical dependence.
- *Schedule III:* Drugs with accepted medical use, which if abused may lead to moderate psychological or physical dependence.
- *Schedule IV*: Drugs with accepted medical use and lower potential for abuse than drugs in Schedule III.
- *Schedule V*: Drugs with accepted medical use and lower potential for abuse than Schedule IV drugs.

Dry Blend   A dry, free-flowing powdery mixture of resin and plasticizer, prepared by blending at high shear and temperature, below the fluxing point. PVC dry blends are frequently used in the extrusion of vinyl tubing for extracorporeal applications.

Dry Coloring   The compounding process of adding dyes and pigments to resins in particulate form. This process enables manufacturers to color match different products, without carrying large inventories of colored resins.

Dry Strength   The strength of an adhesive interface immediately after drying under specified conditions, as opposed to wet strength where the strength of the interface is measured immediately after joining.

Ductility   The maximum amount of strain that a material can withstand, before undergoing ductile fracture. Ductile materials usually exhibit a yield point in the stress-strain curve.

Durometer Hardness   See INDENTATION HARDNESS.

Dye   An intensely colored organic substance that imparts color to a plastic. Dyes used for coloring plastics usually dissolve in the plastic melt, resulting in transparent products, as opposed to pigments that remain as undissolved particles, resulting in opaque products.

EB   (Sterilization)   Abbreviation for *Electron Beam*. Used in conjunction with Electron Beam sterilization. See also STERILIZATION.

EC   Abbreviation for *Ethyl Cellulose*.

ECG (EKG)   Abbreviation for *Electrocardiogram.*

Echocardiograph   A Class II device that uses ultrasonic energy to create images of cardiovascular structures. It includes phased arrays and two-dimensional scanners.

Echoencephalograph   A Class II device that uses noninvasive transducers for measuring intracranial interfaces and blood flow velocity to and within the head.

Ecology   The study of the interactions between plants and animal organisms and their environment. Though primarily a biological phenomenon, ecology involves chemistry in respect to animal nutrients, metabolism, toxicity, etc.

Ectopic   Out of place, e.g., ectopic beat, an arrhythmic contraction not initiated in the sinoatrial node.

Edema   An abnormal accumulation of fluid in the cells, tissues, or cavities of the body.

EDTA   Abbreviation for *Ethylenediamine Tetraacetic* acid, used as an anticoagulant and chelating agent.

EEA   Abbreviation for *Ethylene Acrylate Copolymers.*

EEG   Abbreviation for *Electroencephalogram.*

Efflorescence   Loss of combined water molecules by a hydrate when exposed to air, resulting in partial decomposition indicated by presence of a powdery coating on the surface of the material.

Ejector Pin   (Knockout Pin). A pin driven into the rear of a mold cavity, forcing out the finished product as the mold opens.

Ejector Rod   In injection molding, a bar that actuates the ejector assembly when the mold is opened.

Elaboration   A term used in biochemistry to describe chemical transformations within an organism resulting in formation of specific types of substances; for example, animals elaborate cholesterol.

Elastic Deformation   A change in dimensions of an object under load that is fully recovered following load removal. Also, that part of the total strain in a stressed body which disappears upon load removal.

Elastic Limit   The maximal stress that a material is capable of withstanding, without resulting in permanent deformation upon release of the applied stress.

Elastic Memory   A characteristic of certain polymers evidenced by the tendency to revert to the original dimensions previously existing during their manufacture. For example, oriented film will, upon reheating, return to its unstretched condition due to elastic memory.

Elastic Modulus   See MODULUS OF ELASTICITY.

Elastic Nylon   A specific member of the nylon family of resins that exhibits some elastic characteristics. See also NYLON 610.

Elastic Recovery   That fraction of a given deformation which behaves elastically. A perfectly elastic material has an elastic recovery of 1; a perfectly plastic material has an elastic recovery of 0.

Elasticity   The fundamental ability of a material to fully and quickly recover its original dimensions upon removal of the load that caused deformation. When the deformation is proportional to the applied load, the material is said to exhibit ideal elasticity, or HOOKEAN ELASTICITY.

Elasticizer   A term used for a compounding polymeric additive that contributes elasticity to a resin. For example, acrylonitrile butadiene styrene (ABS) resins can be blended with rigid polyurethanes for this purpose.

Elastin   A scleroprotein that occurs in connective tissue. Partially digested by pepsin, and wholly by trypsin.

Elastodynamic Extruder   See EXTRUDER, ELASTIC MELT.

Elastomer   (1) A macromolecular material, which at room temperature is capable of repeatedly recovering in size and shape after removal of a deforming force. (2) A polymer which at room temperature can be stretched repeatedly to at least twice its original length, and upon release of the stress will immediately return to its approximate length. Most elastomers are given their final properties by a curing cycle. Examples: silicones, ethylene propylene copolymers, polyacrylates, thermosetting urethanes.

Elastoplastic   A plastic that exhibits a degree of resiliency, and will return to, or almost to, its original size and shape if deformed to some extent below its elastic limit, as opposed to a brittle substance.

Electrets   Discs of polymeric materials that have been polarized so one side has a positive charge and the other side has a negative charge, like permanent magnets. Electrets may be formed of poor electrical conductors such as PMMA, nylon, and polypropylene by alternatively heating and cooling in the presence of a strong electromagnetic field.

Electrical Resistance   See INSULATION RESISTANCE, RESISTIVITY.

Electrical Treating   See CORONA DISCHARGE TREATMENT.

Electrocardiogram   The graphic record of the action currents produced during one heartbeat, caused by depolarization and repolarization of the myocardium. Major waves are: P-wave, deflection caused by depolarization of atria; QRS complex, multiphasic deflection caused by depolarization of ventricular myocardium; T-wave, deflection caused by repolarization of ventricular myocardium.

Electrocardiograph   A Class II device used to process the electrical signal transmitted through two or more ECG electrodes, and to produce a visual display of the electrical signals generated by the heart.

Electrochemistry   That branch of chemistry concerned with the relationship between electrical forces and chemical reactions. This relationship is fundamental, as the structure of matter and many of the body's reactions are basically electrical in nature.

Electroconvulsive Therapy Device   A Class II device used for treating severe psychiatric disturbances, e.g., severe depression, by inducing a major motor seizure through a brief intensive electrical current delivered to the head.

Electrode   A terminal member in an electrical circuit designed to promote an electrical field between it and another electrode.

Electrode, Cutaneous   A Class II device to record physiological signals or to apply electrical stimulation.

Electrode, Depth   A Class II device used for temporary stimulation or recording electrical signals at subsurface levels of the brain.

Electroencephalographic Monitor   A Class III device used to detect, measure, and graphically record the rhythmically varying electrical skin potentials produced by the fetal brain. This is accomplished by placing electrodes transcervically on the fetal scalp during labor.

Electroforming   A process used for making inexpensive molds for plastics processes, usually those employing low or moderate mold pressures.

Electrolyte   A substance capable of conducting an electric current when in solution.

Electromagnetic Adhesive   A mixture of an electromagnetic energy absorbing material and a thermoplastic of the same composition as the substrates to be adhered. The substrates are placed in contact, and then the adhesive is rapidly heated by hysteresis and eddy currents produced by high frequency induction coils placed close to the interphase.

Electromyogram   (EMG). A record that traces the electrical activity of muscles. Used to diagnose muscle diseases.

Electromyograph   A Class II device used to monitor and display the bioelectric signals produced by muscles for the diagnosis and prognosis of neuromuscular disease.

Electron   One of the particles of which the atom is composed, bearing a negative charge. About one-half of one-thousandth the size of a hydrogen atom, which is the smallest atom known. Chemical reactions are based on electron transfer and sharing between atoms.

Electron Microscope   A microscope in which the source of illumination is a stream of electrons emanating from a tungsten cathode in a high vacuum and accelerated by a strong electric impulse. The electrons are focused by a series of magnetic fields which function as conventional glass lenses. Two kinds of electron microscopes are used: transmission, in which the electrons penetrate the specimen, and the scanning type, in which the electrons condensed to a fine beam, repeatedly traverse the surface of the specimen, producing a three-dimensional contour of the surface.

Electronegativity   The tendency of halogens (fluorine, chlorine, bromine, and iodine), nitrogen, sulfur, and oxygen to become negatively charged. This is extremely useful in chemistry, since the attractive forces make possible the formation of covalent, ionic, and secondary bonds, and is thus a fundamental factor in the formation of chemical compounds and segmented polymers.

Electronic Heating   See DIELECTRIC HEATING.

Electronic Treating   An important method of rendering a plastic surface more susceptible to bonding and wetting. This is accomplished by subjecting the polymer to a high voltage corona discharge that oxidizes the surface.

Electrophoresis   Migration of suspended or colloidal particles in a liquid, due to the effect of potential difference across immersed electrodes. The migration is toward electrodes or charge opposites to that of the particles. Electrophoresis is important in the study and analysis of proteins because these molecules act like colloidal particles and their charge is positive or negative according to the acidity or alkalinity of the liquid medium.

Electrophoretic Deposition   A coating process in which the article to be coated forms one electrode of a pair immersed in a liquid suspension of the coating material. Upon application of direct current, charged particles of the suspended material migrate to the article, and coat the surface. This process has been used for depositing thin films of PTFE, polyvinylidene chloride, polyethylene, and PVC.

Electroplating   A method of plating common polymers by conventional processes used for metals, after their surfaces have been rendered conductive by precipitation of silver or other conductive substance. This process has proven successful with ABS, polysulfones, polycarbonates, polyphenylene oxide, nylons, polypropylene, and rigid PVC. See also METALIZING.

Electrostatic Coating/Printing   A process that employs electrical charges to direct the path of atomized particles to the work surface. The charged atomized particles are attracted to the grounded object, which must be at least slightly electrically conductive. The coating or ink is subsequently heated to obtain a smooth, fused homogenous layer.

Element   One of the 106 presently known kinds of substance that comprise all matter at and above the atomic level. All elements above lead are unstable and radioactive. All elements beyond uranium are artificially created by bombardment of other elements with neutrons or other heavy particles.

ELISA   Abbreviation for *Enzyme-Linked Immunosorbent Assay*, a sensitive immunodiagnostic technique for detection and quantification of antigens or antibodies in solution. The name is derived from the fact that the assay uses enzyme-linked antigens or antibodies to significantly amplify an antigen-antibody reaction.

Elongation   In tensile testing, elongation is the maximum increase in length of a specimen at the instant before rupture occurs.

Eluant   A solution used for capturing the eluting species from an adsorbent.

Elution Profile   A diagrammatic representation of the amount of eluant diffused from an adsorbent as a function of time. Extensively utilized in the pharmacokinetic characterization of actives delivered via drug delivery systems.

Embedding   (Encapsulation, Potting). The process of encasing an article in a polymeric mass, performed by placing the article in a mold, pouring a polymeric liquid resin into the mold, curing the polymer and removing the encased article from the mold.

Embolus   A detached clot or other object which, when carried by the bloodstream, occludes a vessel. Artificial organs may produce life-threatening emboli.

Embossing   A manufacturing technique used to create desirable surface patterns on plastic films or sheeting. Films may be embossed during calendaring, extrusion, or by reheating the surface and subjecting it to pressure between embossing rolls.

Emergency Ventilator   A Class II device used to provide emergency respiratory support via a face mask, or a tube inserted in the patient's airway.

Emission Spectroscopy   Study of the composition of substances and identification of elements by observation of the wavelengths of radiation they emit as they return to a normal state after excitation by an external energy source.

Emphysema   A pulmonary disease marked by the enlargement of the air sacs caused by destruction of the natural partitions between them. Marked by the inability to exhale completely.

Emulsifying Agents   (Emulsifiers). A substance used to assist in the formation of an emulsion (a stable, permanent mixture between two incompletely miscible liquids, one of which is dispersed as finite globules in the other). Emulsifiers act as surfactants, by reducing the interfacial tensions between the two liquid phases. They also act as protective colloids to promote stability.

Emulsion   A two-phase, substantially permanent mixture of two incompletely miscible liquids, one of which is dispersed as finite globules in the other. The liquid which is broken up into globules is known as the dispersed, discontinuous or internal phase. The surrounding liquid is called the dispersant, continuous or external phase. In plastics usage, the term is broadened to include colloidal dispersions of solids and resins in liquids.

Emulsion Polymerization   A polymerization technique in which the monomer, or mixture of monomers, is emulsified in a liquid, and subsequently polymerized. Emulsion polymerization results in polymers of higher molecular weight than those produced by bulk or suspension processes. The polymers remain in emulsion, and are recovered by chemical, thermal, drying, or freezing precipitation. Examples of resins produced by emulsion polymerization are PMMA, ABS, PVAc, PVC, and polystyrene.

Enamel   (1) A type of paint employing varnish as the vehicle instead of oil. (2) A dispersion of pigment and thermosetting resin that forms a film upon solvent evaporation, and then cures by oxidation, polymerization, or other chemical reaction. (3) A fused ceramic surface coating on a metal substrate, for protective or decorative purposes.

Enantiomer   (Enantiomorphs). (1) One of a pair of optical isomers containing one or more asymmetric carbon atoms, whose molecular configurations have left- and right-hand (chiral) forms. (2) Molecules that are identical in every way except that one is the mirror image of the other.

Encapsulation　The process of applying a thin coating (conformal coating) onto a substrate, which conforms to the external geometry of the article being encapsulated. Medical devices may be encapsulated in silicone, urethane, and other resins to render the products more hemocompatible, resistant to chemical degradation, etc.

Endo　A prefix used in chemical names to indicate an inner position, specifically (1) in a ring rather than in a side chain or (2) attached as a bridge within a ring.

Endocrinology　The science dealing with internal secretions and their physiologic and pathologic reactions.

Endogenous　Refers to a body process that begins, or is produced, within the body. Endorphins, neurotransmitters, and epinephrine are examples of endogenous substances.

Endometrial　Pertaining to the ENDOMETRIUM.

Endometrial Aspirator　A Class II device designed to remove tissue from the endocervix by suction with a syringe, bulb, pipette, or catheter. Used to evaluate the endocervical tissue to detect malignant and premalignant lesions.

Endometrial Brush　A Class III device designed to remove samples of the endometrium by abrading its surface, thus permitting the study of endometrial cytology.

Endometriosis　A condition in which cells that normally line the uterine cavity begin to grow on the surface of other organs within the pelvic structure, and sometimes also in distant areas of the body.

Endometrium　The mucous membrane that lines the normal uterine cavity.

Endorphin　Any group of polypeptides formed in the brain tissue and pituitary gland, which are believed to control the transfer of signals at nerve junctions, thus insuring normal behavior patterns. Imbalance of endorphins result in irrational acts, violence, epilepsy, emotional disorders, and memory lapses.

Endoscope　A device used to provide access, illumination, observation, and manipulation of body cavities, hollow organs, and canals. Examples are: endoscopes, anoscopes, pneumoperitoneoscopes, choledoscopes, colonoscopes, cystoscopes, cystourethroscopes, esophagogastroduodenoscopes, esophagoscopes, pancreatoscopes, proctoscopes, resectoscopes, nephroscopes, sigmoidoscopes, transcervical scopes, urethroscopes and accessories.

Endoscopy　The naked eye inspection of body cavities, by means of tubular illuminated optical instruments. The most frequently used types of endoscopes are listed below:

TYPE	RANGE OF USE	EXAMPLE
Bronchoscope	Trachea	Tumors
Cardioscope	Heart cavities	Valvular and septal defects

TYPE	RANGE OF USE	EXAMPLE
Cystoscope	Urinary bladder	Tumors, stones, inflammation
Esophagoscope	Esophagus	Bleeding, tumors
Gastroscope	Stomach	Gastritis, ulcers, tumors
Laparoscope	Abdomen	Tumors
Laryngoscope	Larynx	Inflammation, tumors
Ophthalmoscope	Eye fundus	Retinal detachment, vessels
Otoscope	Tympanic membrane	Infections, perforations
Proctoscope	Rectum	Hemorrhoids, tumors
Sigmoidoscope	Rectum, colon	Diverticulosis, tumors
Thorascope	Pleural cavity air	Tumors

Endothermic   Referring to a chemical reaction that is characterized by the absorption of heat, as opposed to EXOTHERMIC reactions, which result in the spontaneous evolution of heat.

Endotoxin   Toxins present as a structural part of the cell wall of gram negative bacteria.

Endurance Limit   (Fatigue Limit). The stress level below which a polymer will withstand indefinite cyclic stress without undergoing fatigue failure. Most crystalline thermoplastics and rigid thermoset resins do not exhibit an endurance limit.

Energy   The capacity to do work. It is designated as the product of the force and the distance through which the force is moved.

Engineering Plastics   (Engineering Resins). Polymers characterized by high ratings for mechanical, thermal, electrical, and chemical properties. Engineering plastics are less costly to fabricate than those conventional materials that they replace, such as metals and glass. Engineering Plastics were only identified as a separate distinct category in the 1960s; until then they were merely included with all other plastics. As applications grew, it became apparent that their value lay in "structural" or load-bearing use, with exceptional heat-deflection characteristics. In 1988, the U.S. production of these plastics exceeded 3 billion pounds, and included ABS, acetals, polycarbonates, polyimides, polyphenylene oxide, polysulfone, nylon, epoxies, styrenics, olefinics, fluorinated polymers, and some polyurethanes.

Enthalpy   (Heat Content). A thermodynamic quantity of heat, equal to the sum of the total internal energy of a system, plus the product of the pressure-volume work performed on the system.

Entrainment   The mist or fog of material carried from a liquid through which bubbles or gas are being passed rapidly.

Entropy   A mathematical quantity to measure the "degraded" or unavailable energy in a thermodynamic system, expressed in terms of its changes on an arbitrary scale, the entropy of water being zero at room temperature. The increase in entropy of a body is equal to the amount of heat absorbed divided by the absolute temperature of the body.

Environmental Chemistry   That aspect of chemistry concerned with air and water pollution, chemical, pesticides, and radioactive waste disposal, codified in the Toxic Substances Control Act of 1976.

Enzyme   A complex organic substance formed in the living cells; catalysts for chemical reactions of biological processes, such as digestion. Enzymes are classified by the kind of substance (substrate) consumed in the catalyzed reactions, thus enzymes that break down protein by hydrolytic cleavage are called proteolytic.

Enzyme, Activity   The international unit of activity, U, is the amount of enzyme that will convert 1 μmol of substrate to product in one minute at 25°C, and the optimal enzyme pH.

Enzyme(s), Commercial   Commercial enzymes account for over $1 billion in annual sales in the U.S. Analytical and diagnostic applications are the largest use, generating about $700 million through value enhancements with formulated enzyme-containing products. Therapeutic applications are the second largest category amounting to approximately $275 million. Further growth is expected in the $20 million medical use, particularly utilizing new enzymes derived from biotechnology. Chemical applications are the fourth largest, although most enzyme-based processes remain captive by the companies developing them.

EPA   Abbreviation for the *Environmental Protection Agency*.

EPDM   Abbreviation for *Ethylene-Propylene-Diene Terpolymers*.

Epi   A prefix denoting an intramolecular bond or the presence of condensed double closed chain nucleus substituted in position 16.

Epichlorohydrin Rubbers   A family of elastomers comprising polymers and copolymers of epichlorohydrin. These elastomers are noted for high temperature resistance, low temperature flexibility, and good resistance to solvents and ozone.

Epidemic   A contagious disease that spreads through a large area of a community, a country, and sometimes an entire continent.

Epimer   An isomer that differs from the compound with which it is being compared only in the relative positions of an attached hydrogen and hydroxyl.

Epithelium   Cellular tissue that covers surfaces, forms glands, and lines most cavities of the body.

Eponym   The name of a disease, procedure, principle, or structure derived from the name of the person who discovered or described it first. Many medical devices carry eponymous names, e.g., Swan-Gans catheters, Jarvik artificial heart, etc.

Epoxidation   A chemical reaction in which an oxygen atom is joined to an olefinically unsaturated molecule to form a cyclic, three-membered structure. The chemical moiety resulting from epoxidation is known as an oxirane linkage.

Epoxides   Compounds containing the oxirane structure, a three-membered ring containing two carbons and one bridging oxygen atom. ETHYLENE OXIDE, the most widely used sterilizing gas is an important member of this family.

Epoxy (Oxirane). A prefix denoting an oxygen atom bridging two other atoms that are already united in some way.

Epoxy Plasticizers A family of plasticizers obtained from the epoxidization of vegetable oils or fats. These plasticizers have a heat stabilizing effect in PVC resins, and display a low order of extraction.

Epoxy Resins Resins containing two or more alpha-epoxide groups. The capability of this group to undergo a large variety of addition and condensation reactions leads to numerous thermoplastic and thermosetting forms of epoxy resins. Epoxy resins are generally formed from low molecular weight diglycidyl ethers of bis phenol A, and modifications thereof. Liquid resins are frequently used in medical devices for casting, potting, and adhesives, and are cured with amines, polyamines, anhydrides, and other catalysts.

Epoxy-Novolak Resins Two component resins made by reacting epichlorohydrin with phenol-formaldehyde resins.

Equilibrium (1) A condition in which a reaction and its opposite (reverse) reaction occur at the same rate, resulting in a constant concentration of reactants. (2) Physical equilibrium is exhibited when two or more phases of a system are changing at the same rate, so the net change of the entire system is zero.

Equilibrium Constant A number that relates the concentrations of starting materials and products of a reversible chemical reaction to one another.

Equivalent Weight The weight of an element that combines chemically with 8 grams of oxygen. Since 8 grams of oxygen combine with 1 gram of hydrogen, the latter is considered equivalent to 8 grams of oxygen. (1) The equivalent weight of an acid is the weight that contains one atomic weight of acidic hydrogen, i.e., the hydrogen that reacts during neutralization of acid with base. (2) The equivalent weight of a base is the weight that will react with an equivalent weight of acid. (3) Equivalent weights of other substances are defined in similar manner, such as isocyanates or epoxies.

Erythrocyte A mature red blood cell, the most numerous type of cell found in the blood. Responsible for carrying oxygen and carbon dioxide between the lungs and the body's tissues.

Erythrocyte Sedimentation Rate A laboratory test that determines the presence of infection in the body.

Erythropoitin (EPO) A protein produced in the kidney that stimulates red blood cell production. It is used to treat anemia linked with renal failure and also may find use in anemia resulting from chemotherapy or therapy for AIDS.

ESC Abbreviation for *Environmental Stress Cracking*.

Esophageal Stethoscope A Class I device, it is an unpowered device inserted into the patient's esophagus to enable the user to listen to heart and breath sounds.

Ester Exchange   A reaction between an ester and another compound in which there occurs an exchange of alkoxy or acyl groups, resulting in the formation of another ester. Ester exchange reactions are used in the manufacture of polyvinyl alcohol, polycarbonates, polyesters, acrylics, and plasticizers.

Esters   Organic compounds corresponding in structure to salts in inorganic chemistry. They are derived from acids by the interchange of the replaceable hydrogen of the acid for an organic alkyl radical. Esters are not ionic, but salts usually are.

Ethenoid Plastics   Plastics made from monomers that contain double bonds, e.g., ethylene. Important commercial resins fitting this category are: acrylics, vinyls, and styrene resins.

Ethers   (1) Compounds in which an oxygen atom is interposed between two carbon atoms in the molecular structure. (2) Compounds of neutral character derived from alcohols by elimination of water from two molecules of alcohol.

Ethyl Acetate   (Acetic Acid, Acetic Ester). A colorless liquid made by reacting acetic acid and ethyl alcohol, in the presence of sulfuric acid followed by distillation. It is a powerful solvent for the cellulosics, polyvinyl acetate, CAB, acrylics, and polystyrene. It is among the least toxic of solvents.

Ethyl Alcohol   An alcohol, used as surface disinfectant and solvent from ethyl cellulose, polyvinyl acetate, and polyvinyl butyrate.

Ethyl Cellulose   An ethyl ether of cellulose formed by reacting cellulose with ethyl chloride in the presence of a base.

Ethyl Hydroxyethyl Cellulose   A cellulose ester, used as film former in the pharmaceutical industry for tablet coatings, as binder and thickening agent.

Ethylene Acrylate Copolymers   Resins possessing elastomeric properties similar to rubber and flexible vinyls. Can be processed by thermoforming means, such as extrusion or injection molding.

Ethylene Carbonate $(CH_2)_2CO$. A high boiling, oxygenated solvent exempt from Rule 66. Is practically nontoxic based on oral and acute toxicity testing, with broad solvent powers replacing Isophorone, N-Methyl Pyrrolidone, Dimethylformamide, Dibasic Esters, and Glycol Ether Acetates. A crystal clear, high purity grade is available for medical and pharmaceutical uses.

Ethylene Oxide (EtO)   A colorless gas, with a flash point below $0°F$, derived from the oxidation of ethylene in air or oxygen with silver catalyst. The most widely used sterilant gas in the devices industry. Must be removed from medical devices after sterilization, since it is considered highly cytotoxic.

Ethylene Oxide Gas Sterilizer   A Class II device that uses EtO to sterilize medical devices. Labelling of the device must include directions for the installation of exhaust systems, and describe the need for periodic performance testing using a sterilization indicator. The FDA has established maximum residual limits and maximum levels of exposure to EtO and its two major reaction products, ethylene chlorohydrin and ethylene glycol.

Ethylene Propylene Rubbers (EPR, EPDM)   A family of elastomers produced from the stereospecific copolymerization of ethylene and propylene, and a third monomer such as diene.

Ethylene Urea Resin   A type of amino resin.

Ethylene Vinyl Acetate Copolymers (EVA)   Copolymers comprising major amounts of ethylene with minor amounts of vinyl acetate, that exhibit many of the properties of polyethylene, but also display increased flexibility, elongation, and impact resistance. These properties are derived from the presence and concentration of the vinyl acetate comonomer. EVA films are commonly used as the rate-controlling membranes in certain drug-delivery devices.

Etiology   The study of the causes of disease.

Eugenol   (Clove Oil). A yellowish liquid, derived by extraction of clove oil with aqueous potash. Used extensively in dentistry as an analgesic.

Euphoria   A feeling of happiness and well being, not necessarily based on reality, that may be caused by a drug or illness.

Eutectic   The lowest melting point of an alloy or solution of two substances (usually metals) that is obtainable by varying the percentage of the components.

EVA   Abbreviation for *Ethylene Vinyl Acetate Copolymers*.

Evaporation   The change of a substance from the liquid phase to the gaseous phase or vapor phase. In the case of such solids as ice, snow, dry ice, and a few others, the substances do not go through a liquid phase, the phenomenon is called SUBLIMATION.

Excipient   An inert substance used in the pharmaceutical industry as a binder, solvent, extender, etc., with no pharmacological properties of its own. The following is a summary of excipients commonly used in aqueous injectables:

ANTIMICROBIAL PRESERVATIVES

Benzalkonium chloride
Benzyl alcohol
Chlorobutanol
Metacresol
Methyl paraben
Phenol
Propyl paraben

BUFFERS

Arginine phosphate
Citric acid/Na citrate
Citric acid/Na phosphate
Monoethanolamine

ANTIOXIDANTS

BHA
BHT
Potassium metabisulfide
Sodium bisulfate
Sodium disulfite
Sodium formaldehyde sulfoxylate
Sodium metabisulfide
Vitamin E acetate

OSMOLARITY-TONICITY AGENTS

Dextrose
Gelatin
Glycerin
Lactose

Excipient

BUFFERS	OSMOLARITY-TONICITY AGENTS
Sodium acetate	Maltose
Sodium citrate	Mannitol
Sodium phosphate	Sodium chloride
Succinate	Sucrose
Trometamol	

SOLUBILIZERS-SOLVENTS	OTHERS
Acetone	Edetate disodium
Butyl alcohol	Glycine
Emulphor EL 620	Hydrochloric acid
Ethanol	Magnesium chloride hexahydrate
Igepal CO 630	Protamine sulfate
Mineral oil	Sulfuric acid
Monothioglycerol	Zinc dioxide
Tween 20	Sesame oil
Tween 80	
Propylene glycol	

Exocrine   A glandular secretion delivered directly, or through a duct, to the linings of body parts or to the skin.

Exotherm   The temperature/time curve of a chemical reaction, during which energy in the form of heat is produced. Although the term has not been standardized with respect to sample size, degree of mixing, etc., it is an important consideration during the casting of many two-component resins, such as polyurethanes.

Exothermic   Referring to a chemical reaction that is characterized by the evolution of heat, as opposed to ENDOTHERMIC reactions, which result in the absorption of heat.

Extender   Any substance added to a polymer to reduce the amount, and thus the cost, of the more expensive polymer. The substance may be a filler, resin, plasticizer, or other low-cost material compatible with the main polymer.

Extensibility   The fundamental ability of a material to extend or elongate upon application of sufficient force. Generally expressed as a percentage of the original length.

External Plasticizer   A plasticizer that is added to a polymer, as opposed to an internal plasticizer that is incorporated in a polymer during the polymerization procedure.

Extraction   The transfer of a constituent of a plastic mass to a liquid with which the mass is in contact. Extractions are generally performed by means of a solvent, selected to preferentially dissolve one or more specific constituents.

Extractive Evaporation   A variety of distillation that always involves the use of a fractionating column, and is characterized by use of a purposely added substance that modifies the evaporation characteristics of the materials undergoing evaporation, to make them easier to separate.

Extrudate   The product or molten material delivered from an extruder, such as film, tubing, or profile.

Extruder   (l) The technology used to transform a polymer, by the action of heat and pressure into the production of continuous form such as tubing, sheet, or section. (2) A machine for producing continuous lengths of plastic sections such as tubing, sheets, rods, or profiles. Extruders are divided into single-screw, twin-screw, and ram types, each having specific advantages.

Extruder, Single-Screw   An extruder with one barrel in which a screw is rotated. One of the most frequently used machines in the production of continuous medical tubing.

Extruder, Twin-Screw   An extruder with two barrels forming a figure 8 cross section, each of which contains a screw with tangential or intermeshing flights. Twin-screw extruders are frequently used to compound radio-opacifying solid agents into medical polymers.

Extruder Barrel   A cylindrical metal tube, which forms the housing around an extruder screw and contains the molten plastic material as it is forced through the extruder. Barrels are heated by external electrical heater bands, induction heaters, or hot fluids circulating through attached jackets.

Extruder Breaker Plate   A heavy metal plate perforated with many holes, which supports a screen pack. The function of the breaker plate/screen combination is to filter contaminants from the polymer melt, thus insuring higher purity of the finished product.

Extrusion   A fundamental processing operation in which a molten thermoplastic is forced through a die, followed by cooling or chemical hardening. The high-viscosity thermoplastic is fed into a rotating screw of variable pitch, which forces it through dies under considerable pressure. Extrusion involves complex rheological principles, critical factors being viscosity, temperature, flow rate, and die design.

Extrusion Coating   The process of coating substrates by extruding a layer of molten thermoplastic onto the substrate with sufficient pressure and temperature to affect bonding without resorting to the use of adhesives.

Extrusion Rheometer   An analytical instrument used to determine the melt index of a polymer or compound. The units expressed in units such as grams per minute give an indication of molecular weight distribution, ease of extrusion, etc.

Exudation   (Bloom). The undesirable frosted appearance of a polymer surface when one or more constituents have exuded (migrated) to the surface. In polyurethanes, such exuded constituents may be lubricants, processing aids, mold release agents, etc.

F   Symbol for fluorine; the molecular formula is F_2.

Fabric   A textile composed of mechanically interlocked fibers or filaments; it may be randomly integrated (nonwoven) or closely oriented by warp and filler strands fabricated at right angles (woven).

Fabrication   The assembly or modification of plastic articles by secondary processes such as welding, heat sealing, machining, mechanical bonding, surface coating, etc. The term is frequently misused to include primary (basic, fundamental) production processes, such as extrusion, injection molding, or calendering.

Fabrication Methods   The most important fabrication methods for polymeric materials used in medical devices are:

- Extrusion 38%
- Injection molding 32%
- Foam molding 13%
- Blow molding 9%
- Compression molding 4%
- All others 4%

Fadeometer   An apparatus used for determining the resistance of polymers to fading or color formation, by subjecting samples to high-intensity ultraviolet rays of the same wavelength as those found in natural sunlight.

Fahrenheit   The temperature scale in which 212 degrees is the boiling point of water at 760 mm Hg, and 32 degrees is the freezing point of water. The scale was proposed by the German physicist G. D. Fahrenheit, who also introduced the use of mercury instead of alcohol in thermometers.

Failure, Adhesive   Rupture of an adhesive bond, such that the separation is determined to originate at the adhesive-substrate interface.

Failure, Cohesive   Rupture of an adhesive bond, such that the separation is determined to originate within the adhesive layer itself.

Fallopian Tube Prosthesis   A Class II device designed to maintain the patency of the fallopian tube, and used after reconstructive surgery.

Family Mold   A multiple cavity mold containing variously shaped cavities, each of which produces a component of an item that is assembled from these components.

Fat   A glyceryl ester of higher fatty acids such as stearic and palmitic. There is no chemical difference between a fat and an oil, the only distinction being that fats are solids at room temperature, and oils are liquids.

Fatigue Failure   The failure or rupture of an article under repeated cyclic stresses, at a point below the normal static breaking strength.

Fatigue Life   The number of cycles of deformation required to produce failure of a test specimen under a given set of repeated stresses.

Fatigue Limit   The stress below which a material can be stressed cyclically for an indefinite number of times without failure.

Fatigue Ratio   The ratio of fatigue strength to tensile strength. The mean stress and alternating stress must also be stated.

Fatigue Strength   The maximum cyclic stress a material can withstand for a given number of cycles before failure occurs.

Fatty Acids   Monobasic acids derived from natural oils and fats, such as stearic, palmitic, or oleic. Salts of these acids are frequently used as stabilizers, processing aids, and plasticizers.

Fatty Alcohols   Straight-chain primary alcohols, produced synthetically by the Oxo and Ziegler methods. The most important commercial saturated alcohols are: octyl, decyl, lauryl, myristyl, cetyl, and stearyl. The most important unsaturated alcohols are: oleyl, linoleyl, and lynolenyl.

Fatty Amine   A normal aliphatic amine derived from fats and oils, used as lubricants, mold release agents.

Fatty Ester   A fatty acid with the active hydrogen replaced by the alkyl group of a monohydric alcohol.

FDA   Abbreviation for *Food and Drug Administration*, the agency formed in 1931 under the Department of Health Education and Welfare (HEW), which is concerned with the safety and efficacy of products marketed for medical use. The FDA also promulgates interstate commerce regulations. Under this broad mandate, the regulatory powers of the FDA have been steadily expanding by congressional acts, such as the Food, Drug, and Cosmetics (FD&C) Act of 1938, the Radiological Products Act of 1971, the Toxicological Research Act of 1972, and the Medical Device Amendment Act of 1976. The most respected regulatory agency in the federal government, it is estimated that in 1988 the FDA's annual operating cost reached $1.85 per consumer.

FDA, Device Statutes   Regulations and their governing statutes that pertain to medical device biomaterials are listed below:

STATUTE	PURPOSE	REGULATION
510	Good laboratory practices	21 CFR 58
510(k)	Premarket notification	21 CFR 807
514	Voluntary standards	21 CFR 861
515	Premarket approval	21 CFR 814
518	Recall	21 CFR 7
519	Records and reports	21 CFR 803
520(f)	Good manufacturing pract.	21 CFR 820
520(g)	Invest. dev. exemption.	21 CFR 812.27
		21 CFR 813 812.25(d)
		21 CFR 50 and 56
726	Color additives	21 CFR 70 and 73

FD&C Colors   A series of colorants permitted in food products, medical devices, marking inks, etc., certified by the FDA. Among the most important are: Blues No. 1 and 2; Greens 3 and 6; Reds 2, 3, and 4; Violet 1; and Yellows 5 and 6.

Feed Zone   The first zone of an extruder screw which is fed directly from the hopper, terminating at the beginning of the compression zone.

Felt   A fibrous material composed of interlocked fibers held together by mechanical or chemical action, heat, or moisture.

FEP   Abbreviation for *Fluorinated Ethylene Propylene*.

Fermentation   A chemical change induced by a living organism or enzyme, specifically bacteria or the microorganisms occurring in unicellular plants such as yeast, molds, or fungi. Antibiotics are produced by various forms of microorganisms active in molds, particularly bacteria and actinomycetes.

Fiber   A single homogeneous filament of material having a length of at least 5 mm, which can be spun into a yarn, or made into fabrics by interlocking in a variety of methods.

Fiber Optics   A process, based on newer optical instruments, that allows the visualization of many internal parts of the body.

Fibrillation   Rapid-fire, uncoordinated contractions of separate muscle fibers, e.g., as in the atrial or ventricular muscle.

Fibrin   A body protein essential in the clotting of blood when blood is exposed to foreign surfaces or air.

Fibrinogen   A high molecular weight protein (340,000) occurring in plasma in quantities of 100 to 700 mg/dl. Under the influence of activated thrombin, fibrin monomer molecules polymerize rapidly into long fibrin threads, which form the reticulum of a clot. During this polymerization, calcium ions and another factor called fibrin stabilizing factor enhance bonding between fibrin monomer molecules, as well as cross-linking between the polymerized chains themselves, thus adding stability and strength to the fibrin threads. This reticulum traps additional platelets and leukocytes to form a blood clot.

Filament Winding   A method of forming reinforced plastic articles comprising winding continuous strands of resin-coated material onto a rotating mandrel. In medical devices, epoxies are frequently used in conjunction with carbon to produce a variety of prostheses for orthopedic use.

Filler   A low-cost, relatively nonreinforcing substance added to polymers and adhesives, to reduce the concentration, and thus the cost, of the more expensive material.

Film   A continuous, unsupported thin skin of plastic material no thicker than 10 mils (0.010″). A skin thicker than 10 mils is called a SHEET.

Film Blowing   The primary process of forming thermoplastic film, wherein a vertically extruded plastic tube is continuously inflated by internal air pressure, cooled, collapsed by rolls, and wound up on rolls.

Film Casting   The primary process of making unsupported film by casting a fluid resin or solution on a temporary carrier, followed by solidification, and removal of the solidified film from the carrier.

Fine Chemicals   A generic term signifying chemicals purchased based on specifications and performance, rather than price. They usually meet some standard such as the USP (U.S. Pharmacopeia) or N.F. (National Formulary). Fine chemicals are generally pharmaceutical, agricultural, reagent-grade chemicals, or intermediates.

Finished Device   (Regulatory). A device, or an accessory to a device, which is suitable for use, whether or not it is packaged or labelled for commercial distribution.

Finishing   (1) The secondary operation involving the removal of flash, gate marks, and surface defects from plastic articles. (2) The development of desired surface textures, ranging from smooth to embossed.

Fish Eye   A fault in transparent plastics, appearing as a globular mass of polymer caused by incomplete melting or blending with the bulk. In polyurethanes, fish eyes may also occur as a result of incomplete drying of the resin prior to extrusion.

Fistula   An abnormal passage connecting one hollow organ with another hollow organ.

Flame Retardant   A substance having the ability to resist combustion. A flame-retardant polymer is considered to be one that will cease burning or glow, after the ignition source is removed.

Flame Retardants   Substances usually incorporated as additives into polymers that reduce the tendency of plastics to burn. Nonreactive flame retardants include: antimony trioxide, phosphate esters, and chlorinated paraffins. Reactive flame retardants include: bromine or phosphorous containing polyols and a variety of chlorinated compounds.

Flammability   The extent to which a material will support combustion after ignition. Flammable liquids are those having a flash point below 100°F (37.7°C), and a vapor pressure lower than 40 psi at 100°F. Among flammable liquids (and flash points) are: acetone (-4°F); methyl ethyl ketone (24°F); toluene (45°F). Among nonflammable liquids: methylene chloride, perchloroethylene, trichloroethylene, 1,1,1 trichloroethane.

Flammable Liquids   In general, liquids having a flash point below 100°F. OSHA further classifies flammable liquids into three subcategories:

(1) *Class 1A*—liquids with flash point <73°F and boiling point <100°F.
(2) *Class 1B*—liquids with flash point <73°F and boiling point >100°F.
(3) *Class 1C*—liquids having flash point of 73–100°F.

Flash   Surplus material that is forced into crevices between mating molds during molding operations. The flash is usually removed by secondary operations, such as buffing, grinding, tumbling, or blasting.

Flash Point   The lowest temperature at which a combustible liquid will produce a flammable vapor that will burn momentarily.

Flatting Agent   Minute particles of irregular size incorporated into polymers, used to disperse incident light rays, so that a "flat" or dull surface effect is achieved. Flatting agents most frequently used are silica, diatomaceous earths, and heavy metal salts.

Flexible Molds　　Molds made of elastomeric materials, such as silicones, rubbers, or soft thermoplastics, capable of stretching to permit easy demolding of hard cured pieces with undercuts.

Flexural Modulus　　The ratio of the applied stress on a test specimen in flexure, to the corresponding strain in the outermost fibers of the specimen.

Flexural Strength　　The maximum stress in the outer fiber at the moment of failure. In most plastics, this value is usually higher than the calculated ultimate tensile strength.

Flight　　In extrusion, the outer surface of the helical ridge of metal left after machining the screw channels. The clearance between the screw flights and the inner diameter of the extruder barrel provide the desired compression to the molten polymer.

Flocculation　　The combination or aggregation of suspended colloidal particles in such a way that they form clumps or tufts. Flocculation can be reversed by agitation, as the cohesive forces are weak; this is not true of other forms of AGGREGATION (coalescence and COAGULATION) which are irreversible.

Flock　　Short fibers of synthetic polymers such as acrylic, nylon, or polyesters, used to impart functional/decorative characteristics to a surface by the process of FLOCKING.

Flocking　　A method of finishing whereby the surface is coated with an adhesive, then dusted with fibrous flock to give a finish resembling suede. Flocking is used to provide: visual appeal, sound dampening, thermal insulation, increased surface for evaporation, buffing, polishing, and cushioning.

Flocking　　(Electrostatic). A technique that utilizes a field of static electricity to orient fibers and promote their perpendicular alignment.

Flow　　Movement of an adhesive during the bonding process, before the adhesive is set.

Flow Line　　In injection molding, a blemish on a molded piece caused by the meeting and incomplete fusion of two fronts during molding.

Flow Marks　　Defects in an injection molded article characterized by a wavy surface appearance, caused by improper flow of the molten polymer into the cold mold.

Fluidization　　A gas-solid contacting process in which air is forced through a bed of finely divided resin particles, causing them to lift and separate, behaving like a low-viscosity fluid.

Fluidized Bed Coating　　The process of applying plastic coatings to substrates like metals, wherein the preheated object is immersed in the fluidized resin bed until the desired thickness is obtained. The coated part is subsequently heated to insure particle fusion to a smooth, brilliant layer.

Fluorescence　　A type of luminescence in which an atom or molecule emits visible radiation in passing from a higher to a lower electronic state. Fluorescent dyes are used for labelling molecules in biochemical research.

Fluorescent Pigments Pigments that absorb light at certain frequencies and re-emit light at lower frequencies, thus making polymers containing those pigments appear to possess an inherent glow.

Fluorinated Ethylene Propylene (FEP) A copolymer of tetrafluoroethylene and hexafluoropropylene, displaying most of the characteristics of PTFE, but being a thermoplastic.

Fluorocarbon Resins Thermoplastic resins chemically similar to polyolefins, except that all hydrogen atoms are replaced with fluorine atoms. These modifications result in the formation of polymers with exceptionally low coefficients of friction and high biological stability. The main members of this family are Polytetrafluoroethylene (PTFE), Fluorinated Ethylene Propylene (FEP), and Polyhexafluoropropylene.

Fluorochemical Organic compounds, not necessarily hydrocarbons, in which fluorine has replaced a large percentage of hydrogen atoms. The presence of two or more fluorine atoms on a carbon atom usually imparts stability and inertness. Fluorochemical fluids are used as surfactants, solvents, sealants, and heat transfer media.

Fluoroethylene See VINYL FLUORIDE.

Fluorohydrocarbon Resins Resins made by polymerizing monomers composed of fluorine, hydrogen, and carbon. Examples are Polyvinylidene Fluoride, Polyvinyl Fluoride, Polytrifluorostyrene, and copolymers of halogenated and fluorinated ethylenes.

Fluoroplastics Paraffinic hydrocarbons in which all or some of the hydrogens have been replaced with fluorine or chlorine atoms. These resins exhibit low coefficients of friction, low permeability, negligible water absorption, and chemical/biological inertness.

Foam See CELLULAR PLASTIC.

Foam Casting Any process in which a two-component resin is foamed before or during molding by mechanical frothing, or by a gas dissolved in the mixture or released from a low boiling point liquid.

Foaming Agents See BLOWING AGENTS.

Food and Drug Act Originally passed in 1906 to regulate the purity and safety of foods and drugs. In 1938, Congress passed the Federal Food, Drug, and Cosmetic Act, which required manufacturers of new drugs to prove safety for premarketing approval of new drugs. In 1962, the Act was amended to provide regulatory authority to assure both safety and efficacy of all new drugs.

Foreign Body Reaction A benign variation in normal tissue response, caused by the presence of a foreign material (e.g., an implantable prosthesis). In soft tissue implantations, a "tissue capsule," composed of de novo collagen, multinucleated giant cells, fibroblasts, and blood vessels is normally seen surrounding the prosthesis. See also TISSUE CAPSULE.

Formaldehyde HCHO. (oxymethylene, formic aldehyde, methanal). (1) In polymer chemistry a monomer used to produce acetal resins, phenolics, and urea formaldehyde resins. (2) In biology, a gaseous compound with strongly disinfectant properties. It is used in solution (formol) for surface disinfection.

Forming   A general term encompassing all processes in which the final shape of plastics pieces such as tubing, sheets, etc., is changed to the final desired configuration.

Formula   A list of the ingredients and their amounts required in a product. Such formulas are mixtures, not compounds, used in the plastics, pharmaceutical, and health-care industries.

Formulation   Selection of components of a product to provide optimum specific properties for the desired end use.

Fracture   The separation of a body, characterized as either brittle or ductile. In brittle fracture, the crack propagates rapidly with little plastic deformation. In ductile fracture, the crack propagates slowly, following an irregular pattern along planes on which a maximum resolved shear stress occurred.

Fragrance   An odorant used to impart a pleasant smell to products.

Free Radical   An atom or group of atoms having one unpaired electron. Most free radicals because of their high reactivity and energy are short-lived. They play an important role in many polymerization reactions.

Free Radical Polymerization   A reaction initiated by a free radical derived from a polymerization catalyst. Polymerization proceeds by the chain reaction addition of monomer molecules to the free radical ends of growing chain molecules. Important polymerization methods such as bulk, suspension, emulsion, solution, and photopolymerization reactions are examples of free radical polymerization.

Freeze-Drying   (Lyophilization). A type of dehydration for separating water from heat-sensitive materials, such as biologicals and pharmaceuticals. The material is first frozen and then placed in a high vacuum so that the ice evaporates by sublimation, and the nonwater components are left behind undamaged.

Friction   The resistance to the relative motion of solid body surfaces in contact with each other.

Frozen Strains   (Residual Strains). Strains that remain in an article after it has been shaped and cooled, due to the nonequilibrium configuration of the polymer molecules. Residual strains are often treated by the technique known as ANNEALING.

FTIR   (Fourier Transform Infrared Spectroscopy). A surface analytical technique that determines the chemical composition and bonding of organic, polymeric, and many inorganic materials. FTIR is used to analyze various types of materials in thin film, solid powder, or liquid form. An FTIR spectrum is a plot of infrared light absorbance by the sample as a function of wavelength. Wavelengths from 2.5 to 25 microns (400 to 4000 cm^{-1} wave numbers) are used. FTIR is useful in (1) materials evaluation, (2) failure analysis, and (3) quality control screening.

FTIR, Operation Principle   A beam of infrared light generated by a small furnace in the spectrometer is focused on a sample using special optics. The sample absorbs the light at very specific wavelengths depending on the atomic composition, structure, and thickness of the sample. The reflected or transmitted infrared light is measured at the detector to construct, via fourier transform, the infrared spectrum of the sample mixture. Each substance has a unique infrared spectral fingerprint with the exception of optical isomers and polymers that vary only slightly in molecular weight. The vibrations of atoms in each functional group of a substance have characteristic infrared absorption frequencies that permit substance identification. See also ATR-FTIR.

Fumigant   A toxic agent in vapor form that destroys infectious organisms, insects, and rodents. Commonly used fumigants are ethylene oxide, p-dichlorobenzene, methyl bromide, and formaldehyde.

Fumigation   Disinfection of a contaminated area by means of antiseptic fumes.

Fungicides   Agents incorporated into polymers to control fungus growth by killing the organisms. Most plastics are inherently resistant to fungus, but the cellulosics and many polymers of natural origin are not. Agents that retard fungal growth are called FUNGISTATS.

Fungistats   Agents incorporated into polymers to control fungus growth without killing the fungi.

Fungus   Any of a plant-like group of organisms that do not produce chlorophyll; they derive their food by decomposing organic matter. Examples of fungi are molds, mildews, mushrooms, and the rusts that infect grain and other plants. They grow best in a moist environment at room temperature with little or no light required.

Furane Resins   Dark colored thermosetting resins obtained by condensation polymerization of furfuryl alcohol in the presence of strong acids.

Furnace Black   A type of carbon black, made in a refractory-lined furnace.

Fusion   In plastisol technology, the state attained in the course of heating when all the resin particles have dissolved in the plasticizers present, so that upon cooling a homogeneous solid solution results.

Fusion Temperature   In vinyl plastisols and organosols, the temperature at which fusion occurs.

g (1) Abbreviation for *Gram*. (2) Acceleration due to gravity.

Gamma A prefix denoting the position of atoms or radicals in the main group of a compound.

Gamma Ray Electromagnetic radiation of extremely short wavelength and high energy, originating in the atomic nucleus.

Gamma Ray Spectroscopy An analytical technique involving the use of gamma radiation, which is emitted from radioactive nuclei in discrete energies. The spectrum of energies and the relative intensities of the gamma rays characterize the radionuclide that emits them.

Gangrene Death of a part; necrosis with putrefaction.

Gas A state of matter characterized by very low density and viscosity; comparatively great expansion and contraction in response to pressure and temperature; ability to diffuse into other gases; and ability to occupy with almost complete uniformity any container.

Gas Chromatography An analytical method where the specimen is vaporized and introduced into a stream of carrier gas, which is then delivered through a chromatographic column that separates it into its constituent parts. The constituent parts have characteristic residence rates, and are detected one by one in a temporal sequence as they emerge from the column. The detecting cell responses are recorded on a chart, from which the components are identified both qualitatively and quantitatively.

Gas Transmission Rate The rate at which a given gas diffuses through a stated area of a specimen at standard pressure and temperature. Polymers vary widely in this property, ranging from almost zero GTR for polyvinyl alcohol and fluorocarbons to fairly high rates for polyurethanes, polycarbonates, and some polyolefins.

Gastric Juice A mixture of hydrochloric acid and pepsin secreted by glands in the stomach in response to a conditioned nerve reflex, with a pH of about 2.0.

Gastric Lavage A process of washing the stomach contents, when a toxic substance has been ingested.

Gastrointestinal Tube, and Accessories A Class II device consisting of tubing used for instilling fluids into, and removing them from, the alimentary canal. The device may incorporate an integral inflatable balloon for retention or hemostasis.

Gastroscopy An examination with a lighted tube that enables inspection of the stomach for abnormalities or disease conditions.

Gate In injection molding, the channel through which the molten polymers is forced to flow from the runner system into the injection cavity.

Gel A semisolid system, consisting of a network of solid aggregates in which a liquid is held.

Gel Coat A thin outer layer of a resin, applied to a substrate for protective and decorative purposes. It may also serve as a barrier to liquids, gases, or radiation.

Gel Filtration   A type of fractionation procedure in which molecules are separated from each other according to differences in size and shape; the action is similar to molecular sieves.

Gel Liquid   (Thixotropic Liquid). A liquid formulation that has semi-solid consistency when undisturbed, but which flows readily under shear forces.

Gel Permeation Chromatography   An analytical technique employing as the stationary phase a swollen gel made of cross-linked styrene. The specimen is introduced at the top of a column containing the styrene gel, and then eluted with a solvent, with the molecules of the specimen diffusing through the gel according to their molecular size.

Gel Point   The state at which a liquid begins to exhibit pseudoelastic properties, a stage seen as an inflection point on a viscosity-time graph.

Gelatin   A mixture of proteins obtained by hydrolysis of collagen by boiling skin, ligaments, tendons, etc. Gelatin is strongly hydrophilic, absorbing up to ten times its weight in water, and forming reversible gels of some strength and viscosity.

Gelation   With regard to vinyl plastisols and organosols, the change of state from liquid to solid in the course of heating and/or aging, when the plasticizer has been absorbed by the vinyl resin resulting in a dry, flowing mass.

Gelling Agents   See THICKENING AGENTS.

Genetic Code   Information stored in the genes, which programs the linear sequence of amino acids within the protein polypeptide chain synthesized during cell development.

Genital Vibrator   A Class II device used to vibrate female genitals as a form of massage in the treatment of sexual dysfunction, or as an adjunct to Kegel's exercise (tightening of pelvic muscles).

Geometric Isomer   A type of stereoisomer in which a chemical group or atom occupies different spatial positions in relation to the double bond.

Germicide   Any substance capable of killing germs.

Glacial   A term applied to a number of acids (acetic and phosphoric), which have a freezing point slightly below room temperature when in a highly pure state.

Glass Reinforced Plastics   See REINFORCED PLASTICS.

Glass Transition   (Gamma Transition, Second Order Transition, Rubbery Transition). A reversible change that occurs in amorphous polymers when heated to a certain temperature, characterized by a sudden transition from a hard condition to a rubbery or elastomeric condition. The transition occurs when the normally coiled, motionless polymer chains become free to rotate and slip past each other. This temperature varies widely among polymers, e.g., the T_g of polystyrene is about $100°C$, whereas that of polyurethane elastomers is near $-65°C$.

Glaucoma   An eye disease in which the fluid pressure within the eye rises.

If the condition is not treated it may result in loss of vision.

Globulin   Any group of proteins synthesized by the body when invaded by infective organisms.

Glossmeter   An instrument used for measuring the mar resistance of polymers. As described in ASTM D673, light from a standard source is directed at a 45 degree angle at an abraded specimen, and the reflected light intensity measured by a photoelectric cell.

Glue   Originally, collagen obtained from hides, tendons, cartilage, and bones of animals. In current use, the term is now synonymous with *adhesive*.

Glycocalyx   A general term describing the complex mixture of polysaccharide components found outside the bacterial cell wall. It is generally agreed that bacteria attach themselves to the hydrophobic surface of biomaterials via their glycocalyx, or ''slime layer.''

Glycol   A general term for dihydric alcohols, i.e., alcohols containing two hydroxyl (OH) radicals.

GMP   (Good Manufacturing Practices). The primary basis on which the FDA evaluates a manufacturer's ability to produce a safe and effective device consistently. The Medical Device Amendments of 1976 expressly incorporated into the FDA Act language authorizing the FDA to establish GMPs for the device industry. The FDA has promulgated regulations covering nearly all aspects of manufacturing — device components, production processes, production controls, packaging, storage, labeling, installation, and warehouse distribution procedures. These GMPs are intended to ensure that devices are safe and effective, and that they comply with statutory requirements. Two key documents for GMP compliance are the Center for Devices and Radiological Health (CDRH) May 1987 ''Guidelines on Preproduction Quality Assurance'' and ''Process Validation.'' These documents provide guidance on medical device product manufacturing. The purpose of GMPs is to provide a framework of manufacturing controls. The Agency believes that manufacturers who adhere to these controls increase the probability that their device will conform to their established specifications. This means that if the medical device has been properly designed, following the GMPs will ensure that there is consistent manufacturing of that product with the appropriate quality control checks prior to its distribution and use.

GP   Abbreviation for *General Purpose*.

GPC   Abbreviation for *Gel Permeation Chromatography*.

Grade   Any of a number of purity standards for chemicals established by various specifications. Some of these grades are: U.S.P. (conforms to U.S. Pharmacopeia), N.F. (conforms to National Formulary), C.P. (chemically pure), A.C.S. (analytical reagent quality), and F.C.C. (Food Chemicals Codex specifications).

Gradient Tube Density Test   A simple method for measuring the density of very small samples. A gradient tube is filled with a heterogeneous mixture of liquids; a small drop or particle of sample is dropped into the tube, where it equilibrates at the approximate density, in comparison to known standards.

Graft Copolymer   See GRAFT POLYMER.

Graft Polymer   A heterogeneous polymer comprising a molecular structure where the main backbone has covalently bonded side chains at various points, containing radicals or groups different from those in the main chain. The main chain itself may be a homopolymer or copolymer.

Grafting   A deposition technique whereby organic polymers can be bonded to a wide variety of substrates, both organic and inorganic, in the form of films, tubing, fibers, and other shapes. Grafting occurs at specific catalytic sites on the grafted material.

Gram   One-thousandth of a kilogram. The weight of one milliliter of water at 4°C.

Gram Atomic Weight   The atomic weight of an element expressed in grams, e.g., the gram atomic weight of oxygen is 15.994 grams.

Gram Molecular Weight   The molecular weight of a compound expressed in grams, e.g., the gram molecular weight of carbon dioxide is 44.01 grams.

Gram-Positive, -Negative   A characteristic property of bacteria in reacting to a staining method devised by Gram, circa 1880. The bacteria are stained with crystal violet, treated with Gram's solution, and counterstained with safranine. If the dye is retained, the bacteria is called Gram-positive; and vice versa.

Granular Structure   Nonuniform appearance of plastics due to incomplete fusion, or the presence of coarse particles.

Granulation Tissue   A stage of tissue during repair that includes accumulation of macrophages, fibroblastic ingrowth, deposition of loose connective tissue, and angiogenesis. The term granulation tissue derives from the granular appearance of such tissue when excised and visually examined. The granules are in fact the visible tips of multiple newly formed blood vessels.

Granulators   Equipment comprising rotating knives in close proximity to stationary knives, and a screen through which granulated particles of the desired size are discharged.

Granules   (Granulates). Molding compounds in the form of spheres or small cylindrical pellets.

Granulocyte   A white blood cell.

Granuloma   A nodular inflammatory lesion that contains areas of granulation.

Graphite   A soft, greasy form of carbon, frequently used as a plastic lubricant in fluorocarbon and nylon resins. May also be used in the form of fibers, or whiskers, as a reinforcing agent.

Graphite Fiber   High-tensile fibers made from (1) polyacrylonitrile or (2) rayon, obtained by carbonizing the fibers at high temperatures. Results in fibers with tensile strengths of 50–150,000 psi, resistant to acids and alkalies, self-lubricating, and used in high-strength composites.

GRASE   Abbreviation for *Generally Recognized as Safe and Effective.* Under the FD&C Act, a drug fit for human use must be found safe and effective for indications recommended by its labeling. The safety and effectiveness of the drug must be based primarily on clinical tests using human subjects.

Gravimetric Analysis   A type of quantitative analysis involving precipitation of a compound which can be weighed and analyzed after drying. Also used in determining specific gravity.

Gravure Coating   A coating technique in which the overall amount of coating applied to a substrate is metered by the depressions in the coating cylinder, with excess ink wiped by a doctor blade. Fluid remaining in the cylinder is deposited onto a moving substrate as it passes between the engraved roll and a resilient back-up roll.

Gravure Printing   A printing technique that uses the depressions in an engraved printing cylinder, with excess ink wiped by a doctor blade. Ink remaining in the depressions is deposited onto a moving substrate as it passes between the gravure roll and a back-up roll.

Grit Blasting   A mold finishing technique where abrasive particles are blasted onto a mold surface in order to produce a roughened surface.

Group   (1) One of the major classes or divisions into which elements are arranged in the Periodic Table. (2) A combination of two or more closely associated elements that tend to remain together in reactions, usually behaving chemically as if they were individual entities, e.g., with respect to valence, ionization, etc., such as OH (hydroxyl) and COOH (carboxyl) groups. (3) Any combination of elements that has a specific functional property, for example, a chromophore group in dyes.

Growth Factors   A heterogenous group of substances whose common purpose is to enhance the rate of healing. Growth factors can regulate the migration, proliferation and differentiation of a wide variety of cells. Characteristics of well-characterized growth factors are:

FACTOR	MITOGENIC ACTIVITY	USE
Epidermal (EGF)	Epithelial cells	Skin grafts
Fibroblast (FGF)	Fibroblasts, epithelial cells, smooth muscle, endothelial cells	Angiogenesis, collagen formation
Platelet-derived (PDGF)	Fibroblasts, smooth muscle, glial cells	Chemoattractant, pressure sores
Transforming (TGF)	Fibroblasts	Wound healing
Vaccinia virus (VVGF)	Fibroblasts	Wound healing, pressure sores
Insulin-like (IGF) Type 1	Fibroblasts, osteoblasts	Cell maintenance

GR-S   Abbreviation for *Government Rubber-Styrene*, a rubber copolymer comprising 75% butadiene and 25% styrene, also known as *Buna N* and *Buna SRB*.

Gum   Any class of colloidal substances, exuded or manufactured by plants. These substances are composed of complex carbohydrates and organic acids, which swell in water.

Gutta Percha   (trans-polyisoprene). A geometric isomer of natural rubber obtained from trees native to Malaya, obtained from the milk juice of Palaquium and Payena plants. It is stiff, hard, and inelastic when cold, but softens at 60°C. Present uses are in dentistry, surgical accessories, and as insulating media in electrical devices.

Gynecologic Electrocautery   A Class II device designed to destroy tissue with high temperatures by contact with an electrically heated probe. Used to excise cervical lesions, perform biopsies, or treat chronic cervicitis under direct visual observation.

Gynecology   The branch of medicine that has to do with the diseases peculiar to women, primarily those of the genital tract, as well as female endocrinology and reproductive physiology.

Half-Life   The time during which a radioactive element is reduced to half its original value owing to the disintegration of half its atoms.

Halides   Binary compounds of the halogen family of elements comprising the halocarbons. The term is also used to denote plastics containing these elements, for example polyvinyl chloride is also called polyvinyl halide.

Hallucinogen   Any of a number of drugs acting on the central nervous system causing mental disturbance, imaginary experiences, coma, or even death. Most common are cannabis (marijuana, hashish), lysergic acid (LSD), amphetamines, and morphine derivatives.

Halocarbon   A compound containing carbon, one or more halogens, and sometimes hydrogen. When polymerized they yield polymers characterized by extreme inertness and good heat resistance.

Halocarbon Plastics   A term listed by ASTM for polymers containing only carbon and one or more halogens.

Halogen   An element of the group that includes chlorine, bromine, fluorine, and iodine.

Hammer Mill   A crushing device consisting of metal hammers mounted on a rotating shaft, which makes the hammers impact the material, crushing it against a stationary breaker plate.

Hardener   A substance added to a polymer to promote or control curing reactions. The term is also used to designate a substance added to an oligomer or polymer to control the hardness of the cured product.

Hardness   The resistance of a plastic to indentation, compression, and scratching.

Hazardous Material   Any substance which, if improperly handled, can be damaging to the health and well-being of man. The materials are classified as: (1) poisons or toxic agents, (2) corrosive chemicals, (3) flammable materials, (4) radioactive chemicals, and (5) explosives and strong oxidizing agents. OSHA classifies as a hazardous material, a substance that has one or more of the following characteristics:

1.   PHYSICAL HAZARDS

1.1   Combustible liquid (flash point 100–200°F)
1.2   Compressed gas
1.3   Explosive
1.4   Flammable liquid (flash point < 100°F) >
1.5   Organic peroxide
1.6   Oxidizer
1.7   Pyrophoric
1.8   Unstable (reactive) or water reactive

2 .   HEALTH HAZARDS

2.1   Carcinogen
2.2   Corrosive
2.3   Irritant
2.4   Sensitizer
2.5   Toxic
2.5.1   Oral LD_{50} 50–500 mg/kg; highly toxic < 50 mg/kg
2.5.2   Dermal LD_{50} 200–1000 mg/kg; highly toxic < 200 mg/kg
2.5.3   Inhalation LC_{50} 200–2000 ppm, one hour administration; highly toxic < 200 ppm
2.6   Hepatotoxins, nephrotoxins, neurotoxins, agents affecting blood or hematopoietic system and lungs, reproductive toxins, cutaneous and eye hazards.

Haze   The cloudy or turbid appearance of a transparent specimen due to light scattering from within the specimen, or from its surface.

HDPE   Abbreviation for *High-Density Polyethylene.*

Head-to-Head Polymers   Polymers in which the monomeric units are alternately reversed.

Head-to-Tail Polymers   Polymers in which the monomeric units regularly repeat.

Heart Failure   Mechanical inadequacy of the heart, so that it fails to pump the required amount of blood.

Heat Deflection Temperature   (Polymers with high HDT). For medical device applications, polymers with high HDT's are of interest since they may be suitable for repeated steam-sterilization cycles. Commercially available polymers with high HDT's are listed below:

POLYMER DESCRIPTION	HDT RANGE (°F)
Polyimide	750–600
Polyetherether ketone (PEEK)	675–650
Liquid crystal polymer	675–400
Fluoropolymers	650–425
Polyketone	625–600
Bismaleimide	550–525
Polyamide-imide	540–525
Nylon 4/6	535–515
Phenolics	530–475
Polyphenylene sulfide	525–515
Polycyclohexylene dimethyl terephthalate	505–495
Cyanates	500–475
Bisphenyl-modified polyethersulfone	490–485
Polyethylene terephthalate	440–430
Polyethersulfone	435–420
Polyarylsulfone	420–410
Polyetherimide	415–410
Polyurea	400–350
Polysulfone	340–325
Polycarbonate	325–300

Heat Distortion Point   (Deflection Temperature). The temperature at which a standard test bar deflects .010 inches under the conditions described in ASTM D 648.

Heat Mark   (Sink Mark). A shallow depression in the surface of a molded plastic having practically no depth, and visible because of sharply defined rim, or roughened surface.

Heat Sealing   The process of joining two or more thermoplastic materials by heating areas of contact under pressure. Sealing may be accomplished by (1) thermal sealing, (2) impulse sealing, (3) dielectric sealing, and (4) ultrasonic sealing.

Heat Sink   A device for the absorption or transfer of heat away from a critical part or element.

Heat Stability   The resistance to change in color, or other property, as a result of heat encountered by a polymer during processing or end use. The heat stability of plastics is frequently enhanced by the incorporation of a heat stabilizer.

Heat Sterilizer   A Class II device that uses dry heat to sterilize medical products.

Heating Cylinder   In injection molding, the portion of the machine in which the polymer is heated to a molten condition prior to injection.

Hemagglutination   The agglutination of erythrocytes, especially by antiserum.

Hematologic   Referring to blood, or the study of blood.

Hematology   The medical specialty that pertains to the anatomy, physiology, pathology, symptomatology, and therapeutics related to the blood and blood-forming tissues.

Hematoma   A collection of blood or clotted blood somewhere in the body, usually caused by injury or following surgery.

Hemicellulose   Cellulose having a degree of polymerization of 150 or less.

Hemodiafiltration   A technique of hemodialysis in which blood flow is accelerated to twice the rate of conventional dialysis, also called *high-flux hemodiafiltration*. The speed of blood flow is 500 ml/min; thus the technique requires two dialyzers in series, and replaces the rapid loss of volume with backfiltration from dialysate to blood. Patients who can benefit from this technique must have acceptable blood pressures and fully stable fistulas to accommodate the rapid blood flow rate; these patients can be dialyzed for two rather than the standard four hours per session.

Hemodialysis System   A Class II device used as an artificial kidney system for the treatment of patients with renal failure or toxemic conditions, consisting of an extracorporeal blood system, a dialyzer, a dialysate delivery system, and accessories.

Hemoglobin   The respiratory protein of red blood cells. A conjugated protein consisting of 94% globin and 6% heme.

Hemolysis   Destruction of red blood cells; occurs in infections, due to a toxic substance or drug, or in the laboratory after freezing, thawing, or other activities involving red blood cells.

Hemostasis   The process of stopping bleeding, either with drugs, or mechanically with medical devices. Refers to the combination of processes that account for the cessation of bleeding after injury to the vascular system.

Heparin   A complex mucopolysaccharide, used as an anticoagulant.

Heterocyclic Compounds   Compounds containing molecules whose atoms are arranged in a ring, with the ring containing two or more chemical elements.

Heteropolymer   A copolymer formed by an addition polymerization that involves the combination of two dissimilar unsaturated organic monomers.

Heteropolymerization   A special case of addition polymerization, which involves the combination of two dissimilar unsaturated organic monomers.

Hevea Rubber   A type of natural rubber.

Hexamethylene   See CYCLOHEXANE.

Hexamethylene Adipamides   (Nylon 66). The type of nylon made by the polycondensation reaction of hexamethylenediamine and adipic acid.

Hexamethylenediamine   A colorless solid, which is used primarily in the polycondensation reaction to form Nylon 66.

Hexamethylenetetramine   The reaction product of ammonia and formaldehyde, used as a catalyst and accelerator in the polymerization of phenolic and urea resins.

Hexane   A straight chain hydrocarbon solvent derived from petroleum.

Hexanedioic Acid   Another term for *Adipic Acid*.

Hexyl Methacrylate   One of the monomers used in the polymerization of acrylic resins.

High Frequency   Electrical frequency ranging from 3–30 mc/sec, employed in plastics welding and sealing.

High Polymer   Macromolecular substances consisting of molecules composed of many multiples of the molecular weight of one or more monomer units. Practically all synthetic polymers used in medical devices are regarded as high polymers.

High Technology   Those commercial activities that have a relatively high ratio of research and development expenditures to revenues. Among ''high technology'' industries we can cite:

INDUSTRY	R&D EXPENDITURES AS % OF SALES
Computers	6.3
Semiconductors	6.0
Medical technology	5.6
Drugs	4.9
Instruments	4.2

High-Density Polyethylene (HDPE)   Polyethylene polymers ranging in density from about .94 to .96 and higher. HDPE features longer chains with fewer side branches, resulting in a more rigid material with greater strength, hardness, chemical resistance, and higher softening temperatures.

High-Frequency Sealing   Heating of plastics by dielectric loss in a high-frequency electrostatic field. The material to be heated is placed between electrodes, and by energy absorption from the electrical field, the temperature is raised quickly and uniformly throughout the mass.

High-Frequency Welding   A method of welding confined to thermoplastic materials, in which the parts to be joined are heated by contact with electrodes connected to a high-frequency electrical generator.

High-Load Melt Index   Rate of flow, measured in grams/min of a molten resin forced through an orifice of 0.0825 inches in diameter when subjected to a high load (21,600 grams of force) at 190°C.

High-Pressure Laminates   Laminated molded and cured at pressures of 1000 psi or higher, commonly at 1500 psi.

High-Pressure Molding   According to ASTM D 883, a molding or laminating process in which the pressure is at least 200 psi.

Histochemistry   A branch of biochemistry devoted to studying the chemical composition of tissues. It examines the structures of bone, blood, and muscle using a variety of analytical techniques ranging from microscopic, ultrastructural, radioactive, to instrumental.

HLB   The HLB (Hydrophilic-Lipophilic Balance) of a substance is an expression of the simultaneous attraction of an emulsifier for water and for oil. Low HLB numbers are assigned to lipophilic substances and high numbers are used for hydrophilic materials, with the midpoint being approximately 10.

ACTIVITY	ASSIGNED HLB
Antifoaming	1 to 3
Emulsifiers (w/o)	3 to 6
Wetting agents	7 to 9
Emulsifiers (o/w)	8 to 18
Solubilizers	15 to 20
Detergents	3 to 15

HLB values for some emulsifiers:

AGENT	HLB
Ethylene glycol distearate	1.5
Sorbitan glycol distearate (Span 65)	2.1
Propylene glycol monostearate	3.4
Triton X-15	3.6
Sorbitan monooleate (Span 80)	4.3
Sorbitan monostearate (Span 60)	4.7
Diethylene glycol monolaurate	6.1
Sorbitan monopalmitate (Span 40)	6.7
Sucrose dioleate	7.1
Acacia	8.0
Polyoxyethylene lauryl ether (Brij 30)	9.7
Gelatin	9.8
Triton X-45	10.4
Methyl cellulose	10.5
Polyoxyethylene monostearate (Myrj 45)	11.1
Triethanolamine oleate	12.0
Tragacanth	13.2
Triton X-100	13.5
Polyethylene oxide monostearate (Tween 60)	14.9
Polyoxyethylene sorbitan monooleate (Tween 80)	15.0
Polyoxyethylene sorbitan monolaurate (Tween 20)	16.7
Pluronic F 68	17.0
Sodium oleate	18.0
Potassium oleate	20.0
Sodium lauryl sulfate	40.0

Homeopathy   From the Greek *homoios*, meaning "similar," and *pathos*, meaning "disease." In essence, the basis of homeopathy is that like cures like: that is, a drug that produces in healthy persons the effects or set of symptoms of the illness present will cure the disease. Embodied in this approach are: (1) the testing of the drug on healthy persons to find the effects of the drug so that it may be employed against the same symptoms manifesting a disease in an ill person, (2) the use of only small quantities of drugs in therapy, (3) the administration of only one drug at a time, and (4) the treatment of the entire symptom complex of the patient, not just one symptom.

Homeostasis   The equilibrium maintained by all organisms. In man it is maintained with regards to body temperature, tissue oxygen concentration, water balance, etc.

Homo   A prefix meaning the same or similar.

Homocyclic   A ring structure containing only one type of atom in the ring, such as the ring compound benzene.

Homogeneous   Mixture or solution comprised of two or more substances that are uniformly dispersed in each other.

Homogeneous Reaction   A chemical reaction in which the reacting substances are in the same phases, i.e., solid, liquid, or gas.

Homogenization   A mechanical process for reducing the size of fatty substances of an emulsion to uniform size, thus creating a stable system unaffected by gravity.

Homologous Series   A series of organic compounds identical to each other except for the fact that each successive member has an additional CH_2 group in its chain than the preceding member. An example is methanol, ethanol, propanol, butanol, pentanol, etc.

Homomorphs   Molecules similar in size and shape, needing no other characteristics. The properties of several homomorphs can be predicted by knowing the properties of one.

Homopolymer   (1) A polymer resulting from the polymerization of a single monomer. (2) A polymer consisting substantially of a single type of repeating unit. Examples are: polyethylene, polypropylene, and polystyrene.

Hookean Elasticity   (Ideal Elasticity). The type of elasticity in which the strain (elongation) of the material is proportional to the applied stress, in accordance to HOOKE'S LAW.

Hooke's Law   In an elastic body, the ratio of stress to the strain produced is constant. This may be expressed as:
$$T = E\,[L - L_0]/\,L_0.$$
where T is the imposed tensile strength, E is Young's modulus or modulus of elasticity, L_0 the original length of the specimen, and L is the final length of the specimen at break.

Hoop Stress   The circumferential stress in a material of cylindrical dimensions subjected to internal or external pressure.

Hopper   A container holding a supply of molding material in granulated form to be fed to the screw in a continuous fashion.

Hopper Dryer   A combination of feeding and drying container for extrusion or injection molding of hygroscopic polymers. Preheated air with a low dew point is forced upward through the hopper containing the polymer, thus drying the resin.

Hormone   One of many body substances secreted by various endocrine glands, essential for normal body functioning.

Hormones, General   The following general hormones are of major importance in the regulation of bodily functions:

- Adenohypophyseal hormones: growth hormone, corticotropin, thyrotropin, follicle-stimulating hormone, luteinizing hormone, luteotropic hormone, melanocyte-stimulating hormone
- Neurohypophyseal hormones: antidiuretic hormone, oxytocin
- Adrenocortical hormones: cortisol, aldosterone
- Thyroid hormones: thyroxine, calcitonin
- Pancreatic hormone: insulin, glucagon
- Ovarian hormones: estrogens, progesterone
- Testicular hormone: testosterone
- Parathyroid hormone: parathormone, calcitonin
- Placental hormones: chorionic gondatropin, estrogens, progesterone

Host Response   (to Implantation). A constant aspect of the biological environment is that the introduction of a foreign material will elicit a host response. Nine types of potential responses are recognized: (1) Irritation: the act of stimulation capable of causing discomfort induced by an agent or irritant. (2) Inflammation: a localized protective response elicited by injury or destruction of tissue, characterized by heat (calor), redness (rubor), pain (dolor), and swelling. (3) Pyrogenic reaction: fever produced by endotoxins from gram-positive bacteria. (4) Systemic toxicity: the dosage-related effect on the whole organism form an identifiable agent. (5) Sensitization: a condition of being more susceptible to a specific stimulus involving the immune system. (6) Mutagenic Reaction: an undesirable change in the genetic makeup of the organism induced by a chemical or physical agent. (7) Carcinogenic Reaction: tumor or cancer produced by a chemical or physical agent. (8) Hemolytic Reaction: damage to red blood cells by chemical or physical means, with resultant cell death and release of hemoglobin. (9) Foreign Body Reaction: complex process whereby the body reacts to the presence of a foreign body, and begins a series of steps to encapsulate or dissolve the object.

Host versus Graft Rejection   The usual etiology of graft rejection; the loss of grafted tissue by immunologic responses of the grafted individual toward foreign antigens of the graft.

Hot Manifold Mold   A specialized injection mold with a heated torpedo located in the manifold and nozzle system. This mold is used to handle heat-sensitive resins, such as acetals.

Hot Melts   Thermoplastic compounds that are normally solid at room temperature, but become pourable or spreadable when heated. These compounds are frequently used as adhesives and coatings.

Hot Runner Mold   A specialized mold in which the runners and sprues are maintained hot during the molding cycle and are not ejected during demolding, thus reducing scrap.

Hot Stamping   A method of marking plastics in which a foil is pressed against the plastic by a heated die, thus imprinting selected areas of the foil to the article.

HT-1   A type of nylon made from phenylenediamine and terephthalic acid, with excellent high temperature properties.

Humectant   A substance that helps to preserve moisture in a specific body area, such as skin.

Humidity, Absolute   The pounds of water per pounds of dry air in an air-water vapor mixture.

Humidity, Relative   The percentage relation between the actual amount of water vapor in the air, compared to the maximum amount of water vapor that would be present in that volume if the air were saturated.

Humidity Indicator   A cobalt salt (cobaltous chloride), that changes color as the humidity changes. Cobaltous compounds are pink when hydrated and greenish-blue when anhydrous.

Humoral Immunity   Immunity resulting from immunoglobulins.

Hydration   (1) The reaction of water molecules with a substance in which the $H-OH$ bond is not split. The products are called hydrates. (2) The strong affinity of water molecules for substances due to hydrogen bonding.

Hydride   An inorganic compound of hydrogen with another element. Most common are hydrides of sodium, lithium, aluminum, and boron.

Hydrocarbon Plastics   Plastics derived from monomers containing carbon and hydrogen only. The family includes coumarone-indene resins, cyclopentadiene, terpene resins, etc.

Hydrocolloid   A hydrophilic compound that absorbs water readily, thus increasing viscosity and smoothness even at low concentrations. They are used as mucoadhesives in medical devices. Examples: Karaya gum, alginates, polyacrylonitriles, polyacrylic acid, etc.

Hydrogel   A polymeric material that exhibits the ability to swell in water and to retain a significant fraction (> 20 percent) of water within its structure, but which will not dissolve in water.

Hydrogel Advantages:

- Permeability to small molecules allows initiators, decomposition products, solvents, and other extraneous materials to be efficiently extracted from the gel prior to implantation.
- The soft and rubbery consistency of most hydrogels contributes to their biocompatibility by minimizing irritation to surrounding cells and tissue.
- Low interfacial tension reduces protein adsorption and protein unfolding.

Hydrogen Bond   An attractive intermolecular force, occurring in polar compounds, in which a hydrogen atom of one molecule is attracted to two unshared electrons of another. Hydrogen bonds are only one-twentieth as strong as covalent bonds, but they have pronounced effects as regards to boiling points and crystalline structure.

Hydrogenation   Any reaction of hydrogen with an organic compound. It may be of two types: (1) Hydrogenation, where oxygen is added to the double bonds of unsaturated molecules, resulting in a saturated compound. (2) Hydrogenolysis, where the bonds of organic compounds are ruptured, with subsequent reaction of hydrogen with the molecular fragments.

Hydrolysis   A chemical reaction in which water reacts with another molecule to form two or more new substances.

Hydrophilic   Having an affinity for water.

Hydrophobic   Having a dislike for water; not capable of uniting or mixing with water.

Hydroquinone   A white crystalline material used along with many of its derivatives as an inhibitor in unsaturated polyester resins, and in monomers such as vinyl acetate. Inhibitors are used to prevent the premature gelation of unsaturated compounds, either in storage, or during shipping.

Hydroxyethyl Cellulose (HEC)   A water-soluble film former, created by reacting alkali cellulose with ethylene oxide. Used extensively as a tabletting additive in pharmaceutical applications.

Hydroxyl   A chemical functional group composed of a hydrogen atom bonded to an oxygen atom; $-O-H$.

Hydroxyl Number   In polyurethane terminology a measure of hydroxyl groups present in an organic material capable of reacting with an isocyanate group.

Hydroxypropyl Methacrylate. (HPMA)   A reactive monomer copolymerizable with a wide variety of acrylic and vinylic monomers, used to produce many important resins and surface coatings.

Hygroscopic   Substances that have the tendency to spontaneously absorb moisture from the air. Hygroscopic resins such as the polyurethanes require drying before molding.

Hyperalimentation   A process of providing food to a malnourished person by infusing nourishing fluids directly into a vein (parenteral), or directly into the stomach (enteral).

Hyperbaric Chamber   A Class II device consisting of a chamber that can be pressured above atmospheric pressure, used to increase the environmental oxygen pressure and thus promote the absorption of oxygen by the patient's tissue.

Hypertonic   Refers to a concentration of sodium chloride greater than that present in blood.

Hypo   A prefix used in chemical terminology to indicate a compound (usually an acid) in its lowest oxidation state, or containing the lowest proportion of oxygen in a series of compounds.

Hypoallergenic   A term describing a cosmetic product that is less likely to cause adverse allergenic reactions than competing products. Claims of hypoallergenicity must be substantiated by specific dermatological tests.

Hysteresis, Mechanical   The cyclic noncoincidence of the elastic loading and unloading curves under cyclic stress. The area of the resulting HYSTERESIS LOOP is equal to the heat generated in the system.

Hysteresis Loop   The area between two curves on a graph plotting the results of a changing force, first with ascending values, then with descending values. Hysteresis loops are seen in viscosity curves of thixotropic and dilatant fluids, and in stress-strain curves of elastomeric polymers.

Hysteroscope   A Class II device used to permit direct viewing of the cervical canal and the uterine cavity by means of a telescopic system introduced into the uterus through the cervix. It is used to perform diagnostic and surgical procedures other than sterilization.

I

Iatrogenic   An effect upon the patient that results from suggestions or treatment prescribed by a physician.

Ic   A suffix used in naming inorganic compounds, which indicates the central element is present in its highest oxidation state.

IDE   (Investigational Device Exemptions). The purpose is ". . . to encourage, to the extent consistent with the protection of the public health and safety and with ethical standards, the discovery and development of useful devices intended for human use and to that end to maintain optimum freedom for scientific investigators in their pursuit of that purpose." Without this section of the law, it would be impossible for device manufacturers to be in compliance with the law and at the same time provide for clinical testing to establish the safety and effectiveness of devices.

Idiopathic   Relating to a disease or condition of unknown origin or cause.

Idiosyncrasy   (to Drugs). Unusual sensitivity to certain drugs experienced by susceptible individuals.

Idiotype   An antigen unique to an individual or small group of individuals, as opposed to an allotype, which occurs in most individuals.

Immediate Set   The deformation measured immediately after removal of causative load.

Immiscible   Descriptive of substances of the same phase or state of matter that cannot be uniformly mixed or blended.

Immunity   A condition of being resistant to an infection.

Immunization   The process of developing one's own antibodies against an infectious disease, or being inoculated with inactivated or killed microorganisms that cause a particular disease, in order to develop antibodies and acquire protection against the infection.

Immunoadsorbent   An affinity matrix formed by immobilizing an antibody preparation to an insoluble substrate.

Immunoassay   Any assay method that uses antibodies for the detection and quantification of biological molecules or microorganisms. The two most common methods are: radioimmunoassay (RIA), and enzyme-linked immunosorbent assay (ELISA).

Immunochemistry   The branch of chemistry concerned with the various defense mechanisms against infective agents, particularly the response between the body and foreign macromolecules (antigens).

Immunodiffusion   A laboratory test in which the interactions of specific antigens and antibodies can be observed.

Immunoelectrophoresis   An electrophoretic displacement of antigen(s) or antibodies followed by IMMUNODIFFUSION.

Immunoglobulins   Body proteins that function as antibodies to fight infection.

Immunology   The science dealing with the various phenomena of immunity, induced sensitivity, and allergy.

Immunotherapy   Treating the body to bolster its capacity to fight infection, or the invasion of harmful foreign cells such as cancer cells.

Impact Modifier   A general term for an additive incorporated into a plastic compound, whose main function is to improve the impact resistance of the finished product.

Impact Resistance   The relative ability of plastics to fracture under stresses applied at high speeds. ASTM D 256 uses the Izod pendulum striker swung from a fixed height to strike a notched specimen bar mounted on a cantilever bar. Another test is the Charpy method, which uses a specimen in the form of a beam supported at both ends; the specimen is impacted by a striker under controlled conditions.

Impact Strength   The ability of a material to withstand a sudden impact or shock without fracture, measured by standard impact equipment (Izod, Charpy).

Impalpable   Descriptive of a state of subdivision of particles so fine that individual particles cannot be discerned by pressing the particles between the fingers. Impalpable powders are those whose particle size are 44 μm in diameter, or smaller.

Implantable Biomaterials   Those synthetic polymers and natural macromolecules intended for use as implantable devices. May be grouped into the following categories:

(1) *Reconstructive and Plastic Surgery*

- Soft tissue applications, e.g., mammary reconstruction, trauma repair, cosmetic surgery
- Hard tissue applications, limited to joints with limited forces, e.g., fingers and toes

(2) *Cardiovascular Applications*
- Vascular grafts, particularly small bore
- Bladder surfaces for total hearts and left ventricular assist devices

(3) *Specialized Applications*
- Ear reconstruction, e.g., eustachian tube
- Ureterogenital reconstruction, e.g., artificial sphincters, percutaneous connectors for artificial hearts, Hickman catheters

(4) *Implantable Controlled Drug Release Devices*
- Contraception, growth hormone, chronic pain relief

Implantation   The surgical procedure by which medical devices, or prostheses, are placed permanently in the human body.

Implantology   (1) The combination of biomedical engineering and biomaterials science dealing with implantable medical devices. (2) The study of biomaterials (e.g., tissue or inert material) inserted or grafted into the body for reconstructive or replacement purposes.

Implants, Host Response   A constant aspect of the biological environment is that the implantation of a foreign material will elicit a host response. Nine possible reactions characterize the host response: (1) Irritation: the act of stimulation capable of causing discomfort induced by implant. (2) Inflammation: a localized protective response elicited by tissue destruction. (3) Pyrogenic Reaction: fever produced by endotoxins from gram-positive bacteria. (4) Systemic Toxicity: the dosage-related effect on the whole organism from an identifiable agent. (5) Sensitization: a condition of reacting more vigorously to a specific stimulus that involves the immune system. (6) Mutagenic Reaction: an undesirable change in the genetic makeup of the host induced by a chemical agent. (7) Carcinogenic Reaction: tumor or cancer produced by a chemical or physical agent. (8) Hemolytic Reaction: damage of red blood cells by chemical or physical means with resultant cell death and release of hemoglobin. (9) Foreign Body Reaction: a complex process where the body reacts to the presence of a foreign body and begins a series of steps to encapsulate or dissolve the object.

Impregnation   The process of soaking a porous material with a curable resin. The main difference between impregnation and ENCAPSULATION is that in encapsulation an outer protective layer is formed, with little or no penetration of the resin into the material.

Impression Material   (Dentistry). A Class II device composed of polymers, such as polysulfide or alginate, placed on an impression tray, to reproduce the structure and fine detail of teeth and gums. This provides models for the eventual production of restorative and prosthetic dental devices.

Impulse Sealing   The process of joining (sealing) thermoplastic materials by the application of an intense pulse of thermal energy to the sealing area under pressure, followed immediately by cooling.

Impurity   The presence of one substance in another in such low concentration that it cannot be measured quantitatively or by ordinary analytical methods.

Inclusion   A foreign or impurity phase within a solid.

Indentation Hardness   The surface hardness of materials determined by (1) the size of an indentation made by a tool under fixed load, or (2) the load necessary to produce penetration of an indenter tool to a predetermined depth. In plastics, the Shore durometer is the most widely used, comprising a spring-loaded indentor tool, and a gauge calibrated to register the penetration distance.

Index of Refraction   (Refractive Index). The ratio of the velocity of light in a vacuum to its velocity in a transparent plastic.

Indicator   A dye that indicates the presence or absence of another substance by its color. The most common are acid-base indicators such as litmus, phenolphthalein and methyl orange.

Induction Heating   A method of heating electrically conductive materials, by placing the part in a high frequency electromagnetic field, which induces electromotive forces within the structure, thus resulting in the generation of heat.

Indwelling Oxyhemoglobin Analyzer   A Class III device consisting of a photoelectric cell, used to measure, in vivo, the oxygen-carrying capacity of hemoglobin in blood as an aid in determining the patient's physiological status.

Indwelling Partial Pressure Analyzers   Class III devices consisting of catheter tip transducers used to measure, in vivo, the partial pressure of carbon dioxide, pH, and oxygen in the blood, as an aid in determining circulatory, ventilatory, and metabolic status of patients.

Inert Additive   (Filler). A low-cost material added to a plastic to lower the cost of the finished article, and which does not react chemically with any constituent of the composition.

Infarction   Tissue death due to deprivation of oxygen.

Infection   A disease process caused by the invasion and damaging action of microorganisms, such as bacteria or viruses.

Infiltration   To pass or inject fluid or any other material into the tissues.

Inflammation   The irritation, swelling and other changes of tissue as a result of trauma, pressure, surgery, etc. May also be caused by illness, infection, or drugs. Acute inflammation lasts one or two days, and is characterized by exudation of blood and plasma and the emigration of neutrophils. Chronic inflammation lasts months or years, and is characterized by the presence of monocytes (macrophages) in tissue, fibroblasts that synthesize tissue, and a proliferation of blood vessels.

Infrared Heating   A heating process employing lamps that emit radiation in the infrared wavelength spectrum; the radiation is more penetrating than visible light rays.

Infrared Spectrometry   An important analytical technique, based on the principle that certain natural oscillations occur within any given molecule, and are characteristic of that molecule only; these oscillations, in turn, produce absorbance bands in spectra obtained under infrared radiation.

Infusible   Incapable of melting when heated, as are all thermosetting resins.

Infusion   An aqueous solution obtained by treating drugs with hot water. Generally prepared by pouring boiling water upon a vegetable substance and macerating the mixture in a container until the liquid cools.

Infusion Pump   A Class II device used to pump fluids into a patient in a controlled manner, using a piston pump, roller pump, or peristaltic pump. May include means to detect a fault condition, such as air or blockage of the infusion line.

Inherent Viscosity   The ratio of the natural logarithm of the relative viscosity to the concentration of the polymer in grams per 100 ml of solvent. Inherent viscosity provides a method of measuring the molecular weight of polymers.

Inhibitor   An organic compound that retards or stops an undesired chemical reaction, such as polymerization, oxidation, or corrosion. Inhibitors are used to prolong shelf life, and to control work life. Such substances are sometimes called negative catalysts.

Initiator   In polymerization reactions, agents necessary to cause the reaction to commence. Initiators are frequently used to start emulsion polymerization reactions of vinyls, acrylics, etc.

Injection   Using a needle, attached to a syringe or other sterile container, to infuse liquid material into skin, muscle, or blood vessels to administer drugs, feed, or hydrate an individual.

Injection Blow Molding   A process in which a parison is formed over a mandrel by injection, after which the mandrel and parison are shifted to a blow mold, where the remainder of the cycle is completed. This process produces parts requiring no finishing operations, such as bottles conforming to close tolerances.

Injection Mold   A mold used in the process of injection molding, comprising two sections held together by a clamping device with sufficient strength to withstand the pressure generated by injected molten plastic.

Injection Molding   An important method of forming products from granular or pelletized thermoplastic polymers. The pelletized polymer is fed from a hopper into a heated extruder barrel in which it is molten (plasticated), after which it is forced into a cold mold. The molten thermoplastic is maintained under pressure within the mold cavity until it has hardened sufficiently for removal (demolding).

Injection Molding Pressure   According to ASTM D 883, the pressure applied to the cross-sectional area of the material cylinder, expressed in pounds per square inch (psi).

Injection Nozzle   A metal nozzle that allows the transfer of molten thermoplastic emerging from an injection cylinder into a mold. Typically, it is housed within a sprue bushing, where it terminates in a heated spherical tip.

Inoculation   Injection of a small amount of inactivated or killed microorganisms, or toxin produced by the organisms, to challenge the body to develop antibodies against these organisms.

Inorganic Pigments   Pigments derived from naturally occurring minerals, or synthesized from inorganic substances. Typically they are opaque—as opposed to organic pigments and dyes, which are transparent—and display better resistance to heat and light. In colored medical devices, inorganic pigments such as titanium dioxide, iron oxides, and ultramarine blues are frequently used because of their biocompatibility, but chromate and cadmium compounds are seldom used because of their inherent toxicity.

Inorganic Polymers   Any polymer without carbon in its backbone, with a degree of polymerization sufficient to exhibit mechanical strength, plastic, or elastomeric properties, plus the capability of being formed into finished products by conventional plastic processes. In medical devices, the most important inorganic polymers are the silicones.

Insert   A material incorporated into a molded plastic by (1) pressing the insert into the finished article or (2) placing the insert directly in the molding cavity so it becomes an integral part of the product.

In Situ Foaming   The technique of pouring a foaming composition into the place where it is intended that foaming shall take place.

Instrument   Any device used for one of the following purposes: (1) observation (microscope); (2) measurement (thermometer, thermocouple, flowmeter, balance); (3) chemical analysis (spectrometer). See also INSTRUMENTATION.

Instrumentation   Collective term for sensing devices used to measure, record, and control chemical process variables such as temperature, pressure, flow rate, pH, etc. Such instruments permit automatic correction of variables on a continuous basis.

Insulation Resistance   The electrical resistance between two conductors separated only by an insulating material. Most polymers display good insulating characteristics, making them ideal for use as insulators in pacemaker leads, transcutaneous stimulators, etc. Effective polymers are: polyurethane, polyvinyl chloride, and polystyrene. There are a number of materials called double insulators, since they have both electrical and thermal insulating properties, e.g., polystyrene, PVC, cellulose.

Insulator   Any substance, or mixture of substances, which displays a low dielectric constant, low electrical conductivity, or both. Polymers are effective as electrical insulators, such as vinyls, urethanes, silicones, epoxies, and are widely used in medical devices.

Intensive Mixers   Mixers for dry blending PVC resins with plasticizers and other additives, comprising a propeller rotating at high speed at the bottom of a stationary housing, thus continuously recirculating the compound between closely spaced stationary and rotating pins.

Interface   (1) The junction point, or surface, between two different media. (2) The area of contact between two immiscible phases of a dispersion. Five types are possible: solid/solid (pigment/polymer); liquid/liquid (water/oil); solid/gas (smoke/air); solid/liquid (clay/water); and liquid/gas (water/air). Properties such as wettability of solids, spreading coefficients of liquids, and protective action of colloidal substances are intimately associated with interfacial behavior.

Interfacial Polymerization   A polymerization reaction occurring at the interfacial boundary of two solutions. A classical example is the continuous production of nylon threads from a flask containing a lower layer of sebacyl chloride in carbon tetrachloride, and an upper layer of aqueous hexamethylene diamine. The threads are formed by lowering a pair of tweezers through the top layer, closed on the interfacial layer between the solutions, and then drawn upwards with a continuous strand of nylon.

Interlaminar Strength   The strength of the adhesive bond between adjacent layers of laminated substrates.

Intermediate   An organic compound considered as a chemical stepping stone between the parent substance and the final product; they may be either cyclic (derived from coal tar or petroleum, such as benzene, toluene, naphthalene) or acyclic (such as ethyl and propyl alcohol). Intermediates are the foundation of the modern approach to polymer technology.

Intermittent Positive Pressure Breathing   Artificial respiration via a breathing machine that intermittently inflates the lungs with air or oxygen in cases where a patient is unwilling, due to postoperative pain, or unable to breathe normally.

Internal Lubricant   A lubricating substance added to a plastic prior to extrusion or injection molding to reduce friction and surface tack. Examples are polyglycols, phosphate esters, dibasic acid esters, dibasic acid amides, chlorofluorocarbons, silicone fluids, and polyphenyl ethers.

Internal Mixers   Mixing machines using the principle of cylindrical containers in which the materials are deformed by rotating blades or rotors. Banbury mixers are the best known of the internal mixers, and are used extensively in compounding rubber and plastics, where they have the advantage of keeping dust and fume hazards to a minimum.

Internal Plasticizer   A plasticizing agent incorporated in a resin during polymerization, as opposed to a plasticizer added to the resin during compounding.

Internal Stabilizer   A stabilizer incorporated in a resin during polymerization, as opposed to a stabilizer added to the resin during compounding.

Interpolymer   A type of copolymer in which the two monomer units are so intimately distributed that the plastic is essentially homogeneous in chemical composition. An interpolymer is sometimes referred to as True Copolymer.

Interstitial   Relating to spaces between cells or body organs.

Intra-Aortic Balloon, and Control System   A Class III device consisting of an inflatable balloon, which is placed in the aorta to improve cardiac function during life-threatening emergencies, and a control system for regulating the inflation and deflation of the balloon. The control system, which monitors and is synchronized with the EKG, provides a means for setting the inflation and deflation of the balloon with the cardiac cycle.

Intracranial Pressure Monitor   A Class II device used for short-term monitoring and recording of intracranial pressures and trends. Device includes the transducer, monitor and interconnecting hardware.

Intramuscular   Within the muscle mass. A common route of drug administration, utilizing a hypodermic syringe. Although slower in onset than direct intravenous administration, intramuscular injections exhibit longer duration of action.

Intraosseous Fixation Wire   A Class II device consisting of a metal wire used to stabilize and constrict fractured jaw bone segments by wrapping the wire around the ends of the bone segments.

Intrauterine Device   A Class III device placed high in the uterine fundus with a string extending from the uterus into the vagina, used to prevent pregnancy. This type does not include products that function by drug activity, which are subject to the new provisions of the Federal Food, Drug, and Cosmetic Act.

Intrauterine Pressure Monitor   A Class II device designed to detect and measure intrauterine and amniotic fluid pressure by means of a catheter placed transcervically into the uterine cavity. Used to monitor the strength, duration, and frequency of uterine contractions during labor. Included in this generic category are: ''intrauterine pressure recorder,'' ''intrauterine catheter and introducer,'' and ''intrauterine pressure transducer.''

Intravascular Administration Set   A Class II device used to administer fluids from a container to the vascular system through a needle or catheter inserted into a vein. May include tubing, flow regulator, drip chamber, and infusion line filter.

Intravenous Infusion   The act of introducing fluid, nutritive substances, or drugs directly into veins via needle and syringe, or other sterile apparatus.

Intravenous Pyelogram   A diagnostic procedure in which the patient is given an intravenous injection of contrast agent, allowing diagnostic X-ray studies to be done of the kidneys and the urinary tract.

Intrinsic Viscosity   The limit of the reduced and inherent viscosities as the concentration of the polymeric solute approaches zero, representing the capacity of the polymer to increase viscosity.

Introfaction   The change in fluidity and wetting properties of an impregnating material, produced by the addition of an INTROFIER.

Introfier   A substance capable of converting a colloidal solution into a molecular one, by changing the wetting properties and fluidity of the solution.

Intubation   Insertion of a tube into a body opening or passage.

Intumescence   The foaming and swelling of a plastic when exposed to high surface temperatures or direct flame.

In Vitro   Literally, "under the glass," a biological study performed outside a living body. Opposite of IN VIVO.

In Vitro Diagnostic Products   Those reagents, instruments, and systems intended for use in the diagnosis of disease or other conditions, including a determination of the state of health, in order to cure, mitigate, treat, or prevent disease or its sequelae. Such products are intended for use in the collection, preparation, and examination of specimens taken from the human body. These products are devices as defined in section 210(h) of the Federal FD&C Act, and may also be biological products subject to section 351 of the Public Health Service Act. (21 CFR 809.3[a], 1988).

In Vivo   Within a living organism. A biological study performed inside a living body. Opposite of IN VITRO.

Involuntary   Not subject to voluntary, deliberate, or conscious control. *Autonomic*. Most of the involuntary movements of the body are performed by smooth muscles, which are controlled by the autonomic nervous system, and thus are involuntary.

Iodine Value   The number of grams of iodine that 100 grams of an unsaturated compound will absorb in a given time under arbitrary conditions. Low iodine values in plasticizers are an indication of a high degree of saturation, and vice versa.

Ion   Any atom, molecule, or radical that becomes electrically charged by either gaining or losing an electron. When an electron is gained the ion becomes negatively charged, and is called an ANION. When an electron is lost the ion becomes positively charged and is called a CATION.

Ion Exchange   A reversible interchange of ions between a solid phase and a liquid phase in which there is no permanent change in the structure of the solid phase. In water softening, an ion exchange resin extracts insoluble calcium ions from the water, exchanging them with equivalent amounts of soluble sodium ions, thus "softening" the water. The calcium-loaded resin may be regenerated with sodium chloride to replenish sodium, and make it ready for another cycle of operation.

Ion Exchange Resins   Small spherical resins consisting of a resinous portion, and an ion-active group. Frequently resins are copolymers of styrene and divinyl benzene, whereas the ion-active group may be acidic or basic.

Ionic Initiators   Substances used in ionic polymerization reactions. They act by providing either carbonium ions (cationic initiators), or carbanions (anionic initiators). These substances break the reactive double bonds of vinyl-type monomers and add on, thus regenerating the ion species on the polymerizing chain.

Ionic Polymerization   (Anionic, Cationic Polymerization). An important polymerization process in which monomeric vinyl moieties are added to agents containing electrically charged ions. Vinyl resins, polyvinyl ethers, acrylics, and certain rubbers are generally polymerized in this fashion.

Ionomer   A thermoplastic containing covalent and ionic bonds. The intermolecular ionic forces are very strong, conferring unique characteristics on these polymers. Carboxyl groups provide the anionic portion of the crosslinks, while metal ions constitute the cationic electrostatic links. An example is DuPont's "Surlyn A," which is used in certain medical applications.

IR   Abbreviation for *Infrared*.

Irradiation   A specialized method used for the purpose of cross-linking thermoplastic materials, thus rendering them insensitive to heat (thermosetting).

Irrigation   Bathing a body part or cavity with fluids or medicated fluids, for the purpose of cleaning, healing, or preventing infections.

Irritant   (1) A substance capable of irritating any part of the body, either accidentally or with the intent to produce tissue stimulation. (2) A substance which, by contact in sufficient concentration for a sufficient period of time, will cause an inflammatory response or reaction in the eye, skin, or respiratory system. The contact may be single exposure or multiple exposures.

Ischemic   A body part that is receiving inadequate amounts of blood.

Iso   A prefix denoting an isomer of a compound.

Isocyanate Generator   (Hindered Isocyanate). A compound that thermally decomposes to form isocyanate groups. Used as specialized adhesives for the manufacture of medical devices.

Isocyanates   (Diisocyanates). Important monomers in the synthesis of urethane elastomers, coatings, and adhesives. Isocyanates are generally classified as aromatic (containing benzene rings) or aliphatic, which may be linear or cyclic.

Isocyanurate   A compound closely related to isocyanate, but containing three NCO groups. Used extensively in the production of rigid, thermosetting polyurethanes.

Isolation   Placing a patient who is infected with a communicable disease into a separate area, to prevent spread of the disease to others.

Isomers   Molecules that contain the same number and kind of atoms, but which differ in structure, thus displaying wide differences in properties. Isomers may be classified as: structural, stereo, and optical. Isomeric polymers may be formed by polymerizing isomeric monomers that link together in different ways. Several important elastomeric polyurethanes are polymerized using mixtures of aliphatic isocyanates.

Isomorphism   A state of crystallization characterized by a similar arrangement of geometrically similar structural units.

Isophorone   A powerful solvent for vinyl, acrylic, and cellulosic resins. It displays moderate capacity to dissolve other thermoplastic resins.

Isosterism   Puzzling similarity in physical properties among unrelated elements, ions, or compounds. The similarity can be traced to comparable, or identical, outer shell electron arrangements.

Isotactic   Referring to a type of polymeric molecular structure containing a sequence of regularly spaced asymmetric atoms. Isotactic polymers can be very hard and rigid, due to the high crystallinity possible with this molecular configuration.

Isotonic   A solution displaying the same osmotic pressure (tone) as another solution, e.g., human blood and physiological salt solution.

Isotope   One or more forms of an element that have the same atomic number, but different masses. The difference in mass is generally traced to additional neutrons in the nucleus.

Isotropy   (1) The ability of materials to display similar mechanical reaction regardless of direction of applied stress. (2) Ability to give the same result regardless of the direction of measurement of a physical property.

J   **Jacquet Indicator**   A tachometer frequently used to measure slow linear speeds, such as those encountered in plastics extrusions, calendering, and casting operations.

Jaundice   A condition where the skin and eye sclera appear yellowish due to an abnormal accumulation of bile pigments, usually due to liver or gall bladder disease.

J Chain   A polypeptide chain found attached to secretory IgA and IgM, which may function as a joining chain.

Jejunum   A portion of the small intestine.

Jelly   A modified form of the more correct "gel," used in the chemical literature to refer to the mechanical strength of hydrogels, gelatins, and various natural gums.

Jet Molding   A special modification of the injection molding process designed for thermosetting resins. An elongated nozzle or "jet" is mounted on the front of the molding cylinder, and is provided with a high-intensity heating element to cure the resin.

Jet Spinning   Synonymous with *Melt Spinning*. Jet spinning uses a direct blast "jet" of hot gas to spin molten polymer from a die lip, and extend it into fine monofilaments.

Jetting   Turbulent flow of molten resin from an undersized gate into a thicker mold section. This is in contrast to the laminar flow of molten resin obtained by the gradual progression of the melt from gate to narrower mold extremities.

Jig   (1) Any device used for holding component parts during a manufacture or assembly operation. (2) Any clamping device used to secure a bonded assembly until the adhesive has set.

Jig Welding   The process of welding thermoplastic materials held between suitably shaped jigs. Heat may be applied to the polymer by heating the jigs, or other suitable means.

Joint   The location at which two substrates are held together with a layer of adhesive.

Joint, Lap   A joint made by placing one substrate partly over another, and subsequently adhering the overlapped substrates.

Joint, Scarf   A joint made by sectioning similar angular segments of two substrates, and subsequently adhering the substrates with the angular segments fitted together.

Jugular Vein   Any of four large veins draining blood from the head and neck.

Jugular Vein, External   A prominent vein lying on either side of the neck, which drains blood from face and scalp. Often used as route of insertion for venous catheters.

Jugular Vein, Internal   A large vein lying on either side of the neck, which drains blood from the brain. Can be used for transvenous cardiac pacing leads.

k   Abbreviation for *Kilo-*, as in kilogram or kilocalories.

K   Symbol for the element potassium. Derived from the Latin *kalium*.

Kaolin   A type of clay, consisting primarily of kaolinite, dickite, and nacrite. Kaolin is used as a thickening agent and filler in certain resins.

Karl Fischer Reagent   A solution of iodine, pyridine, and sulfur dioxide dissolved in methanol (or other solvent). Useful in the wet chemistry determination of water contents of resins, plasticizers, monomers, etc.

Karyotype   The characteristic chromosomal pattern in an individual. Usually determined by an array of chromosomes in metaphase from a photomicrograph of a single cell nucleus. The chromosomes are traditionally arranged in pairs of descending size and according to the position of the centromere.

Karyotyping   Chromosomal analysis. Useful in predicting abnormalities in a fetus before birth, using amniotic fluid to study cells.

Kauri-Butanol Value   A measure of the aromatic contents, and thus solvating power, of a hydrocarbon solvent. Based on the fact that kauri resin is soluble in butanol, but insoluble in hydrocarbons.

Keloids   Overgrowth of scar tissue at the site of a skin wound. The scar is elevated, rounded, firm, and irregularly shaped. Often seen following surgery in young women and blacks.

Kelvin Scale   A temperature scale based on the average kinetic energy per molecule of a perfect gas, in which zero is equal to $-273.16°C$, also known as absolute zero.

Keratin   A scleroprotein, present in cuticular structures such as hair, nails, and the outer skin layer. Sometimes used for coating enteric pills intended to be dissolved only in the intestine.

Keratome   A device used for incising the cornea during eye surgery.

Keratoscope   An instrument marked with lines or circles by means of which the corneal reflex can be observed.

Ketimine   A class of curing agent for epoxy resins that makes it possible to use high solid coatings in spray equipment. Reacts very slowly with epoxies, thus delaying curing time.

Ketoacidosis   A serious disorder resulting from a deficiency, or inadequate use of carbohydrates. Seen in diabetes mellitus.

Ketone Bodies   Substances formed when the body metabolizes fats quickly as an energy source.

Ketones   An important group of solvents widely used for polymers, characterized by the presence of one or more carbonyl groups within a hydrocarbon backbone. Examples are acetone, methyl ethyl ketone, and methyl isobutyl ketone.

Ketonuria   Presence of ketone bodies in urine. Usually seen in patients with uncontrolled diabetes mellitus.

Kevlar   Aramid fibers. Generic name for aromatic polyamide fibers, consisting of synthetic polyamides in which at least 85% of the amide linkages are directly attached to the aromatic ring.

K-Factor   A term used to describe the thermal insulation value, or coefficient of thermal conductivity, of foamed plastics.

Kg   Abbreviation for *Kilogram* (1000 grams; 2.2 pounds).

Kidney Machine   (Blood Dialyzer). A device used to remove impurities and waste products from the blood of a patient whose kidney is unable to perform this vital function.

Kidneys   Each kidney contains about 1,000,000 nephrons, each of which is theoretically capable of forming urine by itself. The volume of blood driven through the glomerular capillaries is approximately 1200 ml per minute, thus the whole body water—45 liters on average—is filtered four times in 24 hours. The kidneys perform two major functions: (1) they excrete most of the metabolic end products and (2) they control the concentrations of most of the constituents of the body fluids. Each kidney contains 1 m^2 of dialyzing surface, capable of dialyzing substances up to 2000 daltons in molecular weight. Water is dialyzed by hydrostatic pressure, while solutes are dialyzed by establishing a concentration gradient. The kidneys filter about 180 liters of blood daily, whereas the volume of urine formed is only 1 to 1.5 liters. Blood components normally removed by the kidneys daily are:

Water .1500 gr
Urea . . . . 30 gr
Creatinine . . . . 1 gr
Uric acid . . . . .0.6 gr
Ions . . . . Variable

Kiln A high-temperature furnace used for firing ceramic-based devices.

Kilo Prefix meaning 1000 units.

Kilogram The mass of a liter of pure water at 4°C.

Kinase (1) An enzyme catalyzing the conversion of a proenzyme to an active enzyme. (2) An enzyme that catalyzes the transfer of phosphate groups to form triphosphates.

Kinematic Viscosity (Kinetic Viscosity). The absolute (dynamic) viscosity of a fluid divided by the density of the fluid. The unit of kinematic viscosity is the STOKE, or CENTISTOKE. Silicone fluids are usually classified by their kinematic viscosity.

Kinescope An instrument used to determine the refraction of the eyes.

Kinetics, Chemical The rate of change of a chemical reaction from initial to final stages under nonequilibrium conditions.

Kiss-Roll Coating A coating process by which very thin coatings can be applied to moving substrates. A roll immersed in the coating fluid transfers a layer of fluid coating to a second roll, from which a small portion of the layer is transferred or ''kissed'' onto the substrate.

Kneaders Mixers with a pair of interdigitating blades, often shaped in the form of the letter Z, used for plasticating and compounding plastic masses of high consistency.

Knife Coating A manufacturing method utilizing a knife, or doctor blade, to apply a fluid coating onto a moving substrate. See also SPREAD COATING.

Knockout Pin (Ejector Pin). A pin used to automatically eject a molded article from a mold. It is usually activated simultaneously with mold opening.

K-Polymers Thermoplastic polyimides produced in situ by the reaction of an aromatic diethyl ester with an aromatic diamine dissolved in methyl-pyrrolidone (M-Pyrrol) solvent.

K-Value A number calculated from dilute solution viscosity measurements of a polymer, used to denote the degree of polymerization, or molecular size. Frequently used to describe grades of polyvinyl pyrrolidone (PVP).

L   (1) Prefix indicating the left-handed enantiomer of an optical isomer. (2) Abbreviation for *liter*.

Label   (1) A notice required to appear on medical devices stating any potentially hazardous characteristics. (2) A notice on a pharmaceutical product stating its composition and all contraindications. (3) A warning notice placed on a shipping container transported by air, highway, rail, or water, as follows:

- Corrosive
- Dangerous
- Explosive
- Flammable gas
- Flammable liquid
- Flammable solid

- Irritant
- Nonflammable gas
- Organic peroxide
- Oxidizer
- Poison
- Radioactive

Labeling, FDA   All labels and other written, printed, or graphic matter (1) upon any article or any of its containers or wrappers, or (2) accompanying such article. The term labeling extends to any advertising or corporate promotion relating to medical devices.

Labile   Descriptive of a substance that is susceptible, changed, inactivated, or degraded by high temperature or radiation. Many drugs fall into this category.

Laboratory   A room equipped with specialized apparatus and reagents, for the performance of tests and experiments in physics, chemistry, and biology.

Laboratory Conditions   An ideal set of conditions in which all variables are held constant, except the one under test. Less specifically, it refers to experimental or prototype conditions, as opposed to large-scale production.

Laboratory Machinery   Small-scale, prototype equipment used for experimental purposes in the laboratories of many pharmaceutical and medical device organizations.

Laceration   A break or tear of skin, or other body tissues, usually caused by injury.

Lachrymator   A substance capable of irritating the eyes, thus causing spontaneous tears.

Lacquer   A solution of a film-forming polymer in a volatile organic solvent, which when applied to a surface forms an adherent film that solidifies solely by solvent evaporation. The dried film should have the same physical properties as the polymer used in making the lacquer.

Lactams   Cyclic amides obtained by condensing one molecule of water from an amino acid. An example is Caprolactam.

Lactase   An enzyme that catalyzes the production of glucose and galactose from lactose. Found in intestinal juices and mucosa.

Lactic Acid   (alpha-hydroxypropionic acid). A colorless liquid used as a catalyst for vinyl polymerization, as an additive for phenolic casting resins, and as a coreactant with glycerine to form alkyd resins.

Lactic Dehydrogenase (LDH)   An enzyme in the blood that rises to abnormal levels following a heart attack. Laboratory determination of this and other enzymes helps distinguish a heart attack from other diagnoses

Ladder Polymers   (Double-Stranded Polymers). Polymers comprising chains made up of fused rings. Examples: cyclized (acid-treated) rubbers.

Lake   A type of organic pigment obtained from water-soluble acid dyes, precipitated on an inert carrier. Lakes are seldom used in medical devices, since they can be extracted.

Lambda Chain   An antigenic form of light chain of the immunoglobulins.

Lamellar Structures   Platelike single crystals that can be found in some crystalline polymers.

Laminar Flow   The continuous movement of one fluid layer past another, with no transfer of mass from one to another. The opposite of turbulent flow.

Laminate   (Noun). A manufactured product in which some of the substrate layers are placed at right angles to the remaining layers with respect to the strongest direction of tension. See also REINFORCED PLASTIC and COMPOSITE.

Laminate   (Verb). To adhere two or more layers of substrates.

Laminate, Parallel   A laminate in which all substrate layers are oriented parallel, with respect to the strongest direction of tension.

Lamination   The process or manufacturing sequence used to unite two or more layers of substrate with an adhesive.

Lamp Black   A type of CARBON BLACK, used as pigment.

Lap   In filament winding, the amount of overlay between successive windings.

Lap Joint   A joint made by placing one surface to be joined partly over another surface and bonding the overlapping portions.

Lap Winding   A variation of filament winding, consisting of convolutely winding a resin-impregnated tape (prepreg) onto a mandrel, followed by a curing process.

Laparoscope   A Class II device used to permit direct viewing of peritoneal organs on the female genitalia. May include: trocar and cannula, scope preheater, light source, and component parts.

Laparoscopy   (Abdominoscopy, Peritoneoscopy, Ventroscopy). A percutaneous procedure in which an electrically lighted tubular device is inserted through the abdominal wall to visualize internal organs and structures for diagnostic or therapeutic purposes.

Laser   A device that produces a beam of coherent or monochromatic light as a result of photon-stimulated emissions. Lasers are experimentally utilized to destroy atherosclerotic plaques, and other specialized medical applications.

Latent Heat   The quantity of energy in calories per gram absorbed or emitted as a substance undergoes a change of state. For example, as it changes from liquid to solid (freezes); from liquid to vapor (boils); or from solid to liquid (melts). No change in temperature occurs.

Latent Solvent An organic liquid displaying little or no solvent effect on a polymer at room temperature, but which becomes an active solvent at some elevated temperature.

Latex A stable colloidal dispersion of a polymeric substance in an essentially aqueous medium. Those latices of interest to the medical device industry include vinyl polymers and copolymers, natural rubber, polyurethane, acrylics, etc.

Latices Plural of latex, preferred over the sometimes used "latexes."

Lattice Pattern In filament winding, a pattern with a fixed arrangement of open voids producing a three-dimensional basket-weave effect.

Lauryl Methacrylate One of the monomers used in the synthesis of acrylic resins.

Lavage The washing of an organ or body cavity, such as the stomach, with an appropriate fluid.

LC_{50} (Lethal Concentration, 50%). The quantity of a substance administered by inhalation necessary to kill 50% of test animals exposed to the substance within a specified time. The test applies to gases, vapors, fumes, dust, and other particulates suspended in air.

LCL_0 (Lethal Concentration Low) The lowest concentration of a substance in air reported to have caused death in humans or animals.

LD_{50} (Lethal Dose, 50%). The quantity of a substance administered either orally or by skin contact necessary to kill 50% of test animals exposed to the substance within a specified time. Substances having an LD_{50} of less than 50 mg per kg body weight are rated highly toxic.

LDL_0 (Lethal Dose Low). The lowest dose of a substance introduced by any route, other than inhalation, over any given period of time and reported to have caused death in humans or animals.

LDPE Abbreviation for *Low-Density Polyethylene*.

L/D Ratio In an extruder screw, the ratio of the screw length to screw diameter. In many polymers, L/D ratios of 15:1 and 20:1 are common.

Leaching The process of extraction of one component from a mixture by exposing the mixture to a solvent that will dissolve the component, but has no effect on the remaining portions of the mixture.

Lead Stabilizers A family of highly effective heat stabilizers. Seldom used in medical polymers due to their toxicity.

Lecithin Pure lecithin is a phosphatidyl choline. It is used as an emulsifier, dispersant, wetting agent, penetrating agent, and antioxidant.

Lesion A pathological alteration of tissue more or less circumscribed in nature. Examples: corneal opacity, decubitus ulcer, myocardial infraction.

Leukapheresis A procedure, analogous to PLASMAPHERESIS, in which a certain amount of blood is removed from a donor, so the leukocytes may be removed. The remaining blood is returned to the donor. The separated leukocytes may be used to treat another person, or for various other purposes.

Leukocyte   A white blood cell. Plays a vital part in the defense against disease, foreign substances, and in repair of injured tissue.

Leukocytes, Concentration   The human adult has approximately 7000 leukocytes per cubic millimeter of blood. The normal percentages of the different types of leukocytes are approximately the following:

Polymorphonuclear neutrophils 62.0%
Polymorphonuclear eosinophils 2.3%
Polymorphonuclear basophils 0.4%
Monocytes 5.3%
Lymphocytes 30.0%

Leveling   A term used in coatings to describe the ability of a coating to cover a dry substrate easily, while maintaining its level without sagging, running, or cratering.

Levorotatory   Having the property when in solution of rotating the plane of polarized light to the left. Opposite of dextrorotatory.

Lewis Acid   Any molecule or ion capable of combining with another molecule or ion by covalently bonding with two electrons from the second molecule or ion. A Lewis acid is thus an electron acceptor (electrophile). The simplest Lewis acid is a hydrogen ion, but many compounds such as boron trifluoride and aluminum chloride exhibit the same behavior.

Lewis Base   A substance capable of forming covalent bonds by donating a pair of electrons, resulting in neutralization from an acid-base reaction with formation of a coordinate covalent bond. Lewis bases are also called *Nucleophiles*.

Lewis Electron Theory   A general theory involving acid/base formation, neutralization and related phenomena based on the exchange of electrons between reactants, and the formation of coordinate bonds. Theory advanced in 1923 by Gilbert N. Lewis, for whom it is named.

Ligand   A molecule, ion, or atom attached to the central atom of a coordination compound, a chelate, or other complex. Ligands are also called *Chelators* and *Complexing Agents*.

Light Chain   The smallest of the two types of polypeptide chains (light and heavy) of immunoglobulins, of which two exist in the tetrapeptide unit.

Light Resistance   The fundamental ability of a polymer to resist fading, darkening, or degradation upon exposure to sunlight or ultraviolet light.

Light Scattering   In a dilute polymer solution, light rays are scattered by the solubilized polymer. Measuring the intensity of the light scattered at various angles is an important quantitative method of measuring molecular weights of high polymers.

Light Stabilizer   A compounding agent added to polymers to improve the light resistance of the base polymer.

Limbic System   That part of the nervous system that affects the internal organs of the body.

Limiting Viscosity Number   The IUPAC name for INTRINSIC VISCOSITY.

Linear Polymer   (Thermoplastic). A polymer whose molecules are linked together in the form of chains, with little or no branching or side links. Linear polymers are thermoplastic, as opposed to cross-linked polymers, which are thermosets.

Lipase   Any of a class of enzymes that hydrolyze fats to glycerol and fatty acids.

Lipid   Term for a large group of compounds that include (1) the true fats and fatty acids, (2) the waxy substances known as sterols, e.g., cholesterol and ergosterol, and (3) The phosphorus-containing fats, e.g., lecithin.

Lipoproteins   Body compounds that contain both proteins and fatty substances.

Liposomes   Artificially produced cell-like structures with a multilayered phospholipid "membrane." Like a biologic cell, a liposome is composed of a thin but durable membrane that surrounds an aqueous compartment, protecting it from the environment. Liposomes may be constructed to have a single aqueous compartment surrounded by a lipid layer (unilamellar) or may consist of concentric lipid and aqueous layers (multilamellar). Recently, microfluidization techniques have been used to produce liposomes of well-defined size distribution.

Lipotropic Agent   A substance with high affinity for fats and oil, which helps regulate the metabolism of fat and cholesterol in the body. Example: inositol.

Liquid   An amorphous (noncrystalline) form of matter, intermediate between gases and solids, in which the molecules are much more highly concentrated than in gases, but much less concentrated than in solids.

Lithotomy Position   A position in which the patient is placed on his/her back, with legs and knees raised for examination or treatment.

Lithotryptor, Mechanical   A Class II device consisting of steel jaws, designed for insertion into the urinary bladder through the urethra to reach and crush bladder stones.

Loss Angle   The anti-tangent of the electrical dissipation factor. See also DIELECTRIC LOSS ANGLE.

Loss Factor   The product of the power factor and the dielectric constant of a dielectric material.

Loss Modulus   A damping term indicative of the amount of energy dissipated into heat when a material is physically deformed. Mathematically it is the imaginary portion of the complex modulus. It is calculated by multiplying the storage modulus and the tangent of the loss angle.

Low-Density Polyethylene (LDPE)   Polyethylene resins ranging in density from 0.915 to 0.925. The molecular architecture of LDPE shows the ethylene molecules linked in random fashion, with side branches emerging from the main chain. This branching effectively prevents formation of closely packed

121

chains, reducing crystallinity, and resulting in polymers that are softer and more flexible than High-Density Polyethylene.

Low-Pressure Injection Molding (Liquid Molding, Fluid Molding). A term used for the process of injecting fluid materials into closed molds by means of a low-pressure apparatus. Silicone and polyurethane elastomer articles may readily be produced in this fashion.

Low-Pressure Laminates (Contact Molding). Plastics laminated at pressures ranging from 15 psi to 200 psi (according to ASTM).

Low-Pressure Molding According to ASTM D 883-83T, any molding operation in which the pressure is 200 psi, or less.

Low-Temperature Flexibility Flexible polymers at room temperature become less flexible as they are cooled, finally becoming brittle at the Glass Transition Temperature (T_g). This property can be measured by torsional tests performed over a wide range of temperatures, from which the apparent elastic moduli are calculated.

Lubricant A substance that when interposed between two adjacent solid surfaces tends to make the surfaces slippery, thus reducing friction and preventing sticking. Lubricants are added to medical plastics to (1) assist in processing, (2) prevent sticking of the finished articles, (3) impart lubricity, or (4) aid insertion. Silicone fluids, fluorocarbons, and low molecular weight polyethylenes are used to lubricate medical polymers, because of their inherent biocompatibility.

Lubricant Bloom Cloudy, greasy, irregular, amorphous exudates on the surface of plastics, caused by the migration of lubricants. The term lubricant bloom should only be used when the exudate is caused by a lubricant contained in the plastic compound, or applied to it during processing.

Lubrication The introduction of a substance of low drag between two adjacent solid surfaces, at least one of which is in motion. The ability of a substance to act as a lubricant is known as lubricity.

Lumbar Puncture The insertion of a sterile needle into the spinal canal to (1) withdraw spinal fluid for diagnostic purposes, (2) administer spinal anesthesia, or (3) instill medications.

Lumen (1) The inner space of a tube or catheter. (2) The open inner space in any tubular organ (such as blood vessels or intestines).

Luminescent Pigments (Phosphorescent, Fluorescent Pigments). Pigments that "glow" in darkness or light, producing striking visual effects.

Luminous Transmittance The ratio of transmitted light to incident light.

Luster The appearance of a solid surface in reflected light. Types of luster are: (1) metallic; (2) vitreous, like glass; (3) resinous; (4) adamantine, exceedingly brilliant; and (5) dull, not bright or shiny, like chalk.

Lutein A yellow pigment isolated from the corpus luteum, and found in body fats. Chemically is a carotenoid.

Luteotropin (Lactogenic Hormone, LGH). One of the hormones secreted by the anterior lobe of the pituitary gland. It aids in causing growth of the mammary gland, initiates milk secretion, and influences activity of the corpus luteum, including secretion of progesterone.

Lymph   A colorless body fluid that circulates through lymphatic vessels, eventually joining the general circulation. It consists of white blood cells and tissue fluid.

Lymphadenitis   Inflammation of the lymph nodes, which are located throughout the body along lymphatic vessels.

Lymphatic System   An accessible route by which fluids can flow from the interstitial spaces into the blood. The lymphatics carry proteins and large particulate matter away from the tissue spaces, neither of which can be removed by absorption directly into the lymphatic capillaries. The minute quantities of fluid that return to the circulation (120 ml per hour) are extremely important because high molecular weight substances are incapable of passing through the venous capillary pores, but they can enter the lymphatic capillaries completely unimpeded.

Lymphocyte   An agranular type of white blood cell, with sparse cytoplasm and round nucleus derived from the thymus (T Type) or bone marrow (B Type). Found in lymph, lymph nodes, blood, spleen, etc.

Lymphocyte Transformation   The active nucleic acid metabolism and nuclear enlargement of a lymphocyte in contact with an antigen.

Lyophilic   Descriptive of the ability of a substance to form colloidal suspensions spontaneously. When the suspending medium is water, such ability is called HYDROPHILIC.

Lyophilization   The removal of water from a frozen material via the application of vacuum, where moisture evaporates as a result of sublimation. The method is frequently used to dry heat-sensitive items, such as drugs and cultures.

Lyophobic   Descriptive of a material in the colloidal state that lacks affinity for the suspending medium. Lyophobic suspensions require the presence of stabilizing agents to prevent settling or coagulation.

Lysin   An antibody that causes the disintegration of bacteria or other foreign cells.

Lysosome   An intracellular cytoplasmic structure serving as a concentrated source of hydrolytic enzymes.

Lysozyme   An antibiotic enzyme found in egg white. Capable of hydrolyzing certain sugar linkages in glycoproteins. It can dissolve the mucopolysaccharides found in bacterial walls, hence acting as a mild antiseptic.

MAC *Maximum Acceptable Concentration; Maximum Allowable Concentration.* (Ceiling Value). A limit of concentration not to be exceeded by a toxic substance.

Maceration General term referring to softening due to excessive moisture. Example: skin gets macerated under occlusive dressings.

Machining, of Plastics Operations commonly used for metals that are applicable to plastics, with appropriate variations in tolling and speeds. Examples: Drilling, grinding, threading.

Macro Large or long.

Macromolecular Pertaining to substances consisting of large molecules.

Macromolecule The giant molecules that comprise high polymers. Each macromolecule may contain hundreds of thousands of atoms.

Macrophage Tissue or blood phagocyte, 20 to 80 microns in diameter, containing lysosomes, vacuoles, and partially digested phagocytized debris in their cytoplasm.

Macrophage, Chemotactic Factors The macrophage is a key cell during inflammation and wound repair, as evidenced by the wide variety of chemotactic factors it can produce:

(1) Plasma-Derived Factors
   - *Complement peptide C5a*
   - *Fibrinopeptides*
   - *Ig-G proteolytic fragments*
   - *Macrophage chemotactic factor from skin*
   - *Thrombin*
(2) Extracellular Matrix-Derived Factors
   - *Collagen/collagen fragments*
   - *Elastin/elastin fragments*
   - *Fibronectin fragments*
(3) Cell-Derived Factors
   - *Leukotriene B_4*
   - *Platelet factor 4*
   - *Arterial smooth muscle cell factor*
(4) Bacterial-Derived Factors
   - *Formyl methionyl peptides*
   - *N-acetylmuramyl-L-alanyl-D-isoglytamine*

Macrophage, Involvement in Wound Repair The macrophage is considered a pivotal cell during wound repair. The following is the temporal sequence of events involving macrophages during wound repair: (1) emigration of blood-borne monocyte from the vasculature to the extravascular tissue, under the influence of chemotactic factors; (2) differentiation of monocyte into a macrophage; (3) control tissue debridement by the secretion of proteolytic enzymes; (4) secretion of interleukin-1 which stimulates fibroblasts to synthesize collagen. Fibroblast secretion of collagen is under macrophage control; and (5) secretion of angiogenesis factor(s) that stimulate the directed outgrowth of endothelial cells from adjacent capillaries.

MAF (Master Files for Medical Devices; Device Master File). To distinguish devices from drug master files (DMFs), the FDA's CDRH released a guideline for the submission of MAFs. Both filing systems use a prefix and sequential numbering to identify separate records. MAFs permit holder to: (1) incorporate information regarding facilities, manufacturing procedures, and controls; and (2) incorporate in a customer's application trade secret information by reference only, thereby avoiding disclosure of secrets to the customer. An MAF is reviewed only when a 510(k), IDE, or PMA application is authorized for reference. Only a detailed description of facilities, equipment, manufacturing methods, controls, specifications for in-process materials, and final product constitutes a trade secret and merits this protection.

Magnesium An element present in the body that aids in muscle contraction, bone, and tooth formation. Deficiency may produce irritability of muscles and nerves.

Magnesium Stearate A white, soft powder used as a lubricant and stabilizer in vinyls, polyurethanes, etc.

Malaise A term that describes the general feeling of uneasiness, illness, headache, and other nonspecific pains that occur when a person has the flu or other febrile illness.

Malignant Any condition that is resistant to treatment, is very severe, and may lead to death.

Mammography Visualization and examination of the breast by X-rays.

MAN Abbreviation for *Methacrylonitrile.*

Mandrel (1) The core around which polymers, fabrics, or resin-impregnated fabrics are wound to form tubes. (2) In extrusion terminology, the central member of a tubing die, or of a blow-molding parison die, comprising the inside of the form.

Mania A form of hyperactive behavior, in which an individual becomes hyperexcitable. May be a phase of the mental disorder called manic-depressive psychosis.

Manic-Depressive Psychosis A mental disease characterized by mood swings, in which the patient becomes alternately deeply depressed and deeply excited.

Manifold A channel with multiple inlets or outlets.

Manometer A U-shaped glass tube containing water or mercury, used to measure the pressure of liquids or gases. When pressure is applied, the liquid level in one arm rises while the level on the opposite arm drops. A calibrated scale behind one of the arms permits pressure readings, usually in inches or millimeters. The instrument is frequently used to measure blood pressure.

Manufacturer (Regulatory). Any person, including any repacker and/or relabeler, who manufactures, fabricates, assembles, or processes a finished device. The term does not include any person who only distributes a finished device.

Manufacturing Material   (Regulatory). Any material such as cleaning agent, mold-release agent, lubricating oil, or other substance used to facilitate a manufacturing process and which is not intended by the manufacturer to be included in the finished device.

Mar Resistance   The fundamental ability of a glossy polymer surface to resist abrasive action. ASTM D 673 measures this property by abrading a specimen to a series of degrees, then measuring the gloss of the abraded portions with a Glossmeter, and comparing the results with an unabraded area of the specimen that serves as a control.

Mass   The quantity of matter contained in a particle or body, regardless of its location relative to other gravitational bodies.

Mass Number   The number of neutrons and protons in the nucleus of an atom. Thus the mass number of helium is 4, of carbon 12, of oxygen 16, and so on.

Mass Polymerization   See BULK POLYMERIZATION.

Mass Spectrometry   A method of chemical analysis in which the substance to be analyzed is placed in a vacuum and reduced to low pressure. The resulting vapor is exposed to a beam of electrodes, which causes ionization; the ions are then separated according to their mass, and identified as they emerge from a magnetic field.

Mast Cell   A cell found in connective tissue. These cells produce heparin and histamine, which are stored in cytoplasmic granules.

Mast Cell Degranulation   The release of heparin and histamine during a serologic reaction on the surface of mast cells, or produced by certain chemicals.

Mastectomy   Surgical removal of a diseased breast.

Masterbatch   A general term referring to a previously prepared mixture containing high percentages of an ingredient, to be added in relatively small amounts to a product during compounding. Frequently used to designate color concentrates.

Mastication   Permanent softening of rubbers and thermoplastic elastomers by the application of mechanical energy on a roll mill, or a Banbury intensive mixer. The softening is due (1) to formation of free radicals resulting from the rupture of the polymer chain and the addition of oxygen at these active points, and (2) temporary rupture of hydrogen bonds and other intermolecular forces. The science studying these phenomena is called mechanochemistry.

Mastitis   Inflammation of the breast.

Mat   A fabric or felt of reinforcing material cut to the contour of a mold for use in reinforced plastics processes.

Matched Mold Thermoforming   A sheet thermoforming process in which the heated plastic sheet is shaped between matching male and female molds.

Material　Any synthetic or natural polymer, metal, alloy, ceramic, or other biocompatible substance, including tissue rendered nonviable (via fixation), used as a device or any part thereof.

Matrix　The part of a polymer that surrounds and engulfs embedded material, filaments, or reinforcing particles.

Matter　Anything that has mass or occupies space.

Matter, Levels of　There are a number of different scales upon which matter may be examined, including: (1) subatomic (protons, neutrons, electrons); (2) atomic and molecular (less than ten angstroms); (3) colloidal (10 angstroms to 1 micron); (4) microscopic; (5) macroscopic; and (6) space or celestial.

Matter, States of　There are three accepted phases: solid, liquid, and gas.

Mc　Abbreviation for *Megacycles*, or one million cycles.

MDI　Abbreviation for *Diphenylmethane-4,4' Diisocyanate*, an important intermediate in the synthesis of polyurethane.

Mechanically Foamed Plastic　A cellular plastic in which the cellular structure has been produced by gases introduced by physical means. A typical example is the introduction of Freon gas to a reacting polyurethane to produce foam.

Mechanical Properties　(1) The physical manifestations associated with elastic and inelastic reactions in a polymer when force is applied. (2) Expressing the relationships between stress/strain, tear resistance, abrasion resistance, etc., in a given polymer. (3) Mechanical properties include: elasticity, hardness, impact resistance, friction resistance, stiffness, strength, flexure endurance, etc.

Media　The intermediate and thickest layer of tissue comprising blood vessels.

Mediastinum　The space in the center of the chest, between the lungs, starting at the lower margin of the throat, and extending to the upper surface of the diaphragm. It contains the heart, the major blood vessels, trachea, esophagus, and other nervous structures. On the basis of the organs it contains, it is one of the crucial spaces of the body.

Medical Device Act　The Medical Device Act, signed into law by President Gerald Ford on May 28, 1976, provided the FDA with expanded authority to regulate medical devices. Provisions of the Act determine that the FDA:

- May institute regulatory action without determining that the device was in commerce
- May temporarily detain a device that is in violation of the Act, that presents a substantial deception or unreasonable risk of illness or injury
- May restrict the sale, distribution, or use of a device if its safety and effectiveness cannot be reasonably assured

— Prescribe good manufacturing practices
— Require manufacturers to register, and list their devices semiannually
— Classify devices into one of three categories: Class I (general controls), Class II (performance standards), and Class III (premarket approval)
— Require manufacturers of devices first marketed after May 28, 1976, to notify the agency about the safety and effectiveness of the device

Medical Device Reporting (MDR)   The MDR regulation was enacted in December 1984, and is second only to the Good Manufacturing Practice (GMP) regulation in its significance to medical device manufacturers. The regulations require manufacturers and importers to report to the FDA whenever they have reason to believe that one of their marketed devices may have caused or contributed to a death or serious injury, or malfunctioned. Under the regulation, companies have to report irrespective of the event, whether or not the accident was the fault of the product, or even if the event was caused by product misuse. A "reportable event" must be based on information that reasonably suggests it has caused death, serious injury, or malfunction. Death is the permanent ending of all life in a person. Serious injury is an injury that (1) is life-threatening, (2) results in permanent impairment of a body function or permanent damage to body structure, or (3) necessitates medical or surgical intervention by a health-care professional to prevent permanent impairment or damage, or to relieve unanticipated temporary impairment or damage. Malfunction is a failure of the device to meet any of its performance specifications. It is reportable if the device is likely to cause or contribute to a death or serious injury if the malfunction were to occur.

Medical Emergencies   The most common life-threatening emergencies are listed below in decreasing order of occurrence.

(1) Syncope
(2) Angina Pectoris
(3) Myocardial Infarction
(4) Hypertension
(5) Hypotension/Shock
(6) Insulin Shock/Diabetic Coma
(7) Grand Mal Seizure
(8) Self-Limiting Allergic Reaction
(9) Asthma
(10) Anaphylaxis
(11) Hyperventilation
(12) Cerebrovascular Accident
(13) Hemorrhage

Medicinal Chemistry   A division of chemistry interested in the effects of drugs on the human body, and on infective organisms. It is interested in the synthesis of compounds designed to fight certain human diseases, such as cancer and hypertension. It is also concerned with immunology, hormone activity, and other medical topics.

MEK   Abbreviation for *Methyl Ethyl Ketone*.

MEKP   Abbreviation for *Methyl Ethyl Ketone Peroxide*.

Melamine   A crystalline polymer, derived from cyanuric acid, of which it is the triamide. Frequently used in the manufacture of Melamine Formaldehyde resins.

Melamine-Formaldehyde Resins   Thermosetting resins, widely used for plastic tableware. The lower-molecular-weight resins are water-soluble, and are used to impregnate paper and other hydrophilic materials.

Melamine/Phenolic Resins   Mixtures of melamine and phenolic resins that display the easy coloring characteristics of melamine with the dimensional stability of phenolics.

Melanin   A brownish-black pigment that occurs in skin, hair, and retina of higher animals, with the exception of albinos. It is the cause of darkened skin after sun exposure. Formed by the enzymatic action of tyrosinase on tyrosine.

Melanoma   A tumor that appears on the skin. If malignant, it may spread rapidly to other parts of the body. The lesion derives its name from the presence of the dark brown pigment, MELANIN.

Melasma   A patchy discoloration of the skin, often seen in pregnant women.

Melena   Bowel movement that has a black appearance, caused by bleeding somewhere in the intestinal tract.

Melt   (Noun). A solid thermoplastic that has been heated to a molten condition.

Melt Extractor   A type of injection torpedo, placed in a plasticating system for the purpose of separating fully plasticated melt, from partially molten thermoplastic material. It thus insures a fully plasticated discharge of properly molten resin from the plasticated system.

Melt Flow Index   See MELT INDEX.

Melt Fracture   A flow phenomenon, evidenced by gross irregularities in the shape or surface of the extrudate. Generally assumed to be the result of nonuniform or irregular elastic strains in the material at the die entrance.

Melt Index   As described in ASTM D 1238, the amount in grams, of a thermoplastic resin which can be forced through an orifice of $0.0825''$ diameter when subjected to a force of 2160 grams in ten minutes at 190°C. It is widely used in classifying polyethylene resins, but is equally useful in a number of other thermoplastics. Polymers of low melt index have high molecular weights, while those exhibiting high melt index numbers have correspondingly lower molecular weights.

Melt Instability   An instability in the melt flow through a die starting at the land of the die. It results in surface defects on the finished articles.

Melt Spinning   See SPINNING.

Melt Strength   The physical strength of a polymer while in the molten state.

Melt Zone   The zone of an extruder barrel in which the polymer has been softened (plasticized) by heat and pressure.

Membrane   (1) A region of discontinuity interposed between two phases. (2) A phase that acts as a barrier to prevent mass movement, but allows restricted and/or regulated passage of one or more species.

Membrane, Asymmetric, Anisotropic   A membrane having a different physical characteristic on one side (e.g., a membrane with a fine pore structure on one side, and a large pore size on the other).

Membrane, Organism Retention

PORE SIZE (microns)	ORGANISM	CULTURE MEDIUM
0.22	Pseudomonas diminuta	Saline lactose broth
0.45	Serratia marcescens	Wilson's peptone agar
0.80	Bacillus subtilis	Tryptone glucose extract
1.20	Saccharo. œrevisiae	Tryptone glucose extract

Membrane, Semipermeable   A microporous structure, which acts as a filter in the molecular range, allowing passage of ions, water, and other solvents, but virtually impermeable to macromolecules and colloidal particles. These membranes are used in osmosis, dialysis, etc.

Memory   The fundamental ability of an elastic polymer to revert in dimensions to a size previously existing at some stage during its manufacture. This property is extensively utilized in the production of "stretch film" that has been oriented by stretching, and upon reheating reverts to its original size due to its "memory."

Memory Cell   A cell that responds more quickly to the second challenge of antigen than the primary exposure to antigen and is responsible for the anamnestic response.

Menarche   The onset of the first menstrual period at puberty in females.

Meningitis   Inflammation of the meninges, the membranes covering the spinal cord and the brain.

Meningocele   A body defect in which a portion of the spinal cord membrane protrudes through the spinal column.

Meniscus   The concave curve of a liquid surface in a narrow tube caused by surface tension. In reading the meniscus it is conventional to ignore the higher liquid around the perimeter. Exception: mercury, due to its high surface tension, forms a convex meniscus.

meq   Milliequivalent. The equivalent weight of a compound divided by one thousand.

Mer   The repeating structural unit of any high polymer. One mer is a monomer, two mers form a dimer, three mers form a trimer, several mers form an oligomer, and a great many mers form a polymer.

Meso   A prefix meaning middle or intermediate, specifically: (1) an inactive stereoisomeric form resulting from an even number of dextro and levorotatory isomers; (2) an intermediate hydrated form of an inorganic acid; (3) designating a middle position in certain cyclic organic compounds; or (4) a ring system characterized by a middle position of certain rings.

Metabolism   A general term used to designate all chemical changes that occur to substances within the body, either built-up (anabolism), or breakdown (catabolism).

Metabolite   An intermediate substance produced and utilized in the processes of living organisms. Metabolites function to replace worn tissues, and are a source of energy. Examples: nucleic acids, glucose, cholesterol, enzymes.

Metabolize   To produce a change on a substance by means of the chemical processes continuously happening within living organisms.

Metal   An element that forms positive ions when its compounds are in solution and whose oxides form hydroxides rather than acids with water. Most are crystalline solids with metallic luster, conductors of electricity, and exhibit high chemical reactivity. Exceptions: mercury, cesium, and gallium are liquid at room temperature.

Metallic Fiber   Generic name for any fiber composed of metal, plastic-coated, or metal-coated plastic.

Metallic Flake Pigments   Flake-shaped particles of aluminum or copper that have the ability to reflect light specularly when compounded into a plastic matrix or coating vehicle with their reflecting surfaces approximately parallel.

Metallic Soaps   Salts derived from metals and organic acids, usually fatty acids. They include the sodium and potassium salts, known as soaps, and lead linoleate, calcium resinate, aluminum stearate, etc. Also see SOAPS, METALLIC.

Metallizing   A general term covering all processes by which polymers are coated with a thin layer of metal. Most common are: (1) electroplating; (2) vacuum metallizing; (3) spraying; (4) chemical reduction; (5) gas plating; and (6) vapor pyrolysis.

Metals, Biocompatible   The following metals have been used in orthopedics, maxillofacial instruments, sutures, and other medicinal devices: stainless steels, cobalt/chrome/molybdenum alloys, titanium and titanium alloys, MP35N, nitinol alloys, and tantalum.

Metamerism   The phenomenon where two substances seemingly equal in color when viewed under one light source (e.g., daylight), do not match color when viewed under a different light source (e.g., an incandescent lamp). If the change in color is due to a different viewing angle, the term used is *Geometric Metamerism.*

Metaplasmic Body   One of many small, specialized structures found within the cytoplasm of certain cells. These structures are rich in carbohydrates or other substances secreted or excreted by the cytoplasm, and stored temporarily.

Metastable   An unstable condition of plastics evidenced by changes in physical properties not caused by changes in composition or environment. Example: temporary softening of plastics immediately after molding or mechanical forces. May be due to temporary rupturing of intermolecular bonding forces. See also MASTICATION.

Metathesis Polymerization   A chemical reaction involving a pair of polar compounds in which the positive radical of one reacts with the negative radical of the other. This type of exchange polymerization is the basis for reaction molding of glass-filled olefins, such as dicyclopentadiene, in molding large structural components.

Metering Screw   An extrusion screw used to control the pressure and temperature of the melt.

Metering Zone   The final zone of an extruder barrel, in which the melt advances at a uniform rate toward the die.

Methacrylate Esters   Ester of methacrylic acid. The esters may be derived from methyl, ethyl, isobutyl, or *n*-butyl alcohols. These esters are polymerizable to a family of acrylic resins.

Methacrylate Plastics   See ACRYLIC RESINS.

Methacrylic Acid $CH_2:C(CH_3)COOH$. (Alpha-Methacrylic Acid). A colorless liquid with characteristic odor, widely used in the synthesis of methacrylate resins.

Methacrylonitrile (MAN)   A vinyl monomer containing a nitrile group. Produces homopolymers, which are thermoplastics with good mechanical strength and chemical resistance. MAN may also be used as a replacement for acrylonitrile in the preparation of nitrile elastomers.

Methanal   See FORMALDEHYDE.

Methanol   See METHYL ALCOHOL.

Methyl Acetate   A colorless, volatile liquid with a pleasant odor, used as a solvent for cellulose esters, cellulose nitrate, and acetyl cellulose.

Methyl Acrylate   A colorless, volatile liquid used as a monomer in the synthesis of acrylic resins.

Methyl Alcohol   (Methanol, Wood Alcohol). A colorless fluid used as a solvent for ethyl cellulose, PVAc, polyvinyl butyral, and cellulose nitrate. Also used as an intermediate in the production of methyl methacrylate and formaldehyde.

Methyl Benzene   See TOLUENE–2,4 –2,6 DIISOCYANATE.

Methyl Cellulose   (Cellulose Methyl Ether). Resins ranging in molecular weights from 40,000 to 180,000, with a methoxy group contents of 25–33%. Used as film-formers, binders, protective colloids, dispersing, thickening, and sizing agents.

Methyl Ethyl Cellulose (MEC)   The methyl ether of ethyl cellulose in which both methyl and ethyl groups are attached to the anhydroglucose units by ether linkages. Used as an emulsifier, stabilizer, and foaming agent.

Methyl Ethyl Ketone (MEK)   A powerful solvent for a variety of polymers, such as vinyl, vinyl copolymers, acrylics, and cellulosics.

Methyl Ethyl Ketone Peroxide (MEKP)   A curing agent for silicone elastomers. Produces free radicals when heated to high temperatures.

Methyl Group   The simplest alkyl group, CH$_3$, formed by subtracting a hydrogen atom from methane. It occurs at both ends of paraffinic molecules having two or more carbons in the chain, as well as in many other organic compounds.

Methyl Isobutyl Ketone (MIBK)   A solvent similar to MEK, but with moderate evaporation rate, used as a solvent for vinyl, alkyd, acrylic, phenolic, and cellulosic resins.

Methyl Isopropenyl Ketone   A flammable liquid used as a copolymerizable monomer.

Methyl Lactate   A powerful solvent for several cellulosic polymers.

Methyl Methacrylate   An important monomer used in the synthesis of acrylic resins.

n-Methyl Morpholine (NEM)   A liquid with characteristic pungent odor used as catalyst in urethane foams.

n-Methyl 2-Pyrrolidone (M-Pyrrol)   A low-toxicity solvent for urethanes, vinyls, acrylics, and other resins. Spinning agent for polyvinyl chloride. Miscible with water in all proportions.

Methyl Violet   (Gentian Violet). A green powder, used as biological dye, textile dye, topical antibacterial, antiallergen, and acid-base indicator.

Methylene Chloride   (Methylene Dichloride; Dichloromethane). A colorless, volatile liquid with a penetrating odor. Used as a nonflammable and nonexplosive solvent. Also used as a degreasing solvent, paint remover, blowing agent in foams, and solvent extractor. Is narcotic in high concentrations, and toxic, with a tolerance of 100 ppm in air.

Methylpentene Resin   A clear thermoplastic, based on 4-methylpentene-1, with a melting point over 460°F, and the lowest specific gravity of any plastic. Used to manufacture hard, transparent medical devices. Processable by all thermoplastic methods.

MF   Abbreviation for *Melamine-Formaldehyde Resins.*

mg   Abbreviation for *milligram* (one-thousandth of a gram, or 0.000035 ounces).

mg/m^3   Milligrams per cubic meter; a unit for measuring concentrations of dusts, gases, or mists in air.

MHz   Abbreviation for *MegaHertz*, also known as *Mc.*

MIC   Abbreviation for *Minimum Inhibitory Concentration*, the lowest concentration of an antibiotic in a dilution series that shows no growth of the test organism(s).

Mica   Crystalline silicate-based mineral of varying composition, or synthesized from potassium fluorosilicate and alumina. Used as a filler with good electrical properties and heat resistance.

Micelle   A particle of colloidal dimensions, formed by the irreversible aggregation of dissolved molecules. Soaps and detergents are examples of electrically charged micelles, where the polymerization is thought to commence within the soap micelles.

Microballons   (1) Small hollow spheres used to confer low density to plastics. (2) Tiny vinyl plastic spheres used to reduce evaporation of volatile liquids, by floating on the surface of vessels.

Microcarrier   A small beaded matrix (approximately 100–200 μm diameter) used as a support for the culture of anchorage-dependent cells. Cells grown in this way can be treated as a suspension-cell culture.

Microchemistry   A branch of analytical chemistry that handles very small quantities of chemicals, ranging from 0.1 to 10 mg. Recently, many advances in instrumental chemistry permit analyses below the mg range.

Microcrystalline Structure   A specialized form in which many polymers have been prepared to facilitate handling. Microscopically, the substances are composed of colloidal microcrystals, connected by molecular chains. Examples are nylon, collagen, cellulose, and certain waxes.

Microcurie   One-millionth of a curie.

Microencapsulation   Enclosure of an active ingredient into capsules ranging from 20 to 150 microns in diameter, which act as semipermeable membranes. The capsules are frequently made from polymeric substances such as nylons, polyurethanes, hydrogels, and collagen, and are used as controlled-release agents for pharmaceuticals, cosmetics, etc.

Microfiltration   A filtration process capable of separating substances between 0.02 μm and 10 μm in size. Microfiltration may separate pollen, starch, blood cells, bacteria, DNA, and viruses. Microfiltration applications include separation of microbial cells, media sterilization, and microbiological assays.

Microgels   Small particles of cross-linked polymers containing closed loops. Microgels are present in small amounts due to impurities in monomers, and influence certain polymer properties.

Micromechanics   (Composite). The concepts, mathematical models, equations, and detailed studies used to predict unidirectional composite properties from constituent material properties. These properties may include: stresses, geometric configurations, fabrication variables, etc.

Micron   A unit of length equal to 0.001 millimeter.

Microorganism   (1) A living organism of microscopic size, generally considered to include bacteria, molds, and fungi, but excluding viruses. Found in air, water, and soil. Medical devices are usually sterilized to inactivate or kill microorganisms, thus preventing nosocomial infections. (2) From a biological standpoint, pathogenic microorganisms are divided into protozoa, fungi, bacteria, and viruses. Protozoa are single-celled animals that cause a number of tropical diseases. Fungi have metabolism similar to that of lower animals, but resemble plants externally, causing many skin diseases and some deep infections; fungal diseases are known as mycoses. Bacteria are classified according to shape as: spherical (cocci); rod shaped (bacilli); and spiral (spirilla). Cocci that grow in pairs are called diplococci; streptococci are those that grow in chain-like structures; finally, those that grow in grape-like clusters are called staphylococci. Bacteria are further classified as gram positive or gram negative. Viruses are the smallest living organisms, with a size of 20–300 nm. They can only multiply in living cells, and are grouped according to the symptoms they produce. Several exanthem viruses cause disease accompanied by skin eruptions, such as measles, smallpox, and shingles. Respiratory viruses produce influenza, viral pneumonia, and psittacosis. Neurotropic viruses produce poliomyelitis, encephalitis, rabies, and other diseases of the central nervous system. Hepatitis viruses produce infections of the liver.

Microporous   Solid substances having "pores" of microscopic dimensions. Plastic films and coatings are rendered microporous to permit "breathing" of water vapor, while remaining impervious to water and bacteria.

Microporous Membranes, Manufacturing Methods

PROCESS	MATERIALS
Phase inversion by	Polymers
— solvent separation	— cellulose acetate, polyamide
— temperature change	— polypropylene, polyamide
— precipitant addition	— polyurethane, polysulfone
Stretching sheets of partially crystalline polymers	Polymers (PTFE)
Irradiation and etching	Polycarbonate, polyester Ceramics, metal oxides,
Molding and sintering of fine-grain powders	PTFE, polyethylene

Microscopy, Chemical   Use of microscope for the study and identification of materials. This is specially useful in biological chemistry, medicinal chemistry, and forensic chemistry.

Microspheres   Small, hollow spheres used as fillers and reinforcing agents in low-density plastics. Microspheres are made of polymers, minerals, ceramics, and glass in both solid and hollow forms.

Microwave Heating   A heating process, similar to dielectric heating, but using frequencies in the 10^9 to 10^{10} cps (radar) range. This type of heating has been used to heat and cure thermosetting resins.

Microwave Spectroscopy   A type of absorption spectroscopy, used to analyze substances in the gaseous state, using that portion of the electromagnetic spectrum having wavelengths in the range between the far infrared and the radio frequencies, i.e., between 1 millimeter and 30 centimeters.

Microwaves   Radio-frequency waves generated by electronic devices in which electrons are accelerated and directed toward a target.

Micturition   The conscious act of urination.

Migraine   A severe headache that may appear on only one side of the head and cause secondary symptoms, such as nausea, vomiting, and sensitivity to light and noise.

Migration   The transfer of a constituent of a plastic compound to another contacting substance.

Mil   A unit of length equal to 0.001 inch.

Mildew Preventive   A compound used to prevent the growth of parasitic fungi, usually stain-producing, on such materials as polymers, textiles, and paper.

Mill   A mechanical device used to mix and compound plastics and rubbers. Usually composed of two counter-rotating metal molds, which may be cooled or heated; the shear forces generated in the gap between the rolls transform the raw materials into a condition ready to use.

Milled Fibers   Small particles of glass filaments produced by hammer milling continuous glass strands. Milled fibers are used as anticrazing reinforcing agents for adhesives.

Milli-   Prefix meaning one-thousandth of a part.

Milliequivalent (meq)   One-thousandth of the equivalent weight of a substance. The equivalent weight is the molecular weight divided by the functionality of the substance.

Milligram   One-thousandth of a gram.

Milliliter (ml)   One-thousandth of a liter. The volume occupied by one gram of water at 4°C and 760 mm Hg pressure.

Millimicron   One-thousandth of a micron; 10 Angstrom units; 1 nanometer.

Mineral   Any element, inorganic compound, or mixture occurring in the earth's crust and atmosphere. Includes all metals and nonmetals (except carbon), as well as their compounds and ores. The term has traditionally been used to indicate the "nonliving kingdom" of nature, as opposed to the organic. As used by nutritionists, the term refers to food components such as iron, copper, phosphorus, calcium, iodine, selenium, fluorine, and trace nutrients.

Mineral Black   Black pigments made by grinding and/or heating shale or coal.

Miticide   A pesticide that kills mites, small animals of the spider class.

Mitochondria   Particles of cytoplasm found in most aerobic cells. These organelles synthesize most of the cellular adenosine triphosphate (ATP), thus being the chief energy sources of living cells. Many energy-converting enzymes are located in the mitochondria.

Mitosis   The division of a cell nucleus to produce two cells, each having the same chemical and genetic constitution as the "parent" cell.

Mixers   Mechanical devices used to intimately mix (compound) two or more raw materials to some predetermined state of uniformity. Among the most common types used in the plastics industry are: Ball mills, BANBURY MIXERS, centrifugal mixers, colloid mills, conical mixers, KNEADERS, RIBBON BLENDERS, two-roll mills, and twin-screw extruders.

Mixing   Creating a uniform distribution of liquid, semi-solid, or solid ingredients of a mixture (compound) solely by means of mechanical action. Low-viscosity liquids are mixed with impeller blades; medium-viscosity liquids are mixed with revolving paddles; high-viscosity liquids are mixed with helical rotors and sigma blades, often aided by heat.

Mixture   A physical combination of two or more substances uniformly intermingled with no constant percentage composition, in which each component retains its original properties, and may be separated from the mixture.

mm Hg   Abbreviation for *millimeters of mercury*. A pressure measurement equivalent to the pressure exerted by a column of mercury of the height designated in millimeters. Normal blood pressure is 120/80 mm Hg.

mmpf   (Million Particles Per Cubic Foot). A unit for measuring particles of a substance suspended in air. Exposure limits for dusts (nuisance dusts and others), formerly expressed as mppcf, are now more commonly quoted in mg/m^3.

Mn   Abbreviation for *Number-Average Molecular Weight*; the total weight of all molecules divided by the total number of molecules.

Mobile Intensive Care Unit   An emergency vehicle staffed by EMTs, nurses, or physicians, and equipped to provide care to the ill or injured at the scene of medical emergencies and during transportation to the hospital.

Mobility   The relative ease with which a liquid moves or flows. Nonpolar liquids (e.g., hydrocarbons) due to lower viscosity, surface tension, and specific gravity respond more readily to an applied force, compared to polar (aqueous) liquids.

Modification   A chemical reaction in which some or all the substituent radicals in a polymer have been replaced by other chemical moieties, resulting in a marked change in one or more properties in the polymer, but without destroying its basic structural identity. Examples are the cellulosic resins, which are modified for solubility, viscosity, film-forming abilities, etc.

Modified Resins   A general term referring to any synthetic resin modified by the incorporation of other resins, elastomers, oils, or other compounding ingredient, which alter the processing characteristics or physical properties of the pure resin.

Modifier   Any chemically inert ingredient that when added to a polymer is capable of changing the physical characteristics of the pure polymer.

Modulus   A Latin word meaning "small measure." Modulus is a number that expresses a measure of some property of a material, e.g., modulus of elasticity.

Modulus in Compression   The ratio of the compressive stress to strain within the elastic limits of a material.

137

Modulus of Elasticity (Elastic Modulus, Young's Modulus). The ratio of stress to strain below the proportional limit of a material. Expressed in psi, kg/sq cm, etc. The strain may be a change in length (Young's modulus); a twist or shear (Modulus of rigidity); or a change in volume (bulk modulus).

Modulus in Flexure The ratio of the flexure stress to strain, within the elastic limits of a material.

Modulus in Shear The ratio of shear stress to strain within the elastic limits of the material.

Modulus at 300% The tensile stress necessary to elongate a specimen to three times its original length.

Moisture Absorption The penetration and retention of water vapor into a substance upon exposure to a humid atmosphere. Not to be confused with WATER ABSORPTION, which relates to water acquired by immersion of the substance in water.

Moisture Adsorption The surface retention of moisture by a substance, as opposed to absorption, in which the moisture penetrates into the bulk of the substance.

Moisture Vapor Transmission The rate at which water vapor is capable of permeating through a membrane or film, at a specified temperature and relative humidity.

Molal A concentration in which the amount of solute is measured in moles, and the amount of solvent in kilograms.

Molar A concentration in which the molecular weight (in grams) of the solute is dissolved in enough solvent to make one liter of solution. Molar quantities are proportional to the molecular weights of the solutes.

Mold (Noun). A hollow form or cavity into which a plastic material is placed, and which confers to the plastic its final shape and dimensions.

Mold (Verb). To impart shape and dimensions to a plastic mass by means of a confining form or cavity. The term molding is employed for thermal processes using thermoplastic compounds, e.g., injection, transfer or compression-molding. The term ''casting'' is employed for processes using fluid compounds.

Mold Lubricant See PARTING AGENT.

Mold Release See PARTING AGENT.

Molding The processes involved in shaping articles via the use of molds.

Molding, High-Pressure (ASTM D 883-65T). Molding or laminating operations in which the necessary pressure is greater than 200 psi.

Molding, Low-Pressure (ASTM D 883-63T). Molding or laminating operations in which the necessary pressure is 200 psi or lower.

Molding Compounds Pellets, granules, or powders of resins mixed with additives such as colorants, stabilizers, antioxidants, etc., and ready for final processing into finished or semi-finished products.

Molding Cycle (1) The time necessary to complete the sequence of operations on a molding press for the production of one set of articles. (2) The sequence of operations necessary to produce one set of molded articles without reference to the required time.

Molding Index   According to ASTM D 731-57T, the minimum force (expressed in pounds) necessary to close a standard flash-type cup mold using a thermosetting molding powder under specified conditions.

Molding Powders   See MOLDING COMPOUNDS.

Molding Pressure   The pressure necessary to force a softened plastic to completely fill a mold cavity or cavities. It is expressed in psi of cross-sectional area of the plastic in the cylinder, either in compression, transfer, or injection.

Molding Shrinkage   (Mold Shrinkage, Shrinkage). The decrease in dimensions, expressed in inches/inch, between a molded article and the mold cavity in which it was formed at room temperature.

Mole   The molecular weight of a substance expressed in grams. Equal to the amount of pure substance containing the same number of chemical units as there are in exactly 12 grams of Carbon-12 (i.e, 6.023×10^{23} atoms).

Molecular Biology   A branch of Biology that approaches the subject of life at the molecular level. This applies to phenomena within the cellular nucleus, where chromosomes and genes are found; these are composed of nucleic acids, which control the selection and assembly of amino acids in the dividing chromosomes. Much of life can be understood by the study of DNA and RNA.

Molecular Distillation   (High Vacuum Distillation). Distillation at pressures in the order of 0.001 mm Hg. Process is useful in separation of extremely high boiling and heat-sensitive materials, such as antibiotics, vitamins, and other pharmaceuticals.

Molecular Sieves   Porous mineral particles with the unusual ability to absorb a variety of molecules of other materials. They are used to carry catalysts and blowing agents, to absorb moisture, etc.

Molecular Volume   The volume occupied by one mole; mathematically calculated by dividing the molecular weight by the density of the substance.

Molecular Weight   The sum of the atomic weights of all atoms in a molecule. In most materials, the molecular weight is a constant value; in high polymers, however, the molecular weights of individual molecules vary widely, thus the molecular weights are reported as distributions. Average molecular weights of polymers are reported as NUMBER-AVERAGE MOLECULAR WEIGHT (Mn), or WEIGHT-AVERAGE MOLECULAR WEIGHT (Mw). See also MOLECULAR WEIGHT DISTRIBUTION.

Molecular Weight Distribution   The relative amounts of polymers of different molecular weights that comprise a given specimen of polymer. Two samples of the same polymer with identical weight-average molecular weights may have different physical properties, or process differently, because they have different molecular weight distributions. Two methods are used to measure distributions: (1) fractionation, such as fraction precipitation and fraction solution; and (2) nonfractionation methods, such as light scattering, dilute solution viscosity, gel permeation chromatography, ultracentrifugation and diffusion. The ratio of the weight-average to the number-average molecular weight is called the polydispersivity, and is a measure of the broadness of the distribution.

Molecule   The smallest indivisible unit of matter that can exist by itself, and retain all the properties of the original substance.

Mono   A prefix denoting a single radical.

Monobasic   Pertaining to acids or salts that have one displaceable hydrogen atom per molecule. Substances having two displaceable hydrogen atoms are called DIBASIC, three displaceable hydrogen atoms TRIBASIC.

Monochloroethylene   See VINYL CHLORIDE.

Monocyte   White blood cells, 12–30 microns in diameter, with rounded nucleus. Abundant at sites of medical device implants, due to the normal "foreign body reaction." Also seen in sites of delayed allergic reactions.

Monofilament   A single filament of indefinite length, usually produced by extrusion or solution extrusion. Monofilaments are widely used to produce sutures, vascular grafts, and surgical fabrics by weaving and knitting techniques.

Monomer   A reactive moiety, of low molecular weight, which can react to form a polymer, by combination with itself, or with other reactive moieties.

Monomeric   Pertaining to MONOMER.

Morbidity   State of disease, or calculated ratio of a disease state to the normal state.

Morphology   The study of the physical form and structure of a substance. This includes a wide range of characteristics, extending from the external size and shape of large articles to dimensions and conformations of molecular chains.

Mottle   An irregular distribution or mixture of materials of different colors, giving an appearance of spots, streaks, specks, etc.

MSDS   A *Material Safety Data Sheet* is a written communication concerning a chemical, hazardous or nonhazardous, and prepared according to OSHA Hazard Communication Rule. It supersedes OSHA form 20.

Mu Chain   The heavy chain of immunoglobulin M.

Mucilage   An adhesive prepared from a gum and water.

Mucopolysaccharide   A polymer composed of alternate units of uronic acids and amino sugars (in which a hydroxyl group is replaced with an amino group, which in turn may be *N*-substituted by other groups). The mucopolysaccharides act as structural supports for connective tissue and mucous membranes, holding large amounts of water.

Mucosa   The smooth membranous lining of the interior organs of the body. Present in the intestinal tract, respiratory tract, urinary tract, and the genitourinary tract.

Multifilament   Manufactured fiber yarns composed of a plurality of fine continuous filaments or strands.

Murmur   Cardiac sounds produced by turbulence due to pathological alterations of the valves, such as stenosis (constriction due to scar formation and shrinking) and insufficiency (incomplete valve closure resulting in blood regurgitation). The time when a murmur occurs is determined by whether it is systolic or diastolic as follows:

VALVES	PATHOLOGICAL CHANGE	TIME
Aortic or	Stenosis	Systolic
Pulmonary	Insufficiency	Diastolic
Mitral or	Stenosis	Diastolic
Tricuspic	Insufficiency	Systolic

Mutagenic Agent   (1) Any of a number of chemical compounds able to induce mutations in DNA and in living cells. Alkylating agents, such as the alkyl mustards, dimethyl sulfate, and ethylmethane react with the nitrogen atoms of guanine, leading to mutation in DNA by depurination. Nitrous oxide can deaminate both guanine and cytosine. (2) Ionizing radiation.

Mutation   A distinctive character appearing suddenly in the offspring of an animal, which is transmitted to successive generations, due to change in a gene. A relatively permanent change in hereditary material.

MVTR   Abbreviation for *Moisture Vapor Transmission Rate*.

Mw   (Weight-Average Molecular Weight). The sum of the total weight of molecules of each size, multiplied by their respective weights, and divided by the total weight of all molecules.

Myalgia   Muscular pain.

Myelin   A unique covering of the major nerve trunks, like the insulation around an electrical wire. Comprised of 80% lipid, and the balance proteins, polysaccharides, and water. The breakdown of myelin is characteristic of multiple sclerosis.

Myeloma   A plasma cell neoplasm resulting in the excessive synthesis of one or more immunoglobulins. Causes weakened bone structures and kidney damage.

Myofibroblast   The cell considered to be most responsible for wound contraction. The most striking feature of the myofibroblast cytoplasm is (1) a well-developed microfilamentous system, different from normal fibroblasts, similar to the bundles of parallel actin microfilaments found in smooth muscle; in addition, many electron-opaque areas (dense bodies) thought to be attachment sites are scattered among the actin bundles or located beneath the plasma membrane; (2) another prominent feature of myofibroblasts is the presence of multiple indentations or deep folds in the nucleus, an appearance reminiscent of smooth muscle cells; and (3) gap junctions between neighboring myofibroblasts, capable of generating in vivo forces responsible for wound contraction, a finding inconsistent with normal fibroblasts.

Myoglobin   A protein-iron-porphyrin molecule similar to hemoglobin. The chief difference is that myoglobin complexes one heme group per molecule, whereas hemoglobin complexes four heme groups.

Myoma   Excessive growth of muscular tissue into a tumor.

Myosin   A protein of high molecular weight (>500,000), which is an essential component of muscular tissue and strongly affects its contractile properties.

Myristoyl Peroxide   Soft granular powder, used as polymerization catalyst for vinyl monomers.

N   (1) Symbol for nitrogen, a gaseous element of atomic number 7. It is the presence of nitrogen that constitutes the simplest distinction between protein and carbohydrates or lipids. (2) Abbreviation for *Normal Solution*.

n   Abbreviation for *normal*, designating those hydrocarbons or hydrocarbon radicals whose molecules contain a single unbranched chain of carbon atoms.

Na   Symbol for sodium.

Nanometer (nm)   A term sometimes used in place of millimicron in expressing the wavelength of light.

Narcosis   A reversible condition characterized by stupor or insensitivity; also a state of unconsciousness.

Narcotic   (1) A natural, semisynthetic, or synthetic nitrogen-containing heterocyclic drug that characteristically effects sleep and pain relief, but may also result in addiction. (2) Inducing sleep or coma, i.e., chloroform, barbiturates, benzene, etc.

Nasogastric Tube   (Feeding Tube; Levine Tube). A Class I device inserted through the nose into the upper gastrointestinal tract to provide alimentation, remove air or liquid.

Native Conformation   The spatial conformation of the polypeptide chain of a protein in its normal biological condition, in which it retains its required biological activity.

Native Protein   The spacial conformation of a protein in its native state, without having been subjected to denaturation (inactivation).

Natta Catalysts   Catalysts in stereospecific polymerization reactions, particularly catalysts containing titanium chloride and aluminum alkyl. The agents are ground in a special process to produce an active catalyst surface.

Natural Polymer   Alternative name for *Biopolymer*, such as collagen, fibrin, or elastin.

Natural Rubber   The rubber material obtained from the latex exuded from certain plants, such as hevea brasiliensis, composed essentially of cis-1,4-polyisoprene.

Natural Rubber Latex   The latex obtained from the *Hevea brasiliensis* tree, containing about 35% natural rubber hydrocarbon as particles about 1 micrometer in diameter, and about 5% nonrubber hydrocarbons consisting of protein, lipids, sugar, and salts.

NBR   Abbreviation for *Acrylonitrile-Butadiene Copolymers*.

Nebulizer   A Class II device used to add particulate liquids via a spray to inspired gases that are directly delivered to the airways. Included: gas, heater, venturi, and refillable nebulizers.

Necrosis   Death of cells, tissues or organs due to a lack of oxygen, infection, injury, exposure to cold, or burn.

Negative Catalyst   (Inhibitor, Retarder). A chemical agent that reduces the speed of a reaction.

Neo   (1) Prefix meaning new, and denoting a compound related to an older one. (2) A prefix signifying a hydrocarbon chain in which at least one carbon atom is connected directly to four other carbon atoms.

Neoplasm   An abnormal growth of tissue in the body, which may be benign or malignant.

Neoplastic   Refers to any abnormal growth in the body.

Neoprene   Generic name for polymers of chloroprene, available as gums and latexes.

Nephrology   That branch of medical science that deals specifically with the kidneys.

Nerve   A bundle of many fibers, providing connection between the central nervous system and the rest of the body.

Nerve Gas   One of several toxic chemical warfare agents; they are organic derivatives of phosphoric acid (primarily alkyl phosphates, fluorophosphates, and thiophosphates), which inhibit the enzyme cholinesterase, causing acetylcholine poisoning, and thus cessation of normal nerve transmission.

Nerve Stimulator   A Class II device used to electrically stimulate a peripheral nerve to relieve severe intractable pain. Consists of an implanted receiver with electrodes placed around a peripheral nerve and an external transmitter for transmitting the stimulating pulses across the skin to the implanted receiver.

Nervous System   A system that coordinates and regulates internal functions and governs the response of the body to any external stimuli. In vertebrates, it is composed of the brain, spinal cord, ganglia, peripheral nerves, as well as sensory and motor endings.

Network Polymers   Polymers synthesized from monomers having two or more functional groups, which react together to form interchain bonds to form a large three-dimensional network. The vulcanization of rubber is a prototype formation of a network polymer from a preformed polymer. Network polymers are thermosetting.

Network Structure   An atomic or molecular arrangement in which primary bonds form a three-dimensional network.

Neuralgia   Pain that travels along peripheral nerve tracts.

Neurologic   Refers to an examination or study of the nervous system.

Neurology   That branch of medical science that deals with the nervous system and its disorders.

Neuroma   A tumor arising somewhere in the nervous system.

Neutron   A fundamental particle of matter having a mass of 1.009 but no electrical charge.

Neutrophil Enzymes   Neutrophil products capable of producing tissue liquefaction are:

(1) Oxygen metabolites
   − *Superoxide anion (O_2-)*
   − *Hydrogen peroxide (H_2O_2)*
   − *Hydroxy radical (OH)*
   − *Hypochlorous acid (HOCl)*
   − *N-Chloramines*
(2) Neutral proteases
   − *Collagenase (active on types I, II, and III collagen)*
   − *Elastase*
   − *Gelatinase (active on type V collagen)*
   − *Cathepsin G*
(3) Nonenzymatic cationic proteins

Neutrophils   A type of leukocyte with cytoplasmic granules that are not predominant in their affinity for acid or basic dyes.

Newtonian Flow   A flow characteristic evidenced by a viscosity that is independent of shear rate. That is, the shear rate is directly proportional to shear force. Examples: water and thin mineral oils.

Newtonian Fluid   A liquid material that exhibits NEWTONIAN FLOW characteristics. Such fluids have no yield value.

NIOSH   Abbreviation for *National Institute for Occupational Safety and Health*, a federal agency which, among other activities, tests and certifies respiratory protective devices and air sampling detector tubes, and recommends occupational exposure limits for various substances.

Nip   The v-shaped gap between a pair of calender rolls where the polymer being mixed is ''nipped'' and drawn between the rolls.

Nip Rolls   In film blowing, a pair of rolls situated at the top of the tower that close the blown film envelope, seal air inside, and regulate the rate at which the film is pulled away from the extrusion die.

Nitration   A reaction in which a nitro group replaces hydrogen on a carbon atom by the use of nitric acid or mixed acid. An example is the nitration of cellulose to nitrocellulose.

Nitrile   An organic compound containing the $-CN$ group, for example, acrylonitrile.

Nitrocellulose   A term synonymous with *Cellulose Nitrate*, and other polymers based thereon.

Nitroethane   A colorless liquid used as a solvent for cellulosic, vinyl, alkyd, and other resins.

Nitromethane   A colorless liquid used as a solvent for cellulosic, vinyl, alkyd, and other resins.

Nitrosamines   Any of a series of compounds in which an $-NNO$ group is attached to an alkyl or aryl group. Nitrosamines have been found to be strong carcinogens in experimental animals.

Nitroso Polymer   A flame and heat resistance copolymer derived from trifluoronitrosomethane and tetrafluoroethylene, with methyl-4-nitrosoperfluorobutyrate as the cross-linking agent.

Nitroso Rubber   A copolymer of tetrafluoroethylene and trifluoronitrosomethane.

Nitrous Oxide   A colorless gas used as an anesthetic in dentistry and surgery.

Noble   In chemical terminology the term describes an element that is either completely unreactive or reacts only to a limited extent with other elements. Noble gases are: helium, neon, argon, krypton, xenon, and radon. Nobel metals are: gold, silver, platinum, palladium, iridium, rhodium, mercury, ruthenium, and osmium.

Nominal   The stated value, i.e., the value given as being standard. For example, nominal heart rate is 80 beats per minute.

Nomogram   (Nomograph). A graph containing several (usually three) parallel scales graduated for different variables so that when a straight line is drawn to connect the values of any two, the third value may be read directly at the point intersected by the line. Nomograms assist in estimating data that normally would require intricate calculations.

Nonpolar   A substance displaying no concentrations of electrical charge on a molecular scale, and thus being incapable of significant dielectric loss. Most synthetic polymers are nonpolar.

Nonrigid Plastic   According to ASTM D 883-65T, any plastic that has a modulus of elasticity (either in flexure or tension) of not more than 700 kg per sq cm at 23°C and 50% relative humidity.

Nontoxic Plasticizers   Plasticizers sanctioned by the FDA for use in food-contact applications.

Nonwoven Fabrics   Staple lengths of natural or synthetic fibers, monofilaments, or multifilaments mechanically positioned into a random pattern, then bonded with suitable surface resins to form continuous sheets.

Nonwoven Mat   A mat of glass fibers mechanically positioned into a random pattern, used in reinforced plastics.

Nor   A prefix that stands for normal, used to indicate the parent compound from which a substance may be derived, usually by removal of one or more carbon atoms with attached hydrogen.

Normal   (1) Regarding a hydrocarbon containing a single unbranched chain of carbon atoms. (2) Regarding solutions that contain one equivalent weight of a dissolved substance per liter of solution.

Nosocomial   Refers to an infection or other disorder picked up by a patient while hospitalized. Nosocomial infections are dreaded since hospital-based bacteria are frequently resistant to antibiotic treatment.

Notch Sensitivity   The extent to which the sensitivity of a material to fracture is increased by the presence of surface inhomogeneities or discontinuities. Low notch sensitivity is usually associated with ductile materials, and high notch sensitivity with brittle materials.

Novolacs   (1) A phenol-formaldehyde resin which, unless a source of methylene groups is added, remains permanently thermoplastic. (2) A phenolic-aldehyde resin, which when reacted with methylene groups becomes a cured, thermoset polymer.

Nozzle   In injection or transfer molding terminology, the orifice at the end of the injection cylinder that contacts the mold sprue bushing, and injects the molten resin into the mold under pressure. The nozzle is designed to form a tight seal against the sprue bushing to minimize leakage.

Nozzle Manifold   A series of injection nozzles mounted on a common manifold, where each nozzle feeds a single cavity in the mold.

Nozzles, Mold Gating   In injection molding, nozzles whose tips are parts of mold cavities, feeding molten resin directly into cavities, thus eliminating the use of sprue and runner systems.

NR   Abbreviation for *Natural Rubber*.

Nuclear Chemistry   The division of chemistry that deals with changes or transformations of the atomic nucleus. Nuclear reactions are usually accompanied by large energy changes, far greater than those experienced in conventional chemical reactions.

Nuclear Energy   The energy liberated by (1) the splitting or fusion of an atomic nucleus, (2) the fusion of two atomic nuclei, and (3) the radioactive decay of a nucleus.

Nuclear Reaction   Change in an atomic nucleus, such as fission, fusion, neutron capture, or radioactive decay, as distinct from a chemical reaction, which is limited to changes in the outer electrons that surround the nucleus.

146

Nuclear Reactor   A device in which a fission chain reaction can be initiated, maintained, and controlled.

Nuclear Transformation   The change in an isotope from a less stable to a more stable form, typically involving the emission of alpha, beta, gamma, and/or neutron radiation.

Nucleating Agent   Chemical compounds that form nuclei for the growth of crystals in the polymer melt. Greater crystallinity is obtained in polypropylene by the addition of nucleating agents such as adipic acid and benzoic acids. Colloidal silicas act as nucleating agents in nylons, seeding the material to produce a more uniform growth of spherulites.

Nucleation   The process by which crystals are formed from liquids, super-saturated solutions, or saturated vapors.

Nucleon   General name applied to neutrons and protons, the essential constituents of the atomic nucleus. The study of subatomic particles is called nucleonics.

Nucleophile   An ion or molecule that donates a pair of electrons to an atomic nucleus to form a covalent bond; the nucleus that accepts the electrons is called an electrophile. This occurs in the formation of acid-base reactions according to the Lewis postulate, as well as in covalent carbon bonding in organic compounds.

Nucleoprotein   A special protein found in the nuclei and surrounding cytoplasm of cells. Composed of a protein that is rich in basic amino acids, and a nucleic acid.

Nucleoside   A compound obtained during hydrolysis of nucleic acids, and containing a purine or pyrimidine base linked to either D-ribose, forming ribosides, or D-deoxyribose, forming deoxy ribosides.

Nucleotide   A fundamental unit of nucleic acids. Phosphate monoesters of nucleosides comprise the four nucleotides that are found in nucleic acids: (1) adenylic acid, (2) uridylic acid, (3) guanylic acid, and (4) cytidylic acid.

Nucleus   (1) The positively charged central mass of an atom; it contains essentially the total mass in the form of protons and neutrons. (2) The central portion of a living cell, consisting essentially of nucleoplasm in which the chromatin is found (the hereditary material), thus being responsible for reproduction. (3) The characteristic structure of a group of chemical compounds, e.g., the benzene nucleus.

Nuclide   A general term applicable to all atomic forms of the elements, often mistaken for ''isotope.'' Whereas isotopes are the various forms of a single element, and all have the same atomic number and number of protons, nuclides comprise all the isotopic forms of all elements. Nuclides are distinguished by their atomic number, atomic mass, and energy state. Example: carbon 14 is a radionuclide of carbon.

Nuisance Particulates   Inert dusts that do not cause significant organic disease or toxic effects when exposure is kept under reasonable control.

Permissible exposure levels are as follows: OSHA TWA 15 mg/m^3 of total dust; or 5 mg/m^3 for respirable fraction.

Number-Average Molecular Weight   The total molecular weight of all molecules divided by the number of molecules. See also MOLECULAR WEIGHT, MOLECULAR WEIGHT DISTRIBUTION.

Nutraceutical   Nutritional products that reasonable clinical evidence suggest have a medical benefit. Among these products are: calcium, potassium, magnesium, fiber, and fish oil supplements. These substances occur naturally in plants, animals, and humans.

Nutrient   Any element or compound essential to the life and well-being of plants and animals, either as such or transformed by chemical or enzymatic reactions. In animals, primary nutrients are proteins, carbohydrates, fats, water, and oxygen.

Nutrition   The effects of nutrients on living organisms and the biochemical mechanisms involved.

Nylon   Generic name for all polymers having recurring amide groups in the molecular backbone. Various types of nylons are described by numbers that relate to the number of carbon atoms in the various reactants.

Nylon 1   (Polyurea). The unsubstituted polymer, containing repeating units of $\begin{bmatrix} \text{H} & \text{O} \\ | & \| \\ \text{N} - \text{C} \end{bmatrix}$ in the chain. Synthesized by the anionic chain polymerization of isocyanates.

Nylon 2   Alternative name for *Polyglycine*.

Nylon 4   A type of nylon synthesized from pyrrolidone (which contains four carbons).

Nylon 5   (Polypiperidone). Synthesized by the ring-opening polymerization of piperidone.

Nylon 6   A type of nylon synthesized from caprolactam (which contains six carbons).

Nylon 6/6   A type of nylon made from the condensation of hexamethylene-diamine (which contains six carbons) with adipic acid (which contains six carbons). The most extensively used type of nylon.

Nylon 6/10   A type of nylon made from the condensation of hexamethylenediamine with sebacic acid (which contains ten carbons). Used extensively in the production of monofilaments. If a small amount of alkyl-substituted hexamethylenediamine is added to the mixture, a more elastic polymer known as elastic nylon is obtained.

Nylon 7   A type of nylon synthesized from ethyl aminoheptanoate (which contains seven carbons).

Nylon 9   A type of nylon synthesized from 9-aminononanoic acid (which contains nine carbons).

Nylon 11   A type of nylon derived from 11-aminoundecanoic acid, used in the manufacture of fibers.

Nylon 12   A type of nylon synthesized from either lauric lactam (dodecanoic lactam) or cyclododecalactam, with eleven methylene units between the linking $-NH-CO-$ groups in the polymer chain. This type of nylon displays the lowest water absorption (1.5%) of all nylons.

Nylon Fiber   Generic name for fibers containing a long-chain synthetic polyamide having recurring amide groups ($-CONH-$) as an integral part of the polymer chain.

Nylon Monofilaments   Relatively coarse, continuous strands of nylon used for surgical sutures and other high-strength applications.

Nystagmograph   A Class II device used to measure, record, or visually display the involuntary movements (nystagmus) of the eyeball.

O   Abbreviation for *Ortho*.

Obstetrics   The branch of medicine that deals with the care of the pregnant woman during pregnancy, parturition, and the puerperium.

Occlusion   The isolation of a growing active center during free-radical polymerization from other active centers when it becomes "occluded" within a polymer particle. In this case, termination reactions are reduced, and the rate of polymerization is increased.

Occult Blood Test   A Class II device used to detect occult blood in urine or feces. (Occult blood is blood present in small quantities, detectable only by chemical, microscopic, or spectroscopic tests).

Octyl   The general term for all eight-carbon radicals, often used interchangeably with 2-ethylhexyl.

Offset Printing   A printing process in which the desired image is first applied to an intermediate carrier such as a roll, followed by transfer to a substrate.

Offset Yield Strength   The stress at which the strain exceeds by a specified amount (the offset) an extension of the initial proportional portion of the strain-stress curve. Expressed in force per unit area.

Oil   A term applied to a wide range of substances that are quite different in chemical nature. Petroleum oils are composed of hydocarbon mixtures. Oils derived from animals or plants are chemically identical with fats, the only difference being viscosity at room temperature.

Oil Absorption   The percent increase in weight of a specimen after immersion in oil for a specified time.

Oil-Soluble Resin   A resin capable of dissolving in drying oils at moderate temperatures.

Oleamide   A powder utilized as a lubricant in extruding polymers such as polyethylene and urethanes.

Olefin   (alkene). A class of unsaturated aliphatic hydrocarbons having one or more double bonds, obtained by cracking naphtha or other petroleum fractions at 1500°F. Those containing one double bond are called alkenes, those with two double bonds alkadienes or diolefins.

Olefin Fiber   Generic name for a manufactured fiber composed of a synthetic polymer with at least 85% by weight of ethylene, propylene, or other olefinic units.

Olefin Plastics   See POLYOLEFINS.

Oleoresins   Mixtures of natural resin obtained from a vegetable plant with an essential oil obtained from the same plant. Usually semi-solids and are also called *Balsams*.

Oligomer   A polymer containing no more than ten to twenty monomer units, or their mixtures. Thus, dimers, trimers, tetramers, etc., are considered oligomers. Oligomers are formed during early polymerization of step-growth polymers. Frequently used in UV-curable compositions. The term *telomer* is sometimes used synonymously with oligomer.

Oligopeptide   A peptide composed of not more than ten amino acids.

Oligosaccharide   A carbohydrate containing from two to no more than ten simple sugars.

One-Shot Molding   A urethane-based molding process in which the monomeric reactants are fed as separate streams to a mixing head, and the mixture discharged to a mold where polymerization occurs.

One-Stage Resin   A precursor polymer, which is capable of cross-linking without the use of cross-linking agents, thus resulting in a thermoset resin. The cross-linking reactions result from functional groups present in the precursor polymer. The term is applied particularly to phenol-formaldehyde resins.

Opacity   The optical density of a material; the opposite of transparency. A colorant of high opacity is said to have good covering ability, that is it has the ability to conceal another shade over which it may be applied.

Opalescence   The reduction in clarity through a sheet of transparent plastic at any angle, due to light diffusion within or at the plastic surface.

Open Cell Foam   A cellular plastic in which most cells are interconnected in such a matter that gases or liquids may travel from cell to cell.

Ophthalmology   The branch of medical science that deals with the eye, its diseases and refractive errors.

Opportunistic Infection   An infection that occurs because an individual has lost his natural defence capacity, due to the weakness and incompetence of the immune system, as a result of illness, malnutrition, and other causes.

Opsonin   An antibody which attaches to a cellular or particulate antigen, and preparation for phagocytosis.

Optical Brightener   A colorless fluorescent organic compound capable of absorbing UV light and emitting it as visible blue light, thus masking undesirable yellow tints in polymers, yarns, etc.

Optical Distortion   Any alteration of a geometric pattern seen through a plastic, or as a reflection from a plastic surface.

Optical Isomer   Either of two kinds of optically active three-dimensional isomers, also known as stereoisomers. One kind is a mirror image structure called enantiomer. The other kind is a diastereoisomer, which is not a mirror image.

Oral   Relating to the mouth; one of the most common routes of drug administration, proving slower onset, but greater duration of action than IV or IM.

Orange Peel   An uneven surface texture, resembling the rough surface of an orange.

Ordered Polymer   A copolymer characterized by regularly arranged repeating units. Examples are block copolymers of the $A-B-A-B$ type, and polypeptides where regular amino acid sequences produce ordered macropolymers.

Organ   Organs contain both tissue that furnishes some mechanical strength, and specialized tissue that performs a particular function. Such tissue specific to an organ is called the parenchyma. A number of organs can function in coordination as a system, e.g., the heart, arteries, capillaries, and veins constitute the circulatory system.

Organelle   A portion of a cell having specific functions, distinctive chemical constituents and characteristic morphology; it is a unit subsystem of the cellular cytoplasm.

Organic Chemistry   A major branch of chemistry embracing all compounds of carbon, many found in living systems, thus the name "organic." Does not include binary compounds such as carbon oxides, carbides, carbon disulfide, etc; tertiary compounds such as the metallic cyanides, metallic carbonyls, phosgene, etc; and the metallic carbonates, such as calcium carbonate and sodium carbonate.

Organic Peroxides   Thermally decomposable compounds analogous to hydrogen peroxide, in which one or both hydrogen atoms are replaced by an organic radical. As they thermally decompose, they form free radicals that initiate polymerization reactions and effect cross-linking.

Organic Pigments   Pigments characterized by good brightness, brilliance, and transparency. Generally more resistant to chemicals than inorganic pigments, but are less resistant to heat, light, and solvents.

Organoleptic   A term used to describe consumer testing procedures for medical products, accessories, etc., in which samples of various products are submitted to groups or panels. Such tests aid in determining the acceptance of products by the public, and are thus considered as a marketing technique.

Organometallic Compound   An organic compound comprised of a metal (or nonmetal) attached directly to carbon; except metallic soaps (soaps) of organic acids. Examples: diethylzinc, Grignard compounds, tetraethyl lead.

Organophosphorus Compound   Any organic compound containing phosphorus, classified into (1) phospholipids or phosphatides, (2) esters of phosphinic or phosphonic acids, (3) pyrophosphates, and (4) phosphoric esters of glycerol, glycol, sorbitol, etc.

Organopolysiloxanes   See SILICONES.

Organosilane   (Organosilicone). An organic compound in which silicon is bonded to a carbon atom. The $Si-C$ bond is about as strong as the $C-C$ bonds. This linkage forms the basis for the silicone plastics, which derive their name from the similarity of their formula $(R-SiO-)$ to that of the ketones $(R-C=O)$.

Organosol   A suspension of resin in a plasticizer, together with a volatile organic liquid, the volatile portion comprising at least 5% of the total weight. An organosol is prepared from a plastisol by adding a volatile diluent that serves to lower the viscosity, and evaporates when the compound is heated.

Organotin Compounds   A large family of alkyl tin compounds widely used as stabilizers and catalysts for polymers. These compounds are used in very small amounts since all are highly toxic.

Organotin Stabilizer   A family of high-efficiency vinyl stabilizers, notable for their compatibility and optical clarity.

Orientation   The mechanical process of stretching a hot plastic article to help align the chains in the same direction, thus improving mechanical properties. Orientation may be (1) uniaxial, when the stretching force is applied in one direction, or (2) biaxial, when the stretching is in two directions. Upon reheating, an oriented film will tend to shrink in the direction(s) of orientation, a property useful in shrink-packaging.

Orientation Release Stress   The internal stress remaining in a plastic sheet after orientation, relieved by reheating the sheet to a temperature higher than that at which it was oriented.

Oriented Crystallization   Polymer crystallinity in which the crystallites have some definite three-dimensional relationship.

Orifice   In extrusion terminology, the precision opening in the die formed by the bushing (ring) and mandrel.

Oropharyngeal Airway   A Class II device inserted into the pharynx through the mouth to provide a patent airway.

Orphan Drug   Any drug with a target patient population of less than 200,000 people.

Orphan Drug Act   Congress enacted the Orphan Drug Act in 1983 to provide incentives for industry to make the investment necessary to develop drugs for rare diseases. In 1988, medical devices were added to the provision allowing financial assistance to defray the cost of developing devices for rare diseases or conditions.

Ortho   A prefix denoting a specific position of a substituting radical, or group of radicals, on a benzene ring.

Orthopedic Devices, Usage   In 1990 the following distribution was estimated by body site of implant:

SITE	IMPLANTS
Artificial joints	1,632,000
Hip joints	817,000
Knee joints	525,000
Other	290,000
Fixation Devices*	4,892,000
Head	352,000
Torso	564,000
Upper extremity	646,000
Lower extremity	2,690,000
Other	640,000

*Includes: nails, screws, pins, rods, wires, plates, and spikes.

Orthopedics   The medical specialty dealing with the preservation, restoration, development, form, and function of the extremities, spine, and associated structures.

Orthotopic Graft   A graft placed in its usual anatomic position.

Orthotropic   A substance having three mutually perpendicular planes of elastic symmetry.

OSHA   Abbreviation for the *Occupational Safety and Health Administration*, U.S. Department of Labor.

Osmometer   An apparatus designed for the measurement of osmotic pressure. Composed of a membrane permeable to solvents but impermeable to polymer molecules of a specific size range. Osmometers are used for measuring the NUMBER-AVERAGE MOLECULAR WEIGHT of polymers in the range of 20,000 to 2,000,000 daltons.

Osmosis   (1) The process by which fluid is transferred through a membrane, with water molecules moving in a direction from the less concentrated solution, to the more concentrated. (2) The passage of solvent from a mass of pure solvent into a solution, through a membrane that is permeable to the solvent but not the solute.

Osmotic Pressure   The hydrostatic pressure at which the flow of a solvent through a membrane just stops. Measurement of osmotic pressure provides the most useful method for determining the NUMBER-AVERAGE MOLECULAR WEIGHT of polymers.

Osteology   The anatomy of bones; the science concerned with the study of the bones and their structure.

Ostomy   A Class II device consisting of a bag attached to the skin by a pressure-sensitive adhesive, intended for use as a receptacle for the collection of fecal material or urine following an ileostomy, colostomy, or ureterostomy (a surgically created opening of the small intestine, large intestine, or ureter on the surface of the stomach). Accessories include: pouch, adhesive, disposable appliances, collector, protector, and size selector. It excludes pouches which incorporate arsenic-containing compounds.

OTC   Abbreviation for *Over the Counter*; *Nonprescription*. Medicine available in the pharmacy or other stores without a prescription. An OTC drug is considered safe and effective if the instructions on the label are carefully followed.

Otolaryngology   The combined specialties dealing with diseases of the ear and larynx, often including upper respiratory tract, and many diseases of the head and neck, tracheobronchial tree, and esophagus.

Otology   The branch of medicine treating diseases of the ear.

Outgassing   The evaporation under vacuum of volatile substances, such as moisture, solvents, plasticizers, etc., from a polymer.

Overcoating   (1) Applying a film overlayer for protective or decorative purposes, (2) in extrusion, extruding a web beyond the edge of the substrate web.

Overcure   A thermal decomposition in a thermosetting resin due to overheating or excessive cure time.

Oxetane Resins   See CHLORINATED POLYETHER.

Oxidase   An enzyme whose activity results in the transfer of electrons on the substrate; an oxidizing enzyme.

Oxidation   (1) Traditionally a reaction in which oxygen combines chemically with another substance. More broadly, any chemical reaction in which electrons are transferred. (2) Any degradation in a polymer due to oxygen. DEHYDROGENATION is a form of oxidation, when two hydrogen atoms, each having one electron, are removed from a hydrogen-containing organic compound by a catalytic reaction.

Oxidation Number   The number of electrons that are added to or subtracted from an atom in a compound to convert it to its elemental form.

Oxidation-Reduction Indicator   A substance that changes color between the oxidized and reduced state.

Oxidative Coupling   (1) A polymerization technique for certain types of linear high polymers, such as the formation of polyethers from the oxidation of 2,6-dimethylphenol with an amine complex of a copper salt. (2) A reaction of oxygen with active hydrogen atoms from different molecules producing water and a dimerized molecule.

Oxidative Dehydrogenation   A chemical process used in making monomers such as styrene and vinyl chloride, (1) involving the removal of hydrogen from a hydrocarbon chain by oxygen, with the concomitant formation of water, or (2) removal of hydrogen from a hydrocarbon chain by a halide to form the hydrogen halide, followed by regeneration of the halide with oxygen.

Oximeter   A Class II device used to transmit radiation at a known wavelength through blood in order to measure blood oxygen saturation based on the amount of reflected or scattered radiation.

Oxirane   A synonym for *Ethylene Oxide*, H_2COCH_2.

Oxirane Group   A synonym for *Epoxy Group*.

Oxirane Value   (1) The percent oxygen absorbed by an unsaturated raw material during epoxidation. (2) A measure of the amount of epoxidized double bonds.

Oxy   (1) A prefix denoting the $-O-$ radical (in the U.S.), or (2) the $-OH$ radical in Europe.

Oxygenators   Devices intended to saturate the hemoglobin and ensure gaseous exchange for extracorporeal blood. In oxygenators a mixture of $2-5$ percent carbon dioxide is employed, setting the lower limit for arterial carbon dioxide tension, thus avoiding respiratory alkalosis. There are four types of devices used: bubble oxygenators, film oxygenators, membrane oxygenators and liquid-liquid oxygenators.

Oxymethylene   Another name for *Formaldehyde*.

Ozone Cracking   Surface cracking or crazing in a diene rubber when exposed to low levels of ozone, particularly when the specimen is stressed.

Ozone-Induced Degradation   The chemical reaction occurring between ozone and unsaturated groups in a polymer, resulting in the formation of cyclic ozonide, which subsequently splits, causing chain scission.

Ozonolysis   Degradation caused by the reaction of carbon-carbon double bonds with ozone, which subsequently splits, thus resulting in cleavage of the polymer chain.

P

p   Abbreviation for *Para*.

PAA   Abbreviation for *Polyacrylic Acid*.

Pacemaker   An electronic instrument for stimulating the heart in which the natural pacing mechanism has failed.

Pacemaker, Temporary   Any pacemaker intended for short-term use (usually a few days, and in most cases no longer than 2 weeks). Commonly used in heart block patients, awaiting permanent pacemaker implantation, or in patients recuperating from myocardial infarction.

Pacemaker, Transvenous   The most common type of pacemaker, whose implantation involves inserting the leads through a major vein (subclavian, cephalic, or external jugular). The pulse generator is implanted subcutaneously in the pectoral area, and occasionally under the pectoralis major.

Pacemaker Polymeric Mesh Bag   A Class II device used to hold a pacemaker pulse generator, by encouraging tissue ingrowth, thus creating a stable implant environment for the generator.

Paddle Agitators   A family of plastic mixing equipment, composed of rotating blades driven by a vertical shaft with a set of fixed blades. Frequently used for mixing dispersions, pastes, and doughs.

Paint   A dispersion of pigment in a liquid vehicle, which when applied to a surface forms a protective or decorative film. The liquid vehicle is usually a film-forming resin (acrylic, vinyl, urethane, epoxy) dissolved in a solvent system.

PAN   Abbreviation for *Polyacrylonitrile*. See ACRYLONITRILE.

Pantograph   A Class I device that is attached to the head and is used to duplicate lower jaw movements to aid in the construction of restorative and prosthetic dental devices. A pen is attached to the lower jaw component of the device, and as the mouth opens the pen records on graph paper the angle between the upper and lower jaw.

Paper Chromatography   A type of chromatography where a drop of the liquid to be investigated is placed near one end of a strip of paper. This end is immersed in a solvent, which diffuses down the paper and distributes the materials present in the original drop selectively. Comparison with known substances makes identification possible.

PAPI   Abbreviation for *Polymethylene Polyphenylisocyanate*, also known as *Polymeric MDI*. A brown liquid composed of approximately 50% diphenylmethane diisocyanate (MDI), with the remainder being higher molecular weight fractions.

Para   A chemical prefix from the Greek word meaning beside or beyond, denoting a relation of some kind to another compound such as (1) the specific position of a radical or group on the benzene ring; (2) the relation of the 1 and 4 positions in benzene; (3) a polymeric form, such as paraldehyde; (4) a higher hydrated form of an acid.

Paracentesis   The puncturing of a body cavity for the purpose of removing fluid for diagnostic purposes.

Paraformaldehyde   A low molecular weight polymer of formaldehyde, easily depolymerized by heating to form aldehyde gas and water vapor. It is a convenient form to ship formaldehyde for industrial purposes, such as the manufacture of acetal resins.

Parameter   (1) In mathematics, a variable entering into the mathematical form of any distribution such that the possible values of the variable correspond to different distributions. (2) In plastics, a specified range of variables, characteristics or properties relating to the subject. (3) An arbitrary constant.

Parasite   An organism that lives on and obtains nourishment from another organism, called the host.

Parasitology   The branch of medicine that treats parasitism in all its relations.

Parenteral   (Drug Administration). Any method of administering a drug in a way other than through the alimentary canal.

Parison   The hollow tube or other preformed shape of plastic that is inflated inside the mold in the process of blow molding, with the parison extruded immediately before blowing.

Parison Swell   In blow molding, the physical enlargement of the parison as it emerges from the die.

Paroxysmal   In any context involving arrhythmias, any arrhythmia that begins and ends suddenly.

Particle   Any discrete unit of material structure. Particles are classified according to size as follows: (1) Subatomic: protons, neutrons, electrons, deuterons, etc. (2) Molecular: atoms and molecules with size ranging from a few Angstroms to about half a micron. (3) Colloidal: macromolecules, micelles, and ultrafine particles, with sizes ranging from 1 millimicron up 1 micron, which is the lower limit of the optical microscope. (4) Microscopic: units resolved by optical microscopy. (5) Macroscopic: particles seen by the unaided eye.

Particle Size   A term referring to solid particles used in commerce, such as pigments, colorants, fillers, etc. The smaller the particle size, the greater the total exposed surface of a given volume; since activity is proportional to surface area, the finer the substance, the more efficiently it will react both chemically and physically.

Particulate   Composed of fine particles or droplets.

Parting Agent   (Release Agent, Mole Lubricant, Mold Release). A lubricant that coats the mold cavity to prevent plastic from sticking, thus facilitating product demolding. Parting agents used in the molding of medical-grade products are often based on silicone or fluorocarbon fluids.

Parting Line   (Flash, Flash Line). (1) The line on a molded article caused by flow of molten plastic into the crevices between mold parts. (2) A line established on a 3-dimensional model from which a mold is to be prepared, to precisely define where the mold is to be split into two halves or several components.

Partition Coefficient   The ratio of concentration of a substance in a single defined form between two immiscible or partially miscible phases.

Parylenes   A family of thermoplastics, where polymerization is effected by vapor phase deposition of a dimer of the basic substance onto a substrate. Parylene N is produced from di-*p*-xylene, and Parylene C from mono-chloro-*p*-xylene. Vapor-polymerized films exhibit remarkable thermal stability, chemical and solvent resistance, and excellent dielectric properties.

Paste   (1) An adhesive composition of semisolid consistency, usually water dispersable. (2) More generally, a soft, viscous mass of solids finely dispersed in a liquid medium.

Pasteurization   A term applied to a process for destruction of some microorganisms likely to be present in heat-sensitive materials. Pasteurization is not a sterilization technique.

Patch Test   A skin test performed to detect sensitivity to certain substances (allergens) to which the person may be allergic, or to certain infections.

Pathogen   Any disease-causing microorganism.

Pathology   The science and study of all aspects of disease, with reference to the resulting structural and functional changes.

Pathway   A sequence of reactions, usually of a biochemical nature, in which complex substances are converted to simple end products, as in the digestion of foodstuffs into carbon dioxide, water, and calories. Its course is largely determined by preferential reaction pathways involving enzymes, coenzymes, and other biological catalysts.

PCTFE   Abbreviation for *Polychlorotrifluoroethylene*.

PE   Abbreviation for *Polyethylene*.

Pearlescent Pigments   Crystalline flakes that impart a mother-of-pearl appearance to plastics. Derived from lead or bismuth compounds, the crystals have a high refractive index, so that light reflections from parallel plates reinforce each other, and create a silvery luster.

PEG   Abbreviation for *Polyethylene Glycol*.

Pellets   Granules of uniform size, consisting of pure resins or compounds, prepared for molding operations by shaping in a pelletizing machine, or by extrusion and chopping into short segments.

Pendulum Impact Resistance   See IMPACT RESISTANCE.

Penetrant   Any substance used to increase the speed and ease with which a liquid permeates a material being processed, by reducing the interfacial tension between the liquid and the solid. See also WETTING AGENTS.

Penile Inflatable Implant   A Class III device consisting of two inflatable cylinders implanted in the penis, connected to a reservoir containing radiopaque fluid implanted in the lower abdomen, and a subcutaneous manual pump implanted in the scrotum. The penis becomes rigid (erected) when the cylinders are voluntarily inflated, thus relieving erectile impotence.

PEO   Abbreviation for *Polyethylene Oxide*.

Per   A prefix indicating complete or extreme, and denoting (1) a compound that contains an element in its highest oxidation state, e.g., perchloric acid, (2) presence of the peroxy group, $[-O-O]$, e.g., perchromic acid, (3) complete substitution or addition, e.g., perchloroethylene.

Per-Acids   Derivatives of hydrogen peroxide, containing one or more pairs of oxygen atoms, $[-O-O-]$, e.g., persulfuric, peracetic acids.

Percutaneous   Any device that is introduced through the skin, usually composed of a dilator and a sheath or guide wire.

Perfluoroethylene   See TETRAFLUOROETHYLENE.

Perforating   Processes by which plastic films or sheeting are provided with holes ranging from large diameters for decoration, to very small for performance.

Perfusion   (1) Injection of a liquid or other agent into a blood vessel, so that it may be carried through the body by the circulation. (2) Infiltration of any area of tissue with blood from the supplying artery, so that each cell receives an adequate blood supply.

Pericardium   The tissue around the heart muscle. Continuous with the adventitia of the great vessels, and is composed of two layers: the parietal and the visceral. Provides a friction-free enclosure for the heart by containing the pericardial fluid.

Perineometer   A Class II device, an intravaginal fluid-filled pouch, attached to an external manometer, used to measure the strength of perineal muscles by offering preselected resistance to a patient's voluntary contraction of these muscles. The device may be used in the diagnosis and therapy of urinary incontinence or sexual dysfunction through exercise.

Periodic Table   An arrangement of chemical elements in a pattern designed to represent the periodic law by aligning the elements in "periods," so that the corresponding parts of the several periods are adjacent to each other. When aligned in order of increasing atomic number, they constitute a succession of periods, each beginning with an alkali metal and ending with a noble gas.

Peristaltic Pump   A pumping device that uses a rotating drum with rollers attached to the circumference, rotating within a cylinder. A flexible tube is positioned between the drum and the containing cylinder so that rotation of the drum causes the rollers to squeeze the tube, thus forcing a pumping action.

Peritoneal Dialysis   A Class II device used as an artificial kidney for the treatment of renal failure or toxemic conditions. Consists of peritoneal access device, dialysis administration set, dialysate, and sometimes a water purification system. After installation in the peritoneal cavity, the fluid is allowed to remain, so undesirable substances pass through the lining membranes into the dialysate. These substances are subsequently removed when the dialysate is drained from the peritoneal cavity.

Peritoneo-Venous Shunt   A Class III implantable device consisting of a catheter and pressure-activated one-way valve. The catheter is implanted with one end in the peritoneal cavity and the other in a large vein, thus enabling ascitic fluid in the peritoneal cavity to be drained into the venous system for the treatment of intractable ascites.

Peritoneum   The protective sac lining the interior of the abdominal cavity, and covering most of the abdominal organs. Analogous to the PLEURA in the THORAX.

Permanence   (1) The property of a plastic that describes its resistance to change in characteristics dealing with time and environment. (2) The resistance of an adhesive bond to deteriorating environmental influences.

Permanent Set   The increase in length, expressed as a percentage of the original length, by which an elastic material fails to return to its original length after being stressed for a standard period of time.

Permeability   (1) The passage or diffusion of gas, vapor, liquid, or solid through a barrier without physically or chemically affecting it. (2) The rate of such passage.

Permittivity   The ratio of the capacitance of a given configuration of electrodes with a given material as the dielectric to the capacitance of the same electrode configuration with air as the dielectric.

Peroxide   Recommended cure temperatures:

Dicumyl peroxide	355°F
1-Butyl cumyl peroxide	338°F
2,5 Dimethyl-2,5-bis-(t-butylperoxy)-hexane	325°F
Dicumyl peroxide	320°F
n-Butyl-4,4-bis-(t-butylperoxy)-valerate	315°F
1-Butyl perbenzoate	305°F
1,1-Di-(t-butylperoxy)-cyclohexane	280°F
Benzoyl peroxide	237°F

Peroxides, Organic   See ORGANIC PEROXIDES.

Persorption   The adsorption of a substance in pores only slightly wider than the diameter of absorbed molecules of the substance.

Pesticide   Any substance used to destroy, or inhibit, the action of plant or animal pests. The term includes insecticides, herbicides, rodendicides, miticides, etc.

PETP   Abbreviation for *Polyethylene Terephthalate* (which can also be abbreviated PET).

Petrochemicals   Chemical substances derived directly or indirectly from petroleum or natural gas. Most of the medical plastics are petrochemically derived.

PF   Abbreviation for *Phenol-Formaldehyde Resins*.

pH   A numerical expression of the degree of acidity or alkalinity of an aqueous solution. Originally defined as the logarithm of the reciprocal of the hydrogen ion concentration in gram equivalents per liter. As such, a pH of 7 is neutral, a solution with a pH value of less than 7 is acid, and conversely, more than 7 is alkaline.

Phagocytes   Cells capable of ingesting foreign material, usually by cytoplasmic invagination. Phagocytic cells include: polymorphonuclear leukocytes (PMN), macrophages, and foreign body multinucleated giant cells.

Phagocytosis   From the Greek phagos, "to eat." The engulfment (internalization) of particulate matter, or cells, by leukocytes, macrophages, or other cells.

Pharmaceutical   A generic term that includes drugs, medicinal and curative products, as well as tonics, dietary supplements, vitamins, deodorants, and some cosmetics. See also COSMECEUTICAL.

Pharmaceutics   The science dealing with pharmaceutical systems, such as drug preparation, compounding, and dosage forms.

Pharmacist   A druggist, apothecary. A person trained to prepere, dispense and recommend the safe use of therapeutic drugs by virtue of formal knowledge concerning their properties and interactions.

Pharmacodynamics   The study of the actions and effects of chemicals at all levels of organization of living material and of the handling of chemicals by the organism.

Pharmacokinetics   The kinetics of drug adsorption, distribution, and elimination (i.e., excretion and metabolism).

Pharmacology   The science that deals with drugs, their sources, appearance, chemistry, actions, and uses.

Pharmacopeia   From the Greek *pharmakon*, meaning "drug," and *poiein*, meaning "make." Thus, the combination indicates any recipe, formula, or standard required to make or prepare a drug.

Pharmacy   The preparation, compounding, and dispensing of chemical agents for therapeutic use. It includes (1) pharmacognosy, the identification of the botanical source of drugs; (2) pharmaceutical chemistry , the synthesis of new drugs either as modifications of older or natural drugs or as entirely new chemical entities; and (3) biopharmaceutics, the science and study of the ways in which pharmaceutic formulation of administered agents influence their pharmacodynamic and pharmacokinetic behavior.

Phase Angle   See DIELECTRIC PHASE ANGLE.

Phenol   (1) A class of aromatic compounds in which one or more hydroxyl groups are directly attached to the benzene ring. (2) Carbolic acid, a colorless, hygroscopic material, used as an intermediate in the synthesis of PHENOLIC RESINS.

Phenol-Formaldehyde Resins   An important member in the family of phenolic resins, made by the condensation reaction between phenol and formaldehyde. Historically, the first synthetic thermosetting resin to be commercialized.

Phenolic Foams   Foams produced from phenolic resins. Further subdivided into syntactic and reaction foams. The syntactic foams comprise hollow microspheres of phenolic resins; reaction resins are produced by heating a water containing liquid phenolic resin, a blowing agent, an acid catalyst, and a surfactant.

Phenolic Novolaks   Thermoplastic resins obtained by reacting less than one mole of phenol with one mole of aldehyde, in the presence of an acid catalyst; thermosetting resins are obtained by reacting the methylated resins with diamines or diacids.

Phenolic Resins   A family of thermosetting resins made by the reaction of phenols with aldehydes. Phenolic resins are seldom used in medical devices.

Phenoxy Resins   Thermoplastic polyester resins based on a polyhydrox-yether derived from bisphenol A and epichlorohydrin, thus being similar to epoxy resins, but without epoxy groups. Some grades are FDA approved for food contact.

Phenylethylene   See STYRENE.

Phenylsilane Resins   Thermosetting resins made by the copolymerization of silicone and phenolic resins.

Pheresis   Any procedure in which blood is withdrawn from a donor, a portion (plasma, leukocytes, etc.) is separated and retained, and the remainder is retransfused into the donor. It includes PLASMAPHERESIS, LEUKAPHERESIS, etc.

Phlebograph, Impedance   A Class II device used to provide a visual display of the venous pulse wave by measuring electrical impedance changes in a given region of the body.

Phonocardiograph   A Class II device used to amplify or condition the signal received from a cardiac sound transducer. The device provides the excitation energy for the transducer, and provides a visual or audible display of cardiac sounds.

Phonocardiographic Monitor   A Class II device designed to detect, measure, and graphically record fetal heart sound electronically and nonin-vasively, to ascertain fetal conditions during labor. It includes: signal analysis and display instrumentation, patient and equipment supports, and other ancillary components.

Phosphorescence   A type of luminescence in which the emission of visible radiation occurs after excitation has ceased.

Phosphorescent Pigments   A family of pigments, generally inorganic sulphides, which absorb light energy and reemit it as radiation of a color specific to each pigment.

Phosphorylation   A chemical reaction that combines phosphorus with an organic compound, usually in the form of a trivalent phosphoryl group $[=P=O]$. An important reaction in cellular metabolism, it is particularly important in vitamin activity and enzyme formation.

Photochemistry   The division of chemistry dealing with the effects of radiant energy absorption in producing chemical changes. Includes photochemical polymerization, oxidation, ionization, decomposition, etc., generally involving free radical mechanisms.

Photodegradation   Degradation of plastics due exclusively to the action of light. Absorption by plastics of high-energy radiation in the UV portion of the spectrum activates electrons, leading to oxidation, molecular cleavage, and other degradative reactions.

Photoelasticity   Changes in the optical characteristics of transparent plastics when subjected to mechanical stress.

Photolysis   Decomposition of a chemical compound into smaller molecular weight units as a result of absorbing a quantum of radiation. Photodecomposition also occurs with aldehydes, ketones, azo compounds, and certain organometallic compounds.

Photometric Analysis   A type of analysis relying on the absorption or emission of radiation, primarily in the near ultraviolet, visible, and infrared portions of the electromagnetic spectrum. Includes spectrophotometry, spectrochemical analysis, Raman spectroscopy, colorimetry, and fluorescence.

Photon   The fundamental unit of electromagnetic radiation. Photons are discrete concentrations of energy that have no rest mass and move at the speed of light. Photons are emitted when electrons move among energy states, as in an excited atom.

Photopolymer   Any compound containing a photoinitiator, capable of polymerization and/or cross-linking.

Photopolymerization   A polymerization reaction occurring during exposure of monomers or oligomers to actinic radiation, with or without a catalyst (photoinitiator). Acrylics, vinyls, and styrene are examples of photopolymerizable monomers.

PHR   Abbreviation for *Parts per Hundred of Resins*. In plastic formulations, 10 PHR means that 10 grams of an ingredient should be added to 100 grams of resin.

Phthalocyanine Pigments   Heat- and light-stable organic pigments, frequently used to color medical polymers.

Physical Catalyst   Radiant energy capable of promoting, or modifying, a chemical reaction.

Physical Chemistry   The applications of physical principles to chemical phenomena. For example, application of thermodynamic principles to heats of formation and reaction, theory of rate processes and chemical equilibrium, surface chemistry, electrochemistry, and ionization.

Physiology   The science that deals with living things, and with the normal vital processes of living organisms.

PI   Abbreviation for *Trans-1,4-Polyisoprene Rubber*.

PIA   Abbreviation for *Plastics Institute of America*.

PIB   Abbreviation for *Polyisobutylene*. See POLYBUTENES.

Pigments   Generic term embracing all colorants, organic or inorganic, natural or synthetic, which are insoluble in the medium in which they are used. Pigments are classified as: (1) Toners, or full strength pigments, (2) Lake Pigments, concentrates of organic pigments deposited on an inorganic base, and (3) Reduced Pigments, which are physical mixtures of organic pigments with inorganic bases. See also COLORANTS.

Pink Discoloration   A pink-colored stain that appears on vinyl plastic, attributed to the growth of fungi of the Penicillium species.

PIS   Abbreviation for *Polyisobutylene*. See POLYBUTENES.

Pitch   In extrusion terminology, the distance from a point on a flight of a screw line to the corresponding point on an adjacent flight, measured parallel to the axis of the screw line or threading.

pK A numerical measurement of the completeness of an incomplete chemical reaction, frequently used to express the dissociation of weak acids, such as fatty acids, amino acids, and complex ions. Mathematically it is the negative logarithm of the equilibrium constant K. Thus the weaker the electrolyte, the larger its pK.

pK$_a$ The pH at which a drug (or any other substance) is 50% ionized. For example, phenobarbital has a pK$_a$ of about 7.4, and in plasma it is present in ionized and unionized forms in equal amounts. This is important since the pH of body fluids varies (stomach, pH = 1; lumen of intestine, pH = 6.6; blood plasma, pH = 7.4), and thus the absorption of a drug from various body fluids will differ and may dictate the type of dosage form and the preferred route of administration.

pK$_a$ Values The pK$_a$ values for some acidic and basic drugs are listed below:

ACIDS		BASES	
Acetylsalicilic acid	3.5	Amphetamine	10.0
Barbital	7.9	Apomorphine	7.0
Benzylpenicillin	2.8	Atropine	9.7
Boric acid	9.2	Cocaine	8.4
Phenobarbital	7.4	Codeine	7.9
Theophylline	9.0	Guanethidine	11.8
Thiopental	7.6	Procaine	8.8
Tolbutamine	5.5	Quinine	8.4
Warfarin	4.8	Reserpine	6.6

Placebo From the Latin "I will please," a supposedly inert substance such as a sugar pill or injection of sterile water that can have a beneficial (positive) effect or detrimental (negative) effect on the recipient. It is usually given under the guise of genuine treatment. Placebos are frequently used in controlled clinical trials of new drugs. The patients taking the new drug must have significantly more relief than the control group taking the placebo for the new drug to be considered effective.

Plasmapheresis A procedure in which blood from a donor is externalized, the red blood cells are removed, and are subsequently retransfused into the donor. The remaining blood constituents are then separated, and prepared for administration to patients in need of the various blood fractions or plasma.

Plastic (Adj.). An adjective indicating that the noun modified is made of, consists of, or pertains to plastics.

Plastic (Noun). (1) A material that in its finished state contains as an essential ingredient a synthetic polymer of high molecular weight, which is not an elastomer, and which at some stage in its manufacture can be shaped by flow or by in situ polymerization or curing. (2) A substance that contains as an essential ingredient an organic substance of large molecular weight, solid at room temperature, and at some stage in its manufacture can be shaped by flow. Note: the terms plastics, resins, and polymers are used synonymously, but resins and polymers often denote the basic materials as polymerized, whereas plastics encompasses pure and compounded materials.

Plastic Deformation   A dimensional change of an object that is not recovered when the load is removed. For example, squeezing a piece of putty results in plastic deformation. The opposite is elastic deformation, in which the dimensions return to their original size when the load is removed.

Plastic Foam   See CELLULAR PLASTIC.

Plasticate   To render a thermoplastic more flexible by heat or mechanical action.

Plasticity   The ability of a polymer to withstand continuous and permanent deformation by stresses exceeding the yield value of the material without rupture.

Plasticize   To render a polymer softer, more flexible, and moldable by the physical addition of a PLASTICIZER. Should not be confused with PLASTICATE and PLASTIFY.

Plasticizer   A nonvolatile liquid, or low melting substance, physically incorporated into a polymer, to increase flexibility, workability, and distensibility. A plasticizer may reduce melt viscosity, lower second-order transition, or lower the elastic modulus. In medical plastics, plasticizers are sparingly used due to their nonpermanence.

Plasticizer-Adhesives   Additives, partially replacing plasticizers, which improve the adhesion of plastic coatings to a variety of substrates.

Plasticorder   See BRABENDER PLASTOGRAPH.

Plastics, Rigid   See RIGID PLASTIC.

Plastics, Semi-Rigid   See SEMI-RIGID PLASTIC.

Plastics Tooling   A general term employed for reinforced thermosets, which are used as tools in the fabrication of cast polymers, metals, etc.

Plastics Welding   See WELDING.

Plastify   The process of softening a thermoplastic resin or compound by heat alone, as during extrusion, injection, etc.

Plastigel   A vinyl compound, similar to a PLASTISOL, but containing sufficient gelling agent(s) to produce a gel.

Plastisol   A suspension of vinyl chloride polymer in a liquid plasticizer that has little or no tendency to dissolve the resin at room temperature, but which becomes a solvent at elevated temperatures. Plastisols are seldom used in medical devices, due to the fugitive nature of the plasticizer(s).

Platelet   (Thrombocytes). One of the cellular constituents of the blood. A clear, fragile, disc-shaped structure, about half the size of a red blood cell. An essential part of the process of coagulation.

Platen   A steel plate used to transmit pressure and heat to a mold assembly in a compression press.

Plate-Out   An objectionable coating found on metal surfaces of molds, due to extraction of compounding ingredients such as lubricants, stabilizers, pigments, plasticizers, etc.

Plethysmograph, Impedance   A Class II device used to estimate blood flow characteristics by measuring electrical impedance changes in a given region of the body.

Plethysmograph, Volume   A Class II device used to determine lung volume changes, while the patient is maintained in an airtight chamber.

Plethysmograph Pressure   A Class II device used to determine the airway resistance and lung volumes, by measuring pressure changes while the patient is in an airtight box.

Pleura   The protective membrane that envelops the lungs. Medially the pleura is continuous with the pericardium, and forms the two walls of the mediastinum, which separates the mediastinal space from the pleural space.

Plunger Molding   A variation of TRANSFER MOLDING, in which an auxiliary hydraulic ram is employed to assist the main ram.

PMAA   (Premarket Approval Application). The medical device PMAA is the cousin of the new drug application (NDA) and results in a determination by FDA that the device is safe and effective for its labeled indications. A PMAA is required for Class III devices, which include:

(1) Pre-1976 devices that were subsequently classified into Class III, and devices that are substantially equivalent to these devices
(2) Pre-1976 devices that were regulated as new drugs
(3) Post-1976 devices that are not substantially equivalent to devices commercially available before the Medical Device Amendments were enacted

PMAC   Abbreviation for *Polymethoxy Acetal.*

PMAN   Abbreviation for *Polymethacrylonitrile.*

PMCC   *Penske-Martin Closed-Cup* flash point procedure.

PMMA   Abbreviation for *Polymethyl Methacrylate.*

PMN   *Premarket Notification*, or *510(k) Provision.* The most used and one of the most critical provisions of the 1976 Medical Device Amendments. Under this process, a manufacturer is required to file with the FDA, 90 days before a new device is to be marketed, a premarket notification demonstrating that the device is substantially equivalent to a device that was on the market prior to 1976, and is therefore marketable without formal FDA approval. In enacting Section 510(k), Congress divided medical devices into two broad categories: (1) preamendment—those introduced into commercial distribution prior to May 28, 1976 and (2) postamendment—those introduced into commercial distribution after May 28, 1976. Section 510(k) is used to notify the FDA in two situations: (1) when first marketing a device that is "substantially equivalent" to a preamendment device and (2) when changing a device in a way that could significantly affect safety or effectiveness. Examples of significant changes would be changes in design, material, composition, energy source, manufacturing process, or intended use. A premarket notification is not an approval. A letter from the FDA clearing a premarket notification is simply a determination by the FDA that the proposed device is substantially equivalent to a preamendment device and thus will be placed in the same class as the preamendment device. The FDA strictly prohibits any manufacturer from representing that a 510(k) is an "FDA approval."

Pneumoencephalogram (PEG)   X-ray studies of the brain following injection of air or gas to aid in the visualization of cephalic structures.

Pock Marks   Imperfections on the surface of blow-molded articles, caused by insufficient contact of the blow parison with the mold surface. Contributing factors are: (1) insufficient blow pressure, (2) entrapment of gases, and (3) moisture condensation on the mold surface.

Poise   The fundamental metric unit of viscosity. Defined as the viscosity of a liquid in which a force of one dyne is necessary to maintain a velocity differential of one centimeter per second per centimeter over a surface of one square centimeter.

Poison   (1) Any substance harmful to living tissue, when applied in small doses. Usually expressed in terms of effective dosage, such as concentration, duration of exposure, physical state, affinity for living tissue, solubility in tissue fluids, sensitivity of tissues or organs. (2) Any substance capable of reducing or destroying the activity of a catalyst.

Poison Gas   A toxic or irritant gas designed for use in chemical warfare or riot control. Varying in toxicity from nerve gases (lethal), to tear gases (lachrymators).

Poisson's Ratio   When a material is stretched, its cross-sectional area changes as well as its length. Poisson's ratio is the constant relating changes in dimension during stretching, and is calculated by dividing the change in width per unit length by the change in length per unit length.

Polar   Generic term describing molecules in which the positive and negative electrical charges are permanently separated, as opposed to nonpolar molecules in which the charges coincide. Polar molecules ionize in solution, thus creating electrical conductivity.

Polar Winding   A winding method in which the filament path passes tangent to the polar opening at one end of a mandrel, and tangent to the opposite side of the polar opening at the other end.

Polishing Roll   A highly polished chrome-plated roll, utilized to produce a smooth surface on extruded or calendered film and sheet.

Poly   A prefix denoting many. The term polymer literally means "many mers," a MER (also known as a monomer) being a repeating structural unit of any high polymer.

Polyacetylenes   Dark-colored polymers of acetylene. They have limited use in medical plastics.

167

Polyacrylamides   A water-soluble solid, used as a thickening agent, a suspending agent, and in the synthesis of hydrogels.

Polyacrylate   A thermoplastic resin made by the polymerization of an acrylic compound, such as methyl methacrylate. See also ACRYLIC RESINS.

Polyacrylic Acid (PAA)   A polymer of acrylic acid, used as a sizing agent.

Polyacrylic Esters   See ACRYLIC RESINS.

Polyalcohols   See POLYOL.

Polyalkylene Amides   See AMINO RESINS.

Polyallomers   Crystalline thermoplastic copolymers of ethylene and propylene, synthesized by a unique polymerization process that produces a high degree of crystallinity, conferring high impact strength, low density, and flex resistance. The name "polyallomer" is derived from allomerism, meaning similarity of crystalline form with a different composition.

Polyamide-Imide Resins   Aromatic thermosets based on trimellitic anhydride. The imide linkage is formed by heating, producing a resin with thermal stability up to 550°F.

Polyamide Plastics   See NYLON.

Polyamine-Methylene Resin   A lightly colored resin derived from diphenylol and formaldehyde, used as an ion-exchange resin.

Polyaminotriazoles   Fiber-forming polymers made from sebacic acid and hydrazine, with small amounts of acetamide.

Polyarylsilanes   High-temperature polymers made of silicon atoms, oxygen and thermally stable aromatic rings, part organic and part inorganic in nature.

Polyazelaic Polyanhydride   A carboxyl-terminated polymer, used as a curing agent for epoxy resins.

Polybenzimidazoles   Resins made by the condensation of 3,3'diamino-benzidine with diphenylisophthalate or isophthalamide, resulting in a polymer containing recurring aromatic units with alternating double bonds.

Polyblends   A colloquial term, generally used in the styrene field referring to mechanical mixtures of polystyrene and rubber.

Polybutadiene   A synthetic rubber made from butadiene. The trans-1,4 type is similar to natural rubber, while the cis-1,4 type exhibits superior abrasion resistance and resilience.

Polybutadiene Resins   Unsaturated, thermoplastic hydrocarbons cured by peroxides-catalyzed vinyl-type polymerization, or by sodium-catalyzed copolymerization of butadiene and styrene. Liquid resins, used for casting, encapsulation, and potting.

Polybutenes   (Polybutylenes). A family of polymers of isobutene, butene-1, and butene-2. They range from oils through tacky waxes and elastomeric solids. See also BUTYL RUBBER, and POLYBUTYLENE RESINS.

Polybutylene Resins   A family of polymers consisting of isotactic, stereoregular, crystalline polymers based on butene-1. Their properties are similar to polypropylene and polyethylene.

Poly-*n*-Butyl Methacrylate   One of the ACRYLIC RESINS.

Polycaprolactam   See NYLON 6.

Polycarbonate Resins   Polymers derived from aromatic and aliphatic dihydroxy compounds with phosgene, or by ester interchange with phosgene-derived precursors. When the aromatic dihydroxy is bisphenol A, the resulting polymer is thermoplastic – the most commonly used form. Polycarbonate resins are frequently used in extracorporeal applications such as connectors, luer locks, clear containers, etc.

Polychlorotrifluoroethylene (PCTFE)   A family of polymers, derived from chlorotrifluoroethane gas, by mass, emulsion, or suspension polymerization. Unlike PTFE, PCTFE may be processed by extrusion, injection, or compression molding. The polymers are highly biostable, nontoxic, and slippery.

Polycondensation   See CONDENSATION.

Polycyclamide   A generic term for polyamides containing a cycloalkane ring, a series of linear polyamides formed by the condensation of 1,4-cyclohexanebis(methylamine) with one or more dicarboxylic acids. See also NYLON.

Polycyclic   An organic substance containing three or more ring structures, which may be the same or different, e.g., anthracene, naphthalene.

Polyelectrolyte   A natural or synthetic polymer containing ionic constituents, either anionic or cationic.

Polyester   (Alkyd Resins). A general term comprising all materials in which the main backbone is formed by the esterification of polyfunctional alcohols and acids. The term alkyd was coined from the AL in polyhydric aLcohols, and the CID (modified to KID) in polybasic aCIDs. The term polyester is further explained under POLYESTERS, SATURATED and POLYESTERS, UNSATURATED.

Polyester Fiber   Generic name for any fiber in which the fiber-forming substance is any long-chain synthetic polymer composed of at least 85% by weight of an ester of a dihydric alcohol and terephthalic acid. Polyethylene terephthalate is better know as Dacron, and is extensively used in vascular grafts and medical textiles.

Polyester Plasticizers   A family of plasticizers. Characterized by a large number of ester groups in each molecule. Seldom used in medical applications, because of their leaching tendency.

Polyesters, Saturated   A family of polyesters in which the polyester backbones are saturated, and hence unreactive, used as plasticizers, and as reactants in the synthesis of certain polyurethanes, and as high-molecular-weight thermoplastics such as polyethylene terephthalate (''Dacron'' and ''Mylar''). Dacron fiber is frequently used in the production of vascular grafts and medical textiles.

Polyesters, Unsaturated   A family of polyesters characterized by the presence of double bonds in the backbone. Unsaturation enables subsequent curing by copolymerization with reactive monomers, in which the polyester reactant has been dissolved. These unsaturated polyesters are used in reinforced plastics, and as potting and encapsulating compounds.

Polyether, Chlorinated   See CHLORINATED POLYETHER.

Polyether Foams   A type of urethane foam, which is made by reacting an isocyanate with a polyether polyol. In rigid foams, propylene oxide adducts of sorbitol, sucrose, and pentaerythrytol are often used. For flexible foams, polyols with hydroxyl numbers ranging from 40 to 160 are frequently used. Polyether foams are characterized by good hydrolytic stability.

Polyethers   Compounds containing primary (and some secondary) alcoholic hydroxyl groups, used as reactants in the synthesis of urethane elastomers, coatings, adhesives, and foams.

Polyethylene Foams   Low-density foams made by mixing a blowing agent with hot, molten polymer under pressure, then suddenly releasing the pressure and cooling. Cross-linked foams can be made by blending a peroxide cross-linking agent, with subsequent curing.

Polyethylene Glycol Terephthalate   A saturated thermoplastic resin, made by the condensation of ethylene glycol and terephthalic acid, producing a wear-resistant, dimensionally stable, chemically-resistant film, best known for its trade name of "Mylar."

Polyethylene Glycols   Oligomers of ethylene glycol, with molecular weights ranging from 200 to 6000. Used as reactants for urethanes, excipients in pharmaceutical preparations, mold release agents, etc.

Polyethylene Oxide (PEO)   A water-soluble thermoplastic used as a lubricant, and as an intermediate in the formation of hydrogels.

Polyethylene Terephthalate   See POLYETHYLENE GLYCOL TEREPHTHALATE.

Polyethylenes   An important family of polymers, derived by polymerizing ethylene gas. Properties of the finished polymer, such as density, melt index, crystallinity, molecular weight, etc., can be widely changed by varying catalysts and methods of polymerization. Polymers with densities ranging from .910−.925 are called low-density; those with densities from .926−.940 are medium-density; and those with densities from .941−.965 are high-density.

Polyformaldehyde Resins   See ACETAL RESINS.

Polyglycidyl Polyepichlorohydrin Resins   A family of epoxy resins, derived from epichlorohydrin and a hydroxyl compound, possessing some inherent flexibility.

Polyhexafluoropropylene   A fluorocarbon resin. Hexafluoropropylene is copolymerized with tetrafluoroethylene to form the FEP family of fluorocarbons.

Polyhydric Alcohols   See POLYOL.

Polyhydroxyether Resins   See PHENOXY RESINS.

Polyimides   Condensation polymers derived from pyromellitic dianhydride and aromatic amines. Polyimides are heat-resistant, have low thermal expansion, and have good chemical and radiation stability.

Polyisobutylenes   See POLYBUTENES.

Polyisocyanate   A substance containing a number of isocyanate groups attached to a single molecule.

Polyisocyanurate   Isocyante polymer trimer groups formed by the reaction between isocyanate groups.

Polyisoprene   Polymers of isoprene.

Polymer   The product of a polymerization reaction. The product of polymerization of one monomer is called a homopolymer, or simply polymer. When two monomers are polymerized simultaneously the product is called a copolymer. A terpolymer is the product of three monomers. The product of more than three monomers is called a heteropolymer. The terms polymer, resin, macromolecular substance and plastic are often used synonymously.

Polymer, High   An organic macromolecule composed of a high number of monomers, with molecular weights ranging from 5000 into the millions. Molecular weights lower than 5000 constitute low polymers. High polymers are further subdivided into synthetic and natural. Synthetic polymers are classified according to (1) thermal behavior: thermoplastics (urethanes, acrylics) and thermosets (silicones, epoxy); (2) chemical nature: acrylic, vinyl, cellulosic; (3) molecular structure: atactic, linear, cross-linked, block, graft, stereospecific; and (4) homopolymers, copolymers, and terpolymers.

Polymer, Inorganic   A macromolecule containing no carbon in the main chain, and in which behavior similar to traditional organic polymers can be achieved, i.e., covalent bonding and/or cross-linking, as in silicone elastomers. In these polymers, silicon atoms replace carbon in the straight chain, with substituent groups attached to the silicon. Many authorities consider silicone elastomers to be semi-organic, since their substituent groups are organic radicals, such as methyl and aryl groups.

Polymer, Water-Soluble   Any substance of high molecular weight that swells or dissolves in water at room temperature. May be divided into (1) synthetic (polyvinyl alcohol, ethylene oxide, polyvinyl pyrrolidone, polyethyleneimine); (2) semisynthetic (chemically treated cellulose, modified starches; and (3) natural gums (such as karaya, arabic, tragacanth).

Polymer Structure   A general term referring to the relative position, spacial arrangement and freedom of motion of atoms in a polymer molecule. Such details have important effects on polymer properties, such as second-order transition temperature, flexibility, and ultimate tensile strength.

Polymeric   Composed of, or containing, polymer units in its chemical structure.

Polymeric Materials, Health Care Usage   The major types of polymers used in health care applications are shown in the following:

171

Polymeric Materials, Health Care Usage

THERMOPLASTICS		THERMOSETS	
LDPE	33%	Silicones	6%
PVC	20%	Polyesters	3%
Polystyrene	20%	Epoxy	1%
HDPE	12%		
Polypropylene	10%	TOTAL	10%
Polyurethane	2%		
Acrylic	2%		
Nylon	2%		
TOTAL	90%	TOTALS	100%

Polymeric Modifier   A term applied to any polymer that is blended with another polymer to obtain certain desirable characteristics.

Polymeric Plasticizers   A general term referring to plasticizers with molecular chains much longer than monomeric plasticizers, which comprise virtually all other classifications of plasticizers.

Polymeric Polyisocyanate   A generic term for a family of isocyanates derived from aniline-formaldehyde condensation products, used as reactants for the synthesis of elastomers, pressure-sensitive adhesives, coatings, and foams.

Polymerization   A chemical reaction in which monomers are covalently linked to form large chains whose molecular weight is a multiple of that of the monomer. There are three general types of polymerization: (1) addition, where reactive monomers unite without forming any other products, (2) condensation, where there is concomitant elimination of simple molecules, and (3) ring-opening, where a ringed group such as caprolactone is opened, forming a linear polymer. The majority of thermoplastics, and some thermosets, are made by addition polymerization, types of which are described by the following titles: addition, block, bulk, condensation, emulsion, free radical, graft, ionic, isotactic, photo, solution, stereoblock, stereoregular, stereospecific, suspension, syndiotactic, and thermal polymerization.

Polymethacrylonitrile (PMAN)   A polymer obtained from methacrylonitrile, a vinyl monomer containing a nitrile group.

Polymethyl Methacrylate (PMMA)   A transparent solid, with good physiological and optical properties. Widely used to produce hard contact lenses.

Poly-(4-Methylpentene-1)   A polymer obtained by dimerizing propylene, characterized by low density (0.83), high crystalline melting point, and good optical properties.

Poly(Monochloro-*p*-Xylene)   See PARYLENES.

Polymorphism   The ability of a crystalline substance to exist in two or more forms of crystalline structure.

Polymorphonuclear Leukocyte (PMN)   A type of white blood cell with a granular cytoplasm and multilobed nucleus that is very active in phagocytosis.

Polyol   A substance, usually a liquid resin, containing a number of hydroxyl

172

groups attached to a single molecule. The term includes compounds containing alcoholic groups such as polyethers, polyesters, glycols, and castor oil.

Polyolefins The class of polymers made by polymerizing simple olefins, such as ethylene, propylene, butenes, isoprenes, and pentenes. Also included are Polyallomers, Ionomers, and copolymers such as ethylene-vinyl acetate and ethylene-ethyl acrylate.

Polyoxamides Generic name for nylon-type materials made from oxalic acid and diamines.

Polyoxetanes See CHLORINATED POLYETHER.

Polyoxymethylenes Linear polymers with the formula $HO(CH2)_nH$, in which n is above 100. Those with values between 500 and 5000 are called ACETAL RESINS.

Polyoxypropylene Glycols Polyethers derived from propylene oxide, used as monomers in the production of urethane coatings and foams.

Poly-*para*-Xylene (Parylene N). See PARYLENES.

Polyphenylene Oxide (PPO) Thermoplastic, noncrystalline resins, obtained by the oxidative polycondensation of 2,6-dimethylphenol in the presence of a copper-amine complex catalyst. Resins possess unusual resistance to acids and bases.

Polypropylene A thermoplastic resin made by the polymerization of propylene with catalysts such as aluminum alkyl and titanium tetrachloride with solvents. Molding grades have molecular weights of 40,000 or higher, with good resistance to chemicals and heat.

Polysiloxanes See SILICONES.

Polystyrene Polymers of styrene (vinyl benzene). Thermoplastics with good thermal and dimensional stability, and resistance to staining. Being somewhat brittle, it is often copolymerized with other materials, such as rubber or butadiene copolymers. Copolymerizations with methyl methacrylate improve light stability, and copolymerization with acrylonitrile increases environmental resistance.

Polystyrene Foam Lightweight foams, made by injecting a volatile liquid such as methyl chloride into the molten resin.

Polysulfides A family of elastomers made from sodium tetrasulfide and ethylene dichloride, or sodium polysulfide and dichloro compounds. Available as liquids or solids, they exhibit low permeability to gases and vapors, with good resistance to oxidation and solvents.

Polysulfonate Copolymers Transparent polyester thermoplastic copolymers, formed by reaction of a diphenol with an aromatic disulfonyl chloride, and one of the other disulfonyl chlorides or carboxylic acid chlorides. The copolymers have excellent stability to hydrolysis and aminolysis.

Polysulfones A family of thermoplastics, based on benzene rings or phenylene units linked by three different chemical groups – sulfone group, an ether linkage, and an isopropylidene group, each acting as an internal stabilizer. Characterized by excellent resistance to gamma radiation and steam radiation, as well as resistance to solvents and chemicals.

Polyterpene Resins   Thermoplastic resins based on the polymerization of turpentine in the presence of catalysts, used in the manufacture of adhesives, coatings, and varnishes.

Polytetrafluoroethylene (PTFE)   The oldest of the fluoroplastic family, made by polymerizing tetrafluoroethylene, characterized by extreme inertness, low coefficient of friction, and ability to resist adhesion to almost any material. Blown PTFE is successfully used in the manufacture of vascular grafts.

Polytrifluorostyrene   A thermoplastic said to combine the oxidation resistance of PTFE with the ease of fabrication of styrene.

Polyurethane Resins   A family of polymers produced by reacting diisocyanates with organic compounds containing two or more active hydrogens, derived from hydroxyl or amino groups. The reaction of isocyanates with hydroxyl groups results in the formation of urethane groups, whereas the reaction with amines forms substituted urea linkages. These polymers can be formulated into thermoplastic, thermoset, or ''virtually cross-linked'' products.

Polyurethanes   A large family of polymers with widely varying properties, based on the reaction of diisocyanate groups with compounds containing hydroxyl groups. Urethanes can be formulated as thermoplastics, thermosets, casting resins, prepolymers, and rubber-like vulcanizable gums.

Polyvinyl Acetal   A general term for resins formed by partially or completely replacing the hydroxyl groups of polyvinyl alcohol with aldehydes by means of a condensation reaction. Other members of the family are POLYVINYL BUTYRAL and POLYVINYL FORMAL. These materials find use in adhesives, lacquers, coatings, and films.

Polyvinyl Acetate (PVA)   A transparent thermoplastic, prepared by polymerization of vinyl acetate. Available as powder, solution, emulsion, and latex. Major use is in adhesives, latex paints, fabric finishes, and lacquers.

Polyvinyl Alcohol (PVA)   A water-soluble thermoplastic, obtained from the partial or complete hydrolysis of polyvinyl acetate. Films are impervious to oils, fats, and display zero transmission rate for oxygen, nitrogen, and helium, thus frequently used as barrier resins for packaging.

Polyvinyl Butyral   A member of the Polyvinyl Acetal family, made by reacting butyraldehyde with some unreacted groups within a Polyvinyl Alcohol chain.

Polyvinyl Carbazole   A brown thermoplastic resin, obtained by reacting actylene with carbazole. Seldom used in medical applications.

Polyvinyl Chloride (PVC)   The most important member of the vinyl family of polymers, made by the polymerization of the vinyl chloride monomer in the presence of peroxide catalysts. The homopolymer is hard and brittle, but is flexibilized by the addition of plasticizers. It is extensively utilized in medical tubing for extracorporeal applications requiring flexibility and transparency.

Polyvinyl Chloride-Acetate   A copolymer of vinyl chloride and vinyl acetate, usually containing 85–97 % of vinyl chloride. The presence of vinyl acetate confers greater flexibility and solubility to the finished polymer.

Polyvinyl Dichloride   (Chlorinated PVC). A PVC homopolymer, modified by post-chlorination. The presence of an additional chlorine confers higher melting/softening temperature, and better chemical resistance compared to conventional PVC.

Polyvinyl Fluoride (PVF)   The polymer of vinyl fluoride. The presence of the fluorine atom forms a tight bond within the hydrocarbon chain, accounting for high melting point, chemical inertness, and UV stability. PVF may be dissolved in hot "latent" solvents such as dimethyl acetamide, phthalate, glycollate, and isobutyrate esters.

Polyvinyl Formal   A member of the Polyvinyl Acetal family, made by condensing formaldehyde in the presence of polyvinyl alcohol, or by the simultaneous hydrolysis and acetylation of polyvinyl acetate.

Polyvinyl Isobutyl Ether   A white solid polymer, or viscous liquid, based on the polymerization of vinyl isobutyl ether.

Polyvinyl Methyl Ether   A component in pressure-sensitive and hot-melt adhesives.

Polyvinyl Pyrrolidone (VP)   Polymers of N-vinyl-2-pyrrolidone, extensively used in the pharmaceutical industry as a binder, water-soluble resin, excipient, plasma extender, etc.

Polyvinylidene Chloride   A thermoplastic polymer of 1,1-dichloro ethylene. Copolymers with vinyl chloride (15 % or more) are widely used as barrier films.

Polyvinylidene Fluoride   A member of the fluorohydrocarbon family of polymers, a resin with exceptional thermal stability and good abrasion resistance.

Poromeric   A term used as an adjective for materials that have the ability to transmit moisture vapor while remaining essentially waterproof.

Porosity   The ratio of the void volume to the total volume (solid material plus void), expressed as a percentage.

Porous Molds   Molds that are made up of fused aggregates (powdered metals, pellets, etc.) so the resulting mass contains numerous open interstices through which either air or liquids may pass through the mass of the mold.

Positive Mold   A compression mold designed to prevent the escape of molding resin during the molding cycle.

Post Curing   The process of forming an uncured thermosetting resin, then completing the cure after the resin has been removed from its forming mold or mandrel.

Postforming   A term denoting the heating and reshaping of a fully cured laminate. Upon cooling, the laminate retains the contours and shape of the mold over which it has been formed.

Pot Life   See WORKING LIFE.

Pot Plunger   A plunger used to force softened molding material into the closed cavity of a transfer mold.

Potting   The process of encasing an article in a resinous mass, by placing the article into a mold, pouring liquid resin to surround the article, and curing the resin. The mold remains attached to the potted article. The main difference between potting and encapsulation is that in encapsulation the mold is removed from the encapsulated article.

Powder   Any solid, dry material of small particle size. Powders smaller than 43 μm in diameter cannot be detected by rubbing between the fingers, and are called impalpable. Powders may be prepared by (1) comminution (mechanical grinding); (2) combustion (pyrogenic silica, carbon black); (3) precipitation from a chemical reaction (calcium carbonate).

Powder Density   See BULK DENSITY.

Powdered Plastics   Finely pulverized plastic compounds, for use in fluidized bed coatings, rotational molding, and various sintering techniques.

PP   Abbreviation for *Polypropylene*.

PPI   Abbreviation for *Polymeric Polyisocyanate*.

PPO   Abbreviation for *Polyphenylene Oxide*.

Precipitate   Small particles that settled from a liquid or gaseous suspension by gravity, or resulting from a chemical reaction.

Precure   A partial state of cure existing in an elastomer or thermosetting resin prior to its use as a reactive adhesive, or in a forming operation.

Precursor   (1) In polymer chemistry, any intermediate compound or monomeric unit capable of polymerization, either with itself, or with other monomers to form a plastic. (2) In biochemistry, an intermediate compound or molecular complex present in a living organism, which when activated is converted to a specific functional substance.

Predrying   The drying of a resin or molding compound prior to its introduction into a mold or extruder. Many plastics are hygroscopic and require predrying before thermoprocessing.

Preferential   Descriptive of the selectivity of action, either chemical or physicochemical, exhibited by a substance when in contact with other substances, due to chemical affinity or to surface phenomena.

Prefix   Prefixes in medicine are frequently used. The following examples show some common uses:

PREFIX	MEANING	EXAMPLES
a(n)-	Without	Anemia—blood deficiency
	Not	Anesthesia—lack of feeling
		Anoxia—lack of oxygen

PREFIX	MEANING	EXAMPLES
anti-	Against	Antibacterial — against bacteria
		Antispasmodic — prevent spasms
bi-	Double	Bifocal — two powers
	Two	Bipolar — two poles
di-	Double	Dichotomy — cut in two
dys-	Bad	Dysfunction — functional disorder
	Faulty	Dystrophy — faulty growth
endo-	Within	Endogenous — within the body
	Inward	Endocrine — secreting into blood
extra-	Outside	Extraperitoneal — outside the stomach
		Extrasystole — premature beat
hemi-	Half	Hemianoplia — half vision
	Unilateral	Hemiparesis — one-sided paralysis
hyper-	Excessive	Hyperemia — excess of blood
		Hyperopia — farsightedness
		Hypertension — high blood pressure
hypo-	Low	Hypothermia — low body temperature
	Deficient	Hypotrophy — underdevelopment
		Hypoxia — oxygen deficiency
inter-	Between	Intercellular — between cells
		Intercostal — between ribs
		Intermittent — at intervals
		Interstitial — space between tissues
intra-	Within	Intracranial — within the head
		Intravascular — within a blood vessel
macro-	Large	Macrocyte — a large red blood cell
		Macroscopic — visible to naked eye
mega-	Large	Megacolon — excessively large colon
micro-	Small	Microcyte — a small red blood cell
para-	Faulty	Paralysis — faulty muscular function
	Beside	Paratyphoid fever — resembling typhoid
patho-	Morbid	Pathology — study of disease
		Pathogenic — producing disease
per-	Through	Peroral — through the mouth
		Perforation — through a hole
		Permeable — porous, passable
peri-	Around	Pericardium — around the heart
		Periostium — around bones
poly-	Many	Polyarthritis — inflammation of several
		joints at once
		Polysaccharide — many sugars
retro-	Behind	Retrograde — going backwards
		Retrosternal — behind the sternum
sub-	Under	Subacute — somewhat acute
		Subclinical — without clinical sign
toxi-	Poisonous	Toxicity — poisonous
toxo-		Toxicosis — poisoning
		Toxicology — study of poisons

Preheat Roll   In extrusion coating, a heated roll installed between the pressure roll and unwind roll, used to preheat the substrate before it is coated.

177

Preimpregnation   The practice of mixing resin and reinforcement before shipment. The product of this practice is called a prepreg.

Premarket Notification   (510k) See PMN.

Premix   Molding compounds of any thermosetting resin premixed with fillers, reinforcements, or catalysts, prior to shipment.

Preplasticization   In injection molding, the method of premelting molding powders in a separate chamber, then transferring the melt to the injection cylinder, thus shortening the molding cycles.

Prepolymer   (1) A substance prepared by the reaction of a polyol, with an excess of isocyanates, and containing a number of unreacted isocyanate groups. (2) A polymer of low molecular weight, capable of being hardened by further polymerization during or after a forming process.

Prepolymer Molding   In urethane technology, the practice of prereacting a portion of the polyol with the isocyanate to form a low-viscosity liquid prepolymer. The prepolymer is subsequently reacted with additional polyol, chain extenders, catalysts, etc., to form the finished polymer.

Preservative   (Stabilizer). Any substance that effectively prolongs the useful life of a polymer. Polymers are stabilized by antioxidants, antiozonants, antirads, UV absorbers, heat stabilizers, etc. Drugs are preserved by sterilization, ionizing radiation, etc.

Pressure Forming   A thermoforming process wherein pressure is used to push the sheet to be formed against a mold surface.

Pressure Roll   In extrusion coating, a roll used to apply pressure to better consolidate the substrate and the thermoplastic film with which it has been coated.

Pressure Sensitive Adhesive (PSA)   An adhesive that develops maximum bonding power by the application of light pressure.

Primary   Referring to monohydric alcohols, amines, and related compounds, describing the molecular structure of isomeric or chemically similar individuals. (1) Monohydric alcohols are based on the methanol group, in which three of the bonds may be attached to hydrogen atoms or alkyl groups; primary alcohols have one alkyl group and two hydrogens; secondary alcohols have two alkyl groups and one hydrogen, etc. (2) Primary, secondary, and tertiary amines are formed from ammonia when one, two, or three hydrogen atoms, respectively, are replaced by alkyl groups.

Primary Plasticizer   A plasticizer with good compatibility and permanency characteristics, and which may be used as the sole plasticizer.

Primer   A coating applied to a substrate to improve the adhesion, gloss, or durability of a subsequently applied coating.

Proctoscopy   Examination of the rectal structures with a tubular instrument.

Prodrug   A term in pharmaceutical chemistry referring to a compound that is converted into a physiologically active substance by metabolic processes within the body.

Progeny   A biological offspring.

Promoter   (1) A substance that when added in small quantities to a catalyst increases its activity. The promoter may be a feeble catalyst itself. (2) In flotation, a substance that provides particles to be floated with a water-repellent surface that adheres to air bubbles.

Propeller Mixers   Devices comprising a rotating shaft with propeller blades attached, used for mixing relatively low viscosity solutions or dispersions.

Prophylaxis   Preventive treatment, or health care.

Proportional Limit   The greatest stress that a material is capable of sustaining from proportionality of stress and strain (Hooke's Law). Expressed in force per unit area, usually pounds per square inch.

Prosthetic Group   A chemical grouping in which a metal ion is associated with a macromolecule, i.e., coenzymes, hemin, etc. Such groups activate metabolic mechanisms such as phosphorylation and decarboxylation, by coordination reactions with amino acids, proteins, enzymes, and nucleic acids.

Protease   A proteolytic enzyme that attacks and breaks the peptide linkages in proteins. Included in this group are: pepsin, trypsin, ficin, papain, and renin.

Protective Coating   A film applied to a substrate for protective or decorative purposes. Applied to plastics, the films protect against oxidation, abrasion, etc. Applied to metals they protect against corrosion, discoloration, etc.

Protein   A high polymer comprised of a complex mixture of amino acid monomers, connected by peptide linkages ($-CO.NH-$). Proteins occur in the cells of all living organisms and in biological fluids. Proteins have many important functional forms: enzymes, hemoglobin, hormones, viruses, genes, antibodies, and nucleic acids. They also comprise the basic component of connective tissue (collagen, elastin), hair and nails (keratin), skin, etc.

Protein Resins   A generic term applied to resins derived from proteins, constituting casein and zein.

Protocol   A plan for scientific action or treatment.

Proton   A fundamental unit of matter having a positive charge and a mass number of 1. Protons are constituents of all atomic nuclei, their number in each number nucleus called the atomic number of the element. An atom of normal hydrogen contains one proton and one electron. A proton is identical with a hydrogen ion.

Prototype Mold   A temporary or experimental mold used to test designs or obtain market reactions. Such molds are made of silicone, low-temperature metal alloys, or epoxy resins.

PS   Abbreviation for *Polystyrene*.

PSA   Abbreviation for *Pressure Sensitive Adhesive*.

PSA, Medical Applications   Selected medical applications of pressure sensitive skin adhesives are shown next.

PSA, Medical Applications

CLASSIFICATION	APPLICATIONS
Transdermal	Plasters
	Cataplasms
	Reservoir-type patches
	Matrix-type patches
	Dermal tapes
Surgical	Intravenous placement
	Surgical tapes
	Wound dressings
	Affixing tracheotomy tube
	Sports tapes
	Occlusive bandages
Wound Management	Bandages
	Burn dressings
	Wound closure tapes
	Occlusive dressings
Hospital	Ostomy seals
	Colostomy appliances
	Ileostomy appliances
	Stoma appliances
	External prosthesis
	Maxillofacial devices
	Surgical drapes
	Protective pads
	Male incontinence devices
Biomedical Devices	EEG electrodes
	EKG electrodes
	TENS devices
	Intravenous catheter placement tapes
	Electrosurgery grounding pads
Medical – Clinical Tests	Diagnostic test kits

Pseudoplastic Fluid   A fluid whose apparent viscosity decreases instantaneously with an increase in the rate of shear. That is, the initially high resistance to stirring decreases abruptly as the rate of stirring is increased.

Psychiatry   (1) The medical specialty dealing with mental disorders. (2) The medical specialty dealing with the diagnosis and treatment of mental diseases.

Psychology   The science that deals with the emotional and mental processes, consciousness, sensation, ideation, and memory.

Psychotropic Drug   A drug that affects the behavior, emotions, or mental state of psychologically disturbed patients. They are widely known as "tranquilizers." Minor tranquilizers (benzodiapine and glycerol derivatives) are classified as "antianxiety agents"; the major tranquilizers are classified as "antipsychotics" (phenothiazines, thioxanthines, and butyrophenones), and "antidepressants" (monoamine oxidase inhibitors and tricyclic compounds).

PTFE   Abbreviation for *Polytetrafluoroethylene*.

PTFE Vitreous Carbon Material   A Class II device composed of a mixture

180

of PTFE (polytetrafluoroethylene) and vitreous carbon that may be used in maxillofacial alveolar ridge augmentation, (rebuilding the upper jaw area that contains the tooth sockets). It is also used to coat metal surgical implants in the alveoli (tooth sockets), and temporomandibular joints (joints between the upper and lower jaws).

Ptomaine   Highly toxic substances (derivatives of ethers of polyhydric alcohols) resulting from the metabolic decomposition of animal proteins. The term "ptomaine poisoning" is usually a misnomer for other types of food poisoning.

PU   Abbreviation for *Polyurethane*.

Pull Strength   The bond strength of an adhesive joint, obtained by pulling in a direction perpendicular to the surface of the layer.

Pultrusion   In reinforced plastics, the technique in which continuous strands of resin-impregnated reinforcing material are pulled through the orifice of a steel die, then through a heating chamber. This process yields continuous extrudates with high unidirectional qualities.

Purging   In extrusion or injection molding, the cleaning of one material from the machine by forcing it out with a new material to be used in subsequent production, or with another purging material. Purging is best accomplished when the purging material is more viscous than the material being displaced.

Purification   Removal of extraneous materials (impurities) from a substance or mixture, by a variety of separation techniques. A pure substance is one in which no impurity can be detected by any analytical method. Substances are purified by: extraction, precipitation, distillation, adsorption, electrophoresis, crystallization, and thermal diffusion.

PVA   Abbreviation for *Polyvinyl Alcohol*.

PVAc   Abbreviation for *Polyvinyl Acetate*.

PVB   Abbreviation for *Polyvinyl Butyral*.

PVC   Abbreviation for *Polyvinyl Chloride*.

PVCAc   Abbreviation for *Copolymers of Vinyl Chloride* and *Vinyl Acetate*.

PVD   An infrequently used abbreviation for *Polyvinyl Dichloride*.

PVDC   Abbreviation for *Polyvinyl Fluoride*.

PVI   Abbreviation for *Polyvinyl Isobutyl Ether*.

PVM   Abbreviation for *Polyvinyl Methyl Ether*.

PVOH   Abbreviation for *Polyvinyl Alcohol*.

PVP   Abbreviation for *Polyvinyl Pyrrolidone*.

Pycnometer   A flask used for measuring density of liquids, consisting of two capillary arms so it can be filled to a known volume with good precision. A dilatometer is a pycnometer equipped with instruments to study density as a function of temperature or time.

Pyogenic   Refers to an agent or organism that causes the formation of pus.

Pyro   (1) A prefix indicating formation by the sole action of heat, i.e., without oxidation. (2) An inorganic acid derived by loss of one molecule of water from two molecules of an ortho acid, as pyrophosphoric acid.

Pyrogen   Fever-producing organic substances arising from microbial contamination and responsible for many of the febrile reactions that occur in patients following injection. The causative material is thought to be a liposaccharide from the outer cell of the bacteria and endotoxins. The pyrogen is thermostable, thus remaining after sterilization by autoclaving.

Pyrogenic Silica   A type of silica made by treating silicon at very high temperatures, yielding colloidal particles averaging 0.015 microns in diameter. Used as a reinforcing agent in silicones, as a thickener for liquid resins, as an anticaking agent, etc.

Pyrolysis   Transformation of a substance into other substances by heat alone, i.e., without oxidation. It is similar to destructive distillation. Hydrocarbons are subject to pyrolysis, forming carbon black; silica forms pyrogenic silica powder; acetone is converted into ketenes, etc.

Pyrometer   An instrument for measuring heat. For surface measurements, the equipment consists of a thermocouple which when heated at their junction produces a small electrical signal, and a millivoltmeter for measuring the voltage produced, which is proportional to the temperature of the junction.

Q

Q_{10}   Symbol for the increase in rate of a chemical process by raising the temperature 10°C.

q.d.   Abbreviation used in prescriptions for *quaque die*, every day.

q.h.   Abbreviation used in prescriptions for *quaque hora*, every hour.

q.i.d.   Abbreviation used in prescriptions for *quater in die*, four times a day.

q.l.   Abbreviation used in prescriptions for *quantum libet*, as much as desired.

q.s.   Abbreviation used in prescriptions for *quantum sufficit*, as much as needed.

Quadri   Four.

Quadripolymer   An infrequent term for the simultaneous polymerization product of four different monomers. Acrylic and polyurethane hydrogels frequently contain four (or more) monomers.

Qualification Test   A series of tests conducted to determine conformance of polymers, or polymer systems, to the requirements of a specification.

Quality   The degree of accepted excellence of a product, which is subject to determination by comparison against an ideal standard, or against similar products from independent sources.

Quality Assurance   All activities necessary to assure and verify confidence in performance of a finished device, material, or product.

Quality Characteristic   Any mechanical dimension, physical characteristic, functional attribute, or appearance feature that can be objectively used for measuring the unit quality of a product.

Quality Control   An objective system whereby a manufacturer ensures that materials, methods, workmanship, and final product specifications meet the total requirements of a given standard.

Quantum   Unit quantity of energy where the photon carries a quantum of electromagnetic energy, according to the QUANTUM THEORY.

Quantum Theory   The theory proposed by physicist Max Plack positing that energy is not emitted or absorbed continuously, but discontinuously in quanta units. An important corollary is that the energy of radiation is directly proportional to its frequency.

Quasi-Prepolymer Process   A process, intermediate between the one-shot and prepolymer methods, used in the synthesis of polyurethanes, where the polyol is first reacted with a large excess of diisocyanate, to produce a low-viscosity quasiprepolymer. This quasiprepolymer is subsequently reacted with additional polyol, or chain extenders, to produce the final polymer.

Quaternary Carbon Atom   A carbon atom bonded to four other carbon atoms with single bonds.

Quellung Reaction   The precipitation of specific antibody on the capsule of an organism producing the appearance of capsular swelling.

Quench   (1) A process of sudden cooling of thermoplastic materials from the molten state to the solid state. (2) To limit or stop the electrical discharge in an ionization detector.

Quench Bath   The cooling medium (and apparatus) used to suddenly cool molten thermoplastic materials to the solid state.

Quench Tank Extrusion   An extrusion process wherein the extrudate is conducted through a chilled water bath for sudden cooling.

Quencher   A molecule capable of chelating photo-induced states, and thereby acting as ultraviolet stabilizers in a polymer. Many transition metal chelates, especially nickel-based ones, are thought to be effective UV stabilizers.

Quenching   The process by which excess energy of a photo-initiated excited species is lost by transfer to another species (the quencher, or chelator) which dissipates the energy harmlessly, usually as heat. In this fashion, the excited species cannot undergo bond dissociation, thus protecting polymers against photodegradation.

R **Racemization**   Conversion, by either heat or chemical reaction, of an optically active compound, into the optically inactive form, in which half of the optically active substance becomes its mirror image (enantiomer). This change results in an equal mixture of dextro- and levo-rotatory isomers.

Rad   The unit of energy absorbed by a material from ionizing radiation. One rad is equal to 10^{12} joules per kilogram, or 100 ergs per gram.

Radcure   Another name for *Radiation Cure*. Materials that may be cured with electromagnetic radiation, such as UV and IR.

Radcure Markets   U.S. demand for radcure (radiation cure) materials is expected to increase nearly 14% yearly through 1994 to a value of $495 million. Environmental restrictions on volatile organic solvents used in coatings and other products continue to be the driving force behind demand. Coatings represent about 38% of consumption, followed by electronic applications (36%), while inks, adhesives, and miscellaneous uses account for the remaining 26%.

Radcure Technology   The use of electromagnetic radiation to cause a chemical reaction in organic materials such as resin coatings, adhesives, and inks to produce a rapid hardening or cure. Unlike conventional curing, radcure does not depend on the evaporation of volatile organic solvents. Ultraviolet (UV) and Infrared (IR) radiation are the two principal radcure technologies.

Radiant Energy   Energy in the form of photons or electromagnetic waves.

Radiant Energy, Infrared   Energy with wavelengths between $770-1000$ nanometers.

Radiation, Industrial   Chemical changes induced by exposure to radiation, such as (1) polymer cross-linking, (2) rubber vulcanization, (3) acrylic polymerization and cross-linking, (4) curing of organic-based protective and decorative coatings, and (5) hardening of photopolymerizable monomers by exposure to UV radiation.

Radiation, Ionizing   Extremely short wavelength, energetic, penetrating rays of the following types: (1) gamma rays, (2) X-rays, (3) subatomic charged particles, e.g., electrons, protons, deuterons. Called ionizing since such radiation is capable of removing electrons from any atoms in its path, leading to ionization.

Radiation Biochemistry   The systematic study of substances having the ability to protect cells and body tissues against the damaging effects of ionizing radiation. Radiochemically induced reactions that adversely affect living systems are: (1) deprivation of sulfhydryl groups ($-SH$) essential for normal cell division, (2) formation of peroxides, (3) denaturation of proteins, (4) change in substituent groups of amino acids, (5) oxidation of hemoglobin, and (6) depolymerization of DNA.

Radiation Curing   Process for curing (hardening) polymers with high energy electrons or short wavelengths of light.

Radiation Damage A term expressing the unwanted alterations resulting in a polymer following exposure to ionizing or penetrating radiation.

Radiation Polymerization A polymerization reaction initiated by exposure to radiation such as UV rays, gamma rays, etc., rather than by means of traditional chemical catalysts.

Radical A group of atoms, existing in a molecule, which remains unchanged through many chemical reactions. Typical organic radicals are: ethyl, propyl, and benzyl.

Radio Frequency Heating See DIELECTRIC HEATING.

Radio Frequency (RF) Preheating A preheating method for molding resins to facilitate molding, or reduce molding cycle. The most used frequencies are between 10 and 100 Mc/sec.

Radio Frequency Welding A method of welding thermoplastics using a radio frequency field to provide the necessary heat. Also known as *high-frequency welding*.

Radioactivity Natural or artificial nuclear transformation, resulting in the emission of alpha, beta, or gamma rays. Amounts of radioactivity are expressed in units of activity, as Curies, and its metric fractions: milli and microcuries. A curie is defined as 3.73×10^{10} disintegrations per second.

Radiochemistry The division of chemistry that deals with the properties and uses of radioactive chemicals in industry, biology, and medicine.

Radiogram A photographic record by means of X-rays or by a radioactive substance. Typically used to visualize internal structures during diagnostic or therapeutic procedures.

Radiography Medical radiology includes both diagnostic and therapeutic methods, which utilize ionizing radiation. Diagnostic radiography includes: (1) X-rays, (2) Radiography and Fluoroscopy, and (3) Angiography, designated according to the organ examined, e.g., angiocardiography, nephroangiography, arteriography, phlebography, etc. Radiographic images are optimized by means of special techniques such as tomography, substraction, and dodging.

Radioimmunoassay An immunologic test utilizing radiolabeled antigen, complement, or other reactants. May be adapted to radioimmunodiffusion, radioprecipitations, etc.

Radioisotope (Radionuclide). An isotropic form of an element that exhibits radioactivity. Used as curative agents in medicine, pharmaceuticals, biological tracers, etc. Artificial isotopes are manufactured by neutron bombardment in a nuclear reactor.

Radiopaque Exhibiting opacity or impenetrability to X-rays, or other forms of radiation. Medical polymers can be made radiopaque by the addition of barium or bismuth salts.

Radiopathology A branch of radiology, or pathology, that deals with the effects of radioactive substances on the human body.

Radiopharmaceuticals   Radioactive chemical or pharmaceutical substances, used as diagnostic or therapeutic agents.

Random Copolymer   A copolymer consisting of alternating segments of two monomeric units at random lengths, including single molecules. Random polymerization frequently occurs during copolymerization of two monomers in the presence of a free-radical initiator.

Rankine Temperature   The Rankine temperature scale is the absolute Fahrenheit scale, that is the arithmetic sum of absolute zero on the Fahrenheit scale (-459.69) plus the Fahrenheit temperature.

Reagent   Any substance used in a reaction for the purpose of detecting, measuring, examining, or analyzing other substances. Reagents are high-purity compounds, with over 10,000 reagent-grade chemicals commercially available.

Reagent Resistance   (Chemical Resistance). The ability of a polymer to withstand exposure to acids, alkali, solvents, and other corrosive chemicals.

Rearrangement   A chemical reaction in which the atoms of a single compound recombine, to form a new compound having the same molecular weight, but different physical properties.

Reciprocating Screw Injection Molding   An extrusion process where the screw advances and retreats in cycles. The molten plastic is advanced and plasticated by the rotating screw until the injection shot is made. Rotation is then stopped, and the screw is withdrawn to recharge a new resin shot.

Redox   A contraction of the term "reduction-oxidation." Thus a redox catalyst is one participating in an oxidation-reduction reaction. Polymers formed by this method are referred as redox polymers.

Reduced Viscosity   Ratio of the specific viscosity to the concentration. It is a measure of the inherent capacity of a polymer to increase the viscosity of a solution.

Reduction   (1) Any process that increases the proportion of hydrogen, base-forming elements, or radicals in a compound. (2) Increasing the number of electrons in an atom, ion, or element, thereby reducing the positive valence of the moiety that gained the electron(s).

Refractivity   The index of refraction minus 1. Specific gravity is given by $(n-1)/d$, where n is the index of refraction and d is the density.

Reinforced Molding Compound   Compound containing fibrous reinforcements supplied by the producer in the form of ready-to-use material, as distinguished from Premix.

Reinforced Plastic (RP)   A plastic composition in which fibrous reinforcements are imbedded, with strengths greatly superior to those of the pure resin. The reinforcements are usually fibers, rovings, fabrics, or mats of nylon, carbon, metals, etc. Resins most commonly used are epoxies, nylons, polyesters, silicones, and phenolics.

Reinforced Thermoplastics   Reinforced structures in which the base resin is a thermoplastic, rather than a thermoset, thus allowing the use of conventional molding equipment. Resins commonly used are nylon, polycarbonates, acetals, and polystyrene.

Reinforcement   A strong, inert material incorporated into a plastic mass to greatly improve physical properties, such as higher tensile strength, lower deformation under load, improved flexural strength, higher modulus, etc.

Reinforcing Pigment   Pigments that also serve to improve the physical properties of the finished product. Examples are carbon black, treated silicas, etc.

Relative Density   The ratio of the absolute density of a substance at a stipulated temperature to the absolute density of water at $3.98°C$ (its maximum value).

Relative Viscosity   Ratio of the kinematic viscosity of a specified solution of the polymer to the kinematic viscosity of the pure solvent.

Relaxation   A decrease in stress under sustained constant strain, or creep and rupture under constant load.

Relaxation Time   The time required for a stress under a sustained strain to diminish a predetermined fraction of its initial value.

Release Agent   A substance that prevents another substance, such as molded polymers, from adhering to a substrate, such as a mold. See also PARTING AGENT.

Release Paper   (1) A sheet serving as a protectant, carrier, or both, for an adhesive film or mass, which is easily removed from the film or mass prior to use. (2) A layer of paper that can be easily separated from the surface of a polymer, to which it has been applied or against which the plastic article has been formed. Usually the release is provided by a thin coating of silicone to which the polymer cannot adhere.

Research   (1) A critical and exhaustive investigation or experimentation having as its aim the revision of accepted conclusions in the light of newly discovered facts. (2) The discovery of totally new knowledge based on objective and reproducible observations.

Research, Applied   Investigations directed at the discovery of new scientific knowledge about a particular problem or investigation geared to specific commercial objectives with respect to products or processes.

Research, Basic   Original investigations for the advancement of fundamental scientific knowledge without immediate commercial objectives, but which may have a broad range of applications.

Residual Monomer   The portion of unreacted monomer that remains after the polymerization reaction is considered completed. Residual monomer(s) are a frequent cause for the unexplained toxicity seen in biomaterials.

Resilience   The degree to which a body can quickly resume its original shape after removal of a deforming stress. It is expressed as the ratio of energy returned, after recovery from deformation, to the work input required to produce the deformation.

Resin   A solid or pseudosolid material that has an indefinite molecular weight, which exhibits a tendency to deform when subjected to stress, has a softening or melting range, and usually fractures conchoidally. See also RESIN, NATURAL and RESIN, SYNTHETIC.

Resin, Natural   One of a heterogenous family of solid, or semi-solid materials derived from secretions of plants and trees. Common examples are rosin, amber, pitch, pine tar, etc. Because of their variability, natural resins are seldom used in medical devices.

Resin, Synthetic   This term is interchangeable with the terms polymer and plastic. It refers to liquid, semi-liquid, and solid polymers or prepolymers of synthetic origin, which can be transformed into useful articles by thermoforming techniques. The term encompasses both thermoplastics and thermosets. Synthetic resins form the core of modern biomaterials.

Resin Applicator   In filament winding, a device that deposits the liquid resin onto the reinforcement band.

Resinoid   A term used for a thermosetting resin, either in its initial temporarily fusible state (uncured), or its final nonfusible state (cured).

Resonance   The movement of electrons from one atom of a molecule or ion, to another atom of the same molecule or ion. Thus, given atoms may remain in a fixed spatial arrangement with their electrons arranged to simultaneously satisfy two or more classical structural formulas. A prototype resonant structure is a benzene ring.

Reticulated Urethane Foams   Low-density urethane foams characterized by a three-dimensional skeletal structure of fibers and interconnecting nodes, with no membranes between the fibers, and containing up to 97% void volume. They are made by (1) burning the membranes with a flash ignition, or (2) treating the structure with a dilute aqueous solution of sodium hydroxide solution, so the thin membranes are preferentially dissolved, leaving the fibers substantially unaffected.

Reticuloendothelial System   A collective term for cells of varying morphology and tissue residence with the common feature of being actively phagocytic.

Reverse Osmosis   The separation of one component of a solution from another component by means of osmotic pressure exerted on a semipermeable membrane. As more osmotic pressure is applied to the more concentrated solution water will begin to flow from the concentrated solution to the less concentrated solution. Reverse osmosis is capable of separating substances $0.001\ \mu m$ to $0.0001\ \mu m$ in size, which include aqueous salts and certain sugars. (The OSMOTIC PRESSURE is a measure of the potential energy difference between the two solutions). See also OSMOSIS.

Reverse Roll Coating   A method of coating where the coating fluid is premetered between a pair of rolls, one of which deposits the coating onto the substrate.

Reynold's Number   Ratio used to determine if the flow of a viscous fluid through a pipe is streamlined or turbulent. Values below 2100 represent streamlined flow, whereas values above 3000 denote turbulent flow, calculated by the formula: $R = DUP/\mu$, where D = inside pipe diameter, U = average flow velocity, P = density of the fluid, and μ = viscosity.

Rheology   The study of flow and deformation properties in terms of stress, strain, and time. See also CONSISTENCY, DILATANCY, NEWTONIAN FLOW, THIXOTROPY, VISCOELASTICITY, VISCOSITY, and YIELD VALUE.

Rheometer   (Plastometer). A device that continuously measures the viscosity and elasticity of resin solutions and polymer melts at high shear rates. The most common type is the EXTRUSION RHEOMETER for thermoplastic melts, while the VISCOMETER is used for measuring the flow properties of fuids.

Rheometry   The experimental determination of the rheological properties of fluid materials.

Rheopecticity   (Rheopexy). The opposite of THIXOTROPY. The viscosity of rheopectic materials increases with time under a constantly applied stress, and decreases upon removal of the stress.

Rheovibron   A dynamic rheometer in which the specimen is clamped between two strain gauges and subjected to a sinusoidally varying tensile strain at fixed frequency while varying the temperature from extreme cold to warm. A direct reading is obtained, called the tan δ.

Rhesus Factor   (Rh Factor). A substance present in the red blood cells of rhesus monkeys, and of about 85% of humans. Those red blood cells that contain this substance are termed Rh−positive. A negative individual may develop anti−Rh antibodies if Rh−positive red cells are transfused. Such antibodies then agglutinate Rh−positive cells, causing adverse hemolytic reactions.

RIA   Abbreviation for *Radio Immunoassay*, an important method used in clinical laboratories, which employs antibodies to detect small concentrations of antigens. A known amount of radiolabeled antigen is added to the test solution, together with an antibody to the antigen. Both radiolabeled and unlabeled compete for binding to the antibody. The amount of radiolabel that binds to the antibody is determined, being inversely proportional to the amount of test antigen. The amount of antigen present in the specimen is determined by knowing that the greater the amount of test antigen present, the less radiolabeled compound will bind to the antibody, and vice versa.

Ribbon Blenders   Mixing devices comprising helical ribbon-shaped blades rotating close to the edge of a U−shaped vessel. They may be used for mixing high viscosity fluids and PVC dry blends.

Rigid Plastic   A plastic exhibiting a modulus of elasticity in flexure or in tension >7000 Kg/cm^2 (10,000 psi) at 23°C and 50% relative humidity. A new system for vinyls proposes the elastic modulus of rigids at >20,000 psi; semi-rigids between 60,000 and 200,000 psi; and flexibles at <60,000 psi.

Rigidity, Modulus of   (Shear Modulus). The slope of the linear portion of the initial stress-strain curve. The greater the slope, the greater the rigidity of the polymer.

Rigisol   A coined term for a plastisol containing a polymerizable diluent plasticizer that polymerizes and cross-links during gelation. The final product has a very high hardness, as opposed to the soft and elastomeric nature of conventional plastisols.

Ring-Opening Polymerization   Polymerization by the molecular unfolding of a cyclic monomer, producing a polymer chain in which the repeat units are joined together by links similar to those of the starting monomer, but now in a linear fashion.

Risk   The possibility of consequences involving mortality, morbidity, or injury to a person.

Risk Assessment   The scientific process by which the toxic properties of a substance are identified and evaluated in order to ascertain the likelihood that exposed humans will be adversely affected, and to characterize the nature of the effects they may experience.

Risk Communication   The two-way exchange of information, concerns, and preferences about risks between decision makers and the general public.

Risk in Health Care Settings   According to the U.S. Centers for Disease Control, the following represent the risks associated with some medical procedures. Risk is expressed as the number of times the event is likely to occur for each million exposures:

Contracting Hepatitis B from infected needle	300,000
Surgical wound infection in high-risk patient	147,000
Surgical wound infection in low-risk patient	10,000
Contracting HIV virus from infected needle	3000
Contracting Hepatitis B from infected doctor	2400
Dying from anesthesia	100
Contracting HIV virus from blood transfusion	40
Anaphylactic death from penicillin	20
Contracting HIV virus from infected doctor	3

Risk Management   The combination of information about risks with economic, political, legal, ethical, and other considerations to make public or private decisions regarding protective policies.

RNA   Abbreviation for *Ribonucleic Acid*.

RNA Polymerase   An enzyme essential in imparting the DNA genetic code to RIBONUCLEIC ACID (RNA).

Rockwell Hardness   The hardness of a material expressed as a number derived from the net increase in depth of indentation as the load of an indentor is increased from a load of 10 Kg to a major load (60–150 Kg), and then returned to the minor load. Various scales are used, depending on the diameter of the indentor and the maximum value of the major load.

Roentgen   The international unit of quantity or dose for X-rays or Gamma rays, equal to the quantity of rays that will produce one electrostatic unit of electricity of either sign in 1 cc of dry air at $0^{\circ}C$ at atmospheric pressure.

Roll Mill   An apparatus for mixing a plastic ingredient of high viscosity with solid particulate compounding ingredients. The rolls turn at different speeds to produce a shearing action to the materials being compounded. The rolls are usually heated when the mill is used for compounding of thermoplastic resins, such as polyurethane and vinyls. In contrast, the rolls are chilled when compounding thermosetting resins such as rubber.

Roller Coating   The process of coating substrates with fluid resins by means of a roller that spreads and meters the coating. The process is often used to apply a contrasting coating onto raised portions of a substrate.

Rosin   A resin obtained as a residue in the distillation of crude turpentine from the sap of the pine tree (gum rosin), or from the extract of the stumps and other parts of the tree (wood rosin).

Rotary Molding   A term sometimes used to denote a type of injection, transfer, compression, or blow molding utilizing a plurality of mold cavities mounted on a rotating table or dial. Not to be confused with ROTATIONAL MOLDING.

Rotational Casting   The process of forming hollow articles from fluid materials by rotating a mold containing a given mass of fluid about one or more axes at relatively low speeds, until the fluid has hardened by heating, cooling, or curing.

Rotational Molding   A variation of the rotational casting process utilizing dry, sinterable powders, such as polyethylene and PVC, rather than fluid materials.

Roving   A form of fibrous glass used in reinforced plastics comprising from 8 to 120 single filaments or strands gathered in a bundle, surface treated with coupling agents to promote adhesion to the plastic.

RP   Abbreviation for *Reinforced Plastic*.

RTP   Abbreviation for *Reinforced Thermoplastic*.

RTV   Abbreviation for *Room Temperature Vulcanizing*, a special characteristic of some elastomers, such as silicones, which do not require heating to cure.

Rubber, Natural   A polymer consisting of cis-1,4-polyisoprene obtained from the latex of certain trees, particularly the *Hevea brasiliensis* tree. Latex, preserved with ammonia, may be shipped and subsequently coagulated to form sheets ready for milling and compounding.

Rubber, Synthetic   A large family of elastic materials whose properties resemble those of natural rubber. Commercially available rubbers are listed in the following:

Rubber, Synthetic

NAME	CHEMICAL NAME	PROPERTIES
Butyl	Isobutene—isoprene copolymer	Low permeability Good aging
EPDM	Ethylene—propylene diene monomer	Excellent environmental resistance
Hypalon	Chlorosulfonated polyethylene	Abrasion resistance Low friction
Neoprene	Polychloroprene	High resiliency
Nitrile	Polybutadiene—acrylonitrile	Abrasion resistance Chemical stability
Norsorex	Polynorbornene	High tensile strength Resistant to acids
SBR	Styrene—butadiene	Abrasion resistance
Silicone	Polysiloxanes	Biocompatibility Chemical stability
Synthetic Rubber	Polyisoprene	General purpose
PUR	Polyurethane rubber	Abrasion resistance Tear resistance
Teflon Rubber	Fluorocarbon copolymer	Environmental resistance No stick surface

Rubber Elasticity   The elastic behavior of polymers well above their glass transition temperature, where they exhibit high recovery at strains up to several hundred percent of original. Theoretically, if the polymer is perfectly elastic, then all the work done during stretching will be stored as strain energy.

Rubber-Processing Chemicals   Compounding ingredients for the production of rubber-based products. The following are terms for the most important chemicals:

(1) *Rubber Accelerator*—speeds cross-linking of rubber. Example: 2,2′ dithio bis(benzotriazole).

(2) *Rubber Activator*—renders accelerators more potent. Example: zinc oxide with stearic acid.

(3) *Rubber Antidegradant*—inclusive term denoting antioxidants, antiozonants, and stabilizers.

(4) *Rubber Antioxidant*—chemicals that protect rubber products against oxidative degradation. Examples: N-isopropyl, N-phenylene diamine.

(5) *Rubber Antiozonant*—chemicals that coat the surface, thus protecting against ozone. Examples: waxes; N,N' bis(1,4 dimethylpentyl)-1,4 phenylenediamine.

(6) *Rubber Lubricant*—chemicals that ease the flowing of rubber during milling, extrusion, molding, etc. Example: stearic acid.

(7) *Rubber Peptizer*—agents that promote chemical breakdown of rubber during mastication. Example: pentachlorothiophenol.

(8) *Rubber Plasticizer*—a peptizer oil, softener, or extender. Example: bis(butoxyethoxyethyl)glutarate.

(9) *Rubber Retarder* — lengthens the amount of time before onset of the curing process. Example: phthalic anhydride.

(10) *Rubber Stabilizer* — antioxidant that protects rubber between polymerization and curing steps. Example: tris(nonylphenyl) phosphite.

(11) *Rubber Sulfur Donor* — organic polysulfide that replaces some elemental sulfur in rubber compounds, and promotes curing by monosulfide cross-links. Example: tetramethyldithiuram disulfide.

(12) *Rubber Vulcanizer* — chemicals that cure rubber by forming cross-links among polymer chains. Examples: sulfur, organic peroxides, and phenolic resins.

Rubbery Flow   The viscoelastic region of linear amorphous polymers in which the modulus drops rapidly as temperature increases, after the plateau of the rubbery state.

Rubbery Plateau   The relatively flat portion of the modulus versus temperature curve of linear amorphous polymers.

Rubbery State   The viscoelastic state of a linear amorphous polymer, extending from 30°C above T_g to about 80°C above T_g. In this temperature range, a polymer should exhibit rubber elasticity, with a modulus of about 10^6 Pa.

Runner   In injection molding, the feed channel that connects the sprue with the cavity gate.

Runnerless Injection Molding   A molding process in which the runners are kept hot, so the molded parts are ejected with only small gates attached.

S

Sampling   The methods and techniques used in obtaining representative test samples of raw materials, components, and finished products for quality control. Rules for sampling medical devices have been established by the FDA. These rules are periodically reviewed and updated in cooperation with industry.

SAN   Abbreviation for *Styrene-Acrylonitrile Polymers*.

Saponification   The chemical reaction in which an ester is heated with aqueous alkali, such as sodium hydroxide, to form an alcohol (usually glycerol), and the sodium salt of the corresponding acid.

Saturated Compounds   Compounds whose available atomic valence bonds are attached to other atoms of the same compound, and thus cannot react with other elements or compounds.

Saturation   (1) The state in which all available valence bonds are attached to other atoms. This applies particularly to carbon atoms. (2) The state of a solution when it holds the maximum equilibrium quantity of dissolved matter at a given temperature.

Scanning Electron Microscopy (SEM)   Electron microscopy method that utilizes the secondary electronic emissions from a surface when bombarded with an electron beam. SEM is advantageous in the great depth of field even at high magnifications, although at some loss of resolution. Ideal for examination of surface morphologies of both biological and polymeric structures.

Scavenger   Any substance added to a system or mixture to consume, inactivate, or chelate traces of unwanted material.

Scleroprotein   Any of a large class of proteins that have a supporting or protective function in tendons, bones, cartilages, ligaments, etc. They include collagens, elastins, and keratins.

Scleroscope   An instrument for measuring impact resilience by dropping a ram with a flattened cone tip from a specified height onto the specimen, then measuring the height of rebound.

Scope   Suffix generally indicating an instrument for visualizing internal body structures, but including other methods of examination.

"Scotch Tape" Test   A qualitative method for evaluating the adhesion of a coating to a plastic substrate. Pressure-sensitive adhesive tape, "Scotch Tape," is applied to an area of the plastic article, which is sometimes crosshatched with scratched lines. Adhesion is considered adequate if no coating is removed when the tape is forcibly and quickly removed.

Scratch Hardness   The inherent resistance of a material to scratching by another material. The Birnbaum scratch test is performed by moving the specimen laterally on a microscope stage, under a diamond point loaded with 3 grams of force. The width of the scratch is then measured by a screw micrometer piece, and the hardness value is expressed as the load in kilograms divided by the square of the width of the scratch in millimeters. Other tests employ pencils of differing hardnesses.

Screw   In extrusion, the shaft machined with helical grooves that conveys and plasticates the molten plastic from the hopper outlet through the heated barrel and out through the die.

SDS-Gel Electrophoresis   The most widely used method for determination of protein polypeptide chain molecular weight. The protein is treated with sodium dodecyl sulfate (SDS), which associates with the chain to form electrically-charged sulphate species. Upon electrophoresis on a polyacrylamide gel, the rate of migration is proportional to log M of the protein molecular weight.

Secant Modulus   The ratio of total stress to the corresponding strain at any specific point in the stress-strain curve. It is expressed in force per unit area, at the specified strain.

Second Order Transition   See GLASS TRANSITION.

Secondary Plasticizer   A plasticizer that is less compatible with a given resin than the primary plasticizer, and would thus tend to exude or cause surface tackiness if used above a critical concentration.

Secondary Transition   In an amorphous polymer, a transition of smaller magnitude than the main glass transition. It nearly always occurs at a temperature lower than T_g, and is usually labelled as β, τ-transition, with T_g being labelled as the α transition.

Sedative   A natural or synthetic therapeutic agent having the property of inducing relaxation and varying degrees of depression of the central nervous system. The major types are (1) chlorine substitution products, (2) ethyl alcohol derivatives, and (3) certain aldehydes and ketones. Sedatives are almost always prescription drugs.

Seeded Polymerization   A polymerization procedure in which particles of preformed polymer act as nucleating agents (seeds) for further polymerization.

Segmented Polymers   Elastomers with a two-phase macromolecular structure, where hard segments separate to form discrete domains in a matrix of soft segments. In the relaxed state, spatially separated hard and soft segments can be shown to exist by X-ray diffraction. It is theorized that the hard segments are held together in discrete domains through the action of hydrogen bonds and to a lesser extent, VAN DER WAALS FORCES.

Segmented Polyurethanes   Block copolymers containing the recurring urethane $-(NHCOO-)$ linkages. These elastomers consist of alternating hard and soft segments, with the hard segments tending to aggregate into domains, surrounded by a matrix of soft segments, with the hard segments acting as physical cross-links for the soft segment domains. These multiblock polymers exhibit very good hemocompatibility, and have very high physicomechanical properties even at low durometers.

Self-Extinguishing   The inherent ability of a polymer to cease burning once the flame source has been removed. Examples of self-extinguishing polymers are: PVC, PVC-PVAc copolymers, polyvinylidene chloride, nylon, and casein.

Self-Vulcanizing   Pertaining to a polymer (rubber or adhesive) that undergoes vulcanization without the application of heat.

SEM   Abbreviation for *Scanning Electron Microscopy.*

Semi-Interpenetrating Polymer Network   (Semi-IPN). An interpenetrating polymer network in which one of the polymers is linear rather than cross-linked. Example: a linear polyurethane that is reacted with a cross-linking silicone. The physical properties of the semi-IPN are intermediate between the two pure polymers.

Semiconducting Polymers   Most polymers are insulators, with conductivities below 10^{-12} S/cm. Some polymers may be synthesized having electrical conductivities in the range of 10^2 to 10^{-10}, and are thus called semiconducting.

Semicrystalline Polymer   A polymer that is only partially crystalline, usually in the range of 30–80%. See also CRYSTALLINE POLYMERS.

Semipermeable Membrane   (1) A membrane that is only permeable to the molecules of a solution, but not to the solvent. Example: a membrane that is permeable to water vapor, but is impermeable to liquid water. (2) A membrane that is only permeable to the solvent molecules of a solution, but not to the solute. Example: a membrane permeable to water, but impermeable to salt.

Semirigid Plastic   A plastic that displays a modulus of elasticity either in flexure or tension of between 700 and 7000 kg/cm^2 at 23°C and 50 percent relative humidity.

Semisynthetic   A product involving a chemical reaction that is based on or is derived from a natural material, but which rarely if ever occurs in nature. Examples are cellulose modifications (methyl cellulose, cellulose acetate butyrate, carboxymethyl cellulose), and several modified starches.

Septicemia   Blood poisoning. The presence of pathological organisms, or their toxins, in circulating blood.

Sequenator   An automatic determination of the amino acid sequence of a protein. Based on the Edman method of repeated sequential removal and identification of the N-terminus amino acid of a polypeptide chain.

Sequestration   The formation of a coordination complex by certain phosphates with metallic ions in solution so that the usual precipitation reactions of the latter are prevented or retarded. The term may be used for any instance in which an ion is prevented from exhibiting its usual properties due to close combination with an added material. Two groups are important: (1) aminocarboxylic acids, such as EDTA, and (2) hydroxycarboxylic acids such as citric, gluconic, and tartaric acids. See also CHELATING AGENT.

Serological   The branch of medical science dealing with the characteristics of SERUM, especially with regard to its immunity reactions.

Serum   (1) The fluid portion of the blood obtained after removal of fibrinogen and blood cells, distinguished from the plasma in circulating blood. (2) A clear aqueous fluid, especially those that moisten the surface of serous membranes, or is extravasated during inflammation.

Serum Albumin   Blood albumin that comprises 60% of the plasma proteins. The adsorption of plasma albumin onto biomaterials surfaces is generally considered to "passivate" the surface against mural thrombus.

Set   (1) The physicochemical conversion of a polymer into a fixed or hardened state. (2) To convert into a fixed or hardened state by chemical or physical action, such as condensation, polymerization, oxidation, vulcanization, gelation, hydration, cross-linking, or evaporation of volatile components.

Shear   An action or stress resulting from applied forces, which causes two contiguous parts of a body to slide relative to each other in a direction parallel to their plane of contact. Shear is the primary action of mixers, such as:

SHEAR TYPE	QUANTITY (SEC-1)
High-speed dissolver	50–100,000
Low-speed mixer	20–100
Pump	10–200

SHEAR TYPE	QUANTITY (SEC-1)
Brush	5000–20,000
Spray	1000–40,000
Rolling	3000–40,000
Dip	10–100
Flow coating	10·100
Gravity leveling	1/100

Shear Modulus   The ratio of shearing stress to shearing strain within the proportional limit of a material.

Shear Rate   The overall velocity over the cross section of a channel with which molten polymer layers are gliding along each other or along the wall in laminar flow.

Shear Strength   The maximum load necessary to shear the specimen in such a manner that the moving portion completely clears the stationary portion.

Shear Stress   The stress developed in a polymer when the layers in a cross section are gliding along each other or along the wall of the channel (under laminar flow conditions).

Shear Thickening   (Dilatancy). Non-Newtonian flow behavior in which the apparent viscosity increases upon application of shear forces. In some cases, the volume of the fluid increases, thus the material appears to dilate. It occurs principally with suspensions of irregularly shaped particles.

Shear Thinning   (Pseudoplasticity). Non-Newtonian flow behavior in which the apparent viscosity decreases upon application of shear forces. Most polymer melts and solutions behave in this fashion, particularly at low shear rates in the range of 100 to 1000 s^{-1}.

Sheet   A thin, continuous web of plastic of uniform cross section. The terms sheet and film are closely related. Sheets are distinguished from film only according to thickness: A web of $<0.010''$ (10 mils) is called a FILM; a web of $>0.010''$ (10 mils) is called a sheet.

Shelf Life   (Storage Life, Working Life). (1) The length of time over which a product will remain fit for use during storage under specified conditions. (2) The period of time during which a package coating, adhesive, or reactive fluid may be stored under specified temperature conditions, and remain suitable for use.

Shock   A group of symptoms that occur when a person's circulatory system collapses. It is classified depending on cause, such as:

(1) *Hypovolemic Shock*—reduction in blood volume as a result of hemorrhage.

(2) *Cardiogenic Shock*—due to heart failure.

(3) *Septic Shock*—due to overwhelming bacterial infection.

(4) *Neurogenic Shock*—due to unexplained dilatation of capacitance blood vessels.

Shore Hardness   See INDENTATION HARDNESS.

Shortstopping Agent   A substance used in a polymerization reaction to end

197

the chain elongation at a predetermined point, thus controlling the molecular weight. Examples: the use of tetraethylsilanol in silicone rubbers, and the use of monoamines in polyurethanes.

Shot   The yield from one complete injection molding cycle, including any scrap.

Shot Capacity   The maximum weight of extrudate that can be delivered to an injection mold by one stroke of the ram.

Shrink Packaging   A method of wrapping articles utilizing pre-stretched (oriented) films, which when heated shrink tightly around the articles.

Shrinkage Allowance   The dimensional allowance that must be made in molds to compensate for any expected shrinkage of the plastic compound upon cooling.

SI   The *International System of Units*, adopted by the General Conference on weights and measures, an organization dedicated to developing and unifying the metric system. There are seven base quantities in the SI (*Systeme International d'Unites*) and seven corresponding base units, as in the following table:

QUANTITY	SYMBOL FOR QUANTITY	UNIT	SYMBOL FOR UNIT
Length	l	Meter	m
Mass	m	Kilogram	kg
Time	t	Second	s
Electricity	I	Ampere	A
Temperature	t	Kelvin	K
Substance	n	Mole	mol
Luminosity	Iv	Candela	cd

Sigma Blade   A rotating agitator set horizontally in a kneading chamber used for mixing high-viscosity fluids. The blade is shaped resembling a Greek capital sigma lying on its side. Some kneaders have two such blades which overlap as they turn to provide maximum mixing efficiency.

Sigma Bond   A covalent bond directed along the line joining the centers of two atoms. They are the normal single bonds found in organic molecules.

Sigmoidoscopy   Visual examination of the sigmoid colon just above the rectum with a lighted tube.

Silane Coupling Agents   Gaseous or liquid compounds of silicon and hydrogen (Si_nH_{2n+2}), analogous to alkanes or saturated hydrocarbons. Organo-functional silanes coatings are noted for improving the bonding of organic polymer systems to inorganic substrates. The $Si(OR_3)$ portion reacts with the inorganic reinforcement, while the organofunctional (vinyl, amino, epoxy, etc.) group reacts with the resin. Example: improving the wetting and bonding characteristics of pyrogenic silica particles to silicone rubber. Some available silane coupling agents are:

   — N-β(Aminoethyl)-τ-Aminopropyltrimethoxy Silane
   — τ-Aminopropyltriethoxy Silane
   — Bis (β Hydroxyethyl)-τ-Aminopropyltriethoxy Silane

   — β (3,4 Epoxycyclohexyl) Ethyltrimethoxy Silane
   — τ-Glycidoxypropyltrimethoxy Silane
   — τ-Methacryloxypropyltrimethoxy Silane
   — Vinyl Trichloro Silane
   — Vinyl Triethoxy Silane
   — Vinyl-tris (β-Methoxyethyl) Silane

Silica SiO_2. (Silicon Dioxide). A naturally occurring substance found in sand, quartz, opal, agate, etc. In medical polymers, synthetic silicas are frequently used as thixotropic and reinforcing agents. Synthetic (amorphous) silicas are made by heating silicon compounds at high temperatures. See also PYROGENIC SILICA.

Silicone Antifoams   Polydimethylsiloxane fluids compounded with high surface area silica, available as compounds and emulsions. The fluid-coated silica particles create "weak spots" in bubble films, thus acting as defoamers.

Silicone Foams   Foams based on fluid silicone resins made by mixing the resins with a catalyst and blowing agent, pouring the mixture into a mold, and curing at room temperature for about 10 hours.

Silicone Gels   Lightly cross-linked, unfilled polymethylsiloxane gels, characterized by low cohesive strength, which behave as fluids at low distortion, and contain some free silicone fluids not bonded into the cross-linked matrix. Used in breast, testicular, chin, and custom implants.

Silicone-Polycarbonate Copolymers   Thermoplastic copolymers varying from strong elastomers to rigid engineering plastics depending on composition. They can be thermoprocessed into optically clear films.

Silicones   An important family of semi-organic polymers comprising chains of alternating silicon and oxygen atoms (siloxane), modified with various organic groups attached to the silicon atoms. Depending on the nature of the attached organic groups and the extent of cross-linking between the molecules, the polymers may be (1) fluids, (2) gels, (3) gums, and (4) solid resins. In general, the medical-grade silicones are composed of dimethyl siloxane groups, and are among the most stable and biocompatible polymers used in medical devices. Silicones are extensively used in the production of medical devices as: tubing, catheters, surface lubricants, tissue substitutes, penile prostheses, finger joints, and cardiovascular components.

Silicones, Controlled Delivery Products   The following is a list of current controlled delivery products employing silicones:

PRODUCT	DRUG	SYSTEM
ANTIANGINALS		
Nitrodisc	Nitroglycerine (Searle)	Transdermal matrix
Transderm Nitro	Nitroglycerine (Ciba–Geigy)	Transdermal reservoir
Deponit	Nitroglycerine (Pharma Schwartz)	Transdermal adhesive/matrix

Silicones, Controlled Delivery Products

PRODUCT	DRUG	SYSTEM
ANTIFERTILITY		
Progestasert	Progesterone (Alza)	Intrauterine Reservoir
Norplant	Levonorgestrel (Leiras)	Subcutaneous implant reservoir
GROWTH PROMOTANT		
Compudose	17-B-Estradiol (Eli Lilly)	Implant matrix

Silicones, Controlled Delivery Systems   The classes of therapeutic agents successfully delivered through silicones are:

- Contraceptives
- Abortifacients
- Spermicides
- Analgesics
- Antipsychotics
- Antibiotics
- Local anesthetics
- General anesthetics
- Hypnotics
- Sedatives
- Hypotensives
- Antimitotics
- Muscle relaxants
- Antineoplastics
- Anticholinergics
- Anticonvulsants
- Antischistosomals
- Hypoglycemics
- Growth promotants
- Antipyretics
- Antiinflammatories
- Antianginals

Silicones, Medical Grades   The following is a compilation of silicone elastomer selection by biological testing, quality, and manufacturing assurance for various grades:

	GRADES			
	IMPLANT	MEDICAL	CLEAN	COMMERCIAL
BIOTEST DATA AVAILABLE				
2-year implant	Yes	No	No	No
90-day implant	Yes	Yes	No	No
USP Class VI	Yes	Yes	No	No
Pyrogen	Yes	Yes	No	No
Skin sensitization	Yes	Yes	No	No
LOT QA TESTS				
Cell culture	Yes	Yes	No	No
Metals contents	Yes	Yes	No	No
Physicals	Yes	Yes	Yes	Some
MANUFACTURING				
Lots matched	Yes	Yes	No	No
FDA/GMP's	Yes	Yes	No	No
Retained samples	4 yrs.	4 yrs.	4 yrs.	3 mos.
Strained, mesh	200	200	200	120
Lot certification	Yes	Yes	Yes	No

Silicones, Pharmaceutical Uses   The following is a list of current pharmaceutical uses of silicones:

- Medical adhesives
- Powder treatments
- Medical elastomers
- Sheeting
- Fluids/Emulsions/antifoams
- Silylation agents
- Topical personal care products
- Tubing

Silicones, Urology Applications   Silicone elastomers and gels are widely used in the manufacture of foley, mushroom, and ureteral catheters; suprapubic urine drainage systems; testicular and penile implants; and artificial sphincters.

Siliconization   A general term denoting the reversible coating of surfaces with low-viscosity silicone fluids, as an aid in surface lubrication, to produce hydrophobic surfaces (complete drainage), to make surfaces nonadherent (for easier cleaning), and to improve blood compatibility.

Siloxanes   See SILICONES.

Sinter Molding   The process of compacting thermoplastic particles under pressure at temperatures below their melting point until the particles become sintered together, often followed by further heating and/or post forming. Many fluorocarbon resin parts are made by sinter molding or extrusion. Example: blown PTFE, which is used as vascular grafts, and as a tissue ingrowth platform.

Sinter Plastic Coating   A coating process in which the article to be coated is preheated to sintering temperature and immersed in a plastic powder, then withdrawn and heated to a higher temperature to fuse the sintered coating adhering to the article.

Sintering   The welding together of powdered plastic particles at temperatures just below the melting or fusion point. The particles are fused (sintered) together to form a relatively strong mass, but the mass as a whole does not melt. Sintering can be achieved by a combination of any of the following mechanisms: (1) viscous or plastic flow, (2) evaporation and condensation, and (3) volume diffusion and surface diffusion.

Sizing   The process of applying a material on a substrate in order to fill pores and thus reduce adsorption of adhesives, water, or polymers; otherwise to modify surface properties of the substrate to improve adhesion.

Skin Adhesives   Those adhesives, mainly pressure sensitive adhesives, designed for use in conjunction with medical devices and transdermal therapeutic systems. See also PSA and PSA, MEDICAL APPLICATIONS. The major classes are summarized below:

ADHESIVE CLASS	POLYMER TYPE
Rubber-Based	Karaya gum
	Styrenebutadiene
	Polyisoprene
	Polybutene
	Polyisobutylene

Skin Adhesives

ADHESIVE CLASS	POLYMER TYPE
Polyacrylic-Based	Ethyl acrylate
	2-Ethylhexyl acrylate
	Isooctyl acrylate
Polysiloxane-Based	Polydimethyl siloxane
	Polymethylphenyl siloxane
	Siloxane blends
	Polysilicate resins

Slip (1) With reference to adhesives, the ability to position the adherends after an adhesive has been applied to the surfaces. (2) The ability of a surface to display low tack, and a low coefficient of friction.

Slip Agent A modifier that acts as an internal lubricant that exudes to the surface of a plastic during processing, to provide lubricity and reduce the coefficient of friction.

Slippage The movement of substrates with respect to each other during the bonding process.

Slitting The conversion of plastic film or sheeting to several smaller widths by means of knives. The operation may be performed in tandem as the material emerges from a production unit (in-line slitting), or by slitting the rolls (roll slicing). Slitting knives may be flat-blade knives, razor blades, or circular knives.

Slot Extrusion A method of extruding film in which the molten thermoplastic is forced through a straight slot.

Small Manufacturer According to FDA, any entity with fewer than 500 employees, unless there are persuasive arguments against this defined level.

Soaps, Metallic Products derived by reacting fatty acids with metals, widely used as stabilizers and slip agents in plastics. The fatty acids commonly used are: lauric, stearic, ricinoleic, naphthenic octoic. Typical metals are: aluminum, barium, calcium, cadmium, magnesium, tin, and zinc.

Soft Segment The blocks in a block copolymer thermoplastic elastomer which have a T_g and T_m well below room temperature, so they retain molecular flexibility and elasticity at room temperature. These segments thus impart elastomeric properties to the copolymers.

Softening Range (1) For flexible thermoplastics, the range of temperature in which a plastic exhibits a sudden and substantial decrease in hardness. (2) For rigid thermoplastics, the range of temperature in which a plastic exhibits a change from a rigid to a soft state.

Solid Matter in its most highly concentrated form, where atoms are generally more closely packed than in the liquid or gaseous state, and thus more resistant to deformation.

Solid Casting The process of forming solid articles by pouring a fluid resin or dispersion into an open mold, causing the material to solidify by curing or heating at atmospheric pressure, then demolding the formed article.

Solid Content The percentage by weight of the nonvolatile matter in a solution or dispersion.

Solid State Chemistry   Study of the exact arrangement of atoms in solids, especially crystals, with particular emphasis on imperfections or irregularities in the electronic and atomic patterns within a crystal structure, and the effects of these on the physical, electrical, and chemical properties.

Solid State Polymerization   Polymerization with the monomer in the solid crystalline state, especially those involving vinyl monomers initiated by high-energy radiation, such as an electron beam.

Solubility   The inherent ability of one substance to blend uniformly with another. Examples: solid in liquid, liquid in liquid, gas in liquid, gas in gas. Liquids and gases are often said to be miscible in other liquids, rather than soluble.

Solubility Parameter   Symbol δ. Mathematically, the square root of the cohesive energy density of a material. A measure of solvency or a means of predicting whether a particular solvent will dissolve a resin. Practically, it also allows prediction of compatibility among chemicals and resins, since it states that any chemical must have the same affinity for resins, as resins-to-resins themselves. The calculated solubility parameters of some biomaterials and blood components are shown below:

POLYMER OR BLOOD COMPONENT	SOLUBILITY PARAMETER δ
Aromatic polyurethane	
Soft segment	10.5
Hard segment	13.0
Aliphatic polyurethane	
Soft segment	9.4
Hard segment	12.0
Dacron	9.7 – 10.7
Epoxy	11.5
Nylon	13.6
Polyethylene	7.9
Polystyrene	9.1
PTMEG	8.0 – 12.0
PVAc	9.4
PVC	9.5
PVDC	12.2
PMMA	9.4
Silicone oil	6.2
Silicone rubber	7.3 – 7.6
Teflon	6.2
Cholesterol and esters	8.4 – 8.9
Triglycerides	8.0 – 8.3
Phospholipids	> 16.0
Proteins (non-denatured)	> 18.0
Water	23.2

Solubility Parameters (Lubricants, Polymers)   For internal lubrication, the overall solubility parameter of the lubricant should be within $\pm 3\ (MPa)^{1/2}$

of the polymer. If higher, it may be a filler, tackifier, nucleating agent, etc. (Notice that in this table, the solubility parameters are given in MPa units, as well as the more conventional calories. To convert calories to MPa multiply by 2.05). The solubility parameters of commercially important lubricants and some prototype polymers are shown below:

I. LUBRICANTS	CALORIES$^{1/2}$	(MPa)$^{1/2}$
Stearic acid monomer	9.4	19.0
Stearic acid dimer	8.7	17.8
Glycerol monostearate	8.5	17.5
Stearamide	9.7	19.8
Divalent stearates	8.8	18.0
Alkali metal stearates	9.3	19.0
Polyethylene wax	8.3	17.0
Oxidized waxes	8.8−9.3	18.0−19.0
Long chain esters	8.5−9.0	17.5−18.5
II. POLYMERS		
Polyolefins	7.8−8.5	16.0−17.5
Styrenics, SBR	8.8−9.2	18.0−18.8
PVC homopolymers	9.3−9.5	19.0−19.5
PVC copolymers, NBR/PVC	9.0−9.3	18.5−19.0
Cellulosics	10.0−11.2	20.5−23.0

Solute   That constituent of a solution which is considered to be molecularly dissolved in the solvent. The solvent is usually present in larger amounts than the solute.

Solution   A molecularly homogenous mixture of two or more components, such as a polymer dissolved in a solvent, which forms more or less spontaneously, will not settle, and has no fixed proportions of the components. The term also embraces gas dissolved in another gas, and a liquid in a liquid.

Solution, Colloidal   A liquid colloidal dispersion, often called a *sol*. Since colloidal particles are much larger than molecules, it is strictly incorrect to call such dispersions solutions.

Solution Coating   Any coating process employing a solvent solution of a resin, as opposed to dispersion, hot-melt, or uncured thermosetting resin. The film is obtained strictly by solvent evaporation.

Solution Polymerization   A polymerization method in which the monomer or mixture of monomers is dissolved in a nonmonomeric liquid solvent at the beginning of the process. The solution process is most advantageous when the polymers are to be used as coatings, films, or adhesives.

Solutrope   A ternary mixture having two liquid phases between which one component is distributed in an apparent ratio varying with concentration from less than one to more than one. That is, the solute may be selectively dissolved in one or the other of the phases or solvents depending on the concentration. This phenomenon has been compared to azeotropic behavior.

Solvent   A substance capable of molecularly dissolving another substance (solute) to form a uniformly dispersed mixture (solution). Solvents are (1) polar, with high dielectric constants, or (2) nonpolar. Water, the most used solvent is strongly polar, while hydrocarbons are nonpolar. The most widely used organic-based solvents are: alcohols, esters, glycol ethers, ketones, aliphatic hydrocarbons, chlorinated hydrocarbons, and nitroparaffins.

Solvent, Aprotic   A solvent that cannot act as a proton acceptor or donor, i.e., as an acid or base.

Solvent, Classes   Solvents may be classified as: (1) Terpenes: turpentine; (2) Hydrocarbons: aliphatics, aromatics; (3) Oxygenated: alcohols, esters, ketones, ether alcohols; (4) Miscellaneous: chlorinated, nitroparaffins, furans (furfural alcohol, furfural, THF).

Solvent, Latent   (Co-Solvent). An organic liquid that will dissolve a polymer in combination with an active solvent.

Solvent Drying   Removal of water from surfaces by means of an organic solvent that displaces it preferentially. Examples: alcohols, acetone, fluorinated solvents.

Solvent Extraction   A separation operation which may involve three types of mixtures: (1) two or more solids, (2) a solid and a liquid, and (3) a mixture of two or more liquids. One or more of the components are removed (extracted) by exposing the mixture to a solvent, in which the component to be removed is soluble. This procedure is often called leaching, especially if the solvent is water.

Solvent Polishing   A method for improving the gloss of thermoplastic articles by immersion in, or spraying with a solvent that will dissolve surface irregularities, followed by evaporation of the solvent. Plastics such as polycarbonate and polystyrene, which are subject to crazing, are treated by spraying or are exposed to solvent vapors in a vapor degreaser.

Solvent Stress Cracking   A form of environmental stress cracking when the liquid causing the cracking also has a solventing effect on the polymer. This phenomenon occurs primarily with rigid polymers, such as polycarbonate, PMMA, PS, etc.

Solvent Welding   The process of joining articles made of thermoplastic resins by applying a solvent capable of softening the surfaces to be joined, and pressing the softened surfaces together. Adhesion is attained by means of evaporation of the solvent, absorption of the solvent into adjacent material, and/or polymerization of the solvent adhesive.

Sorbent   A substance capable of either absorbing or adsorbing another substance.

Sorption   A general term signifying the binding of one substance to another by any of three mechanisms: (1) adsorption, (2) absorption, and (3) persorption.

SPE   Abbreviation for *Society of Plastics Engineers*.

Specialty Chemicals   In the U.S., specialty chemicals make up a $47 billion market divided into almost fifty categories. Among the categories: agrochemicals are $5.5 billion, biomaterials $2.5 billion, adhesives $1.4 billion, catalysts $1.2 billion, electronic chemicals $3.6 billion, and water management chemicals $1.2 billion. In many of these markets, products have high added value and are routinely sold for between $20 and $100 per pound.

Specific Adhesion   Adhesion between two surfaces that are held together by valence forces of the same type as those that give rise to cohesion, as opposed to mechanical adhesion in which the adhesive holds the parts together by interlocking action.

Specific Gravity   The ratio of the weight of a given volume of a substance to that of an equal volume of water at the same temperature, usually room temperature. The term apparent specific gravity is used to denote the specific gravity of a porous solid when the volume used in the calculation is considered to exclude the permeable voids. The term bulk specific gravity denotes specific gravity measurements in which a volume of a solid includes both the permeable and impermeable voids.

Specific Heat   (1) The ratio of the thermal capacity of a substance to that of water at $15°C$. (2) The amount of heat required to raise a specific mass of substance by one degree at a specific temperature, expressed as $cal/g/°C$, or $Btu/lb/°F$.

Specific Viscosity   The specific viscosity of a polymer solution of known concentration is numerically equal to the relative viscosity minus one. It represents the increase in viscosity that is attributable to the polymeric solute only.

Specific Volume   (1) The volume of a unit of weight of a material. (2) The reciprocal of density. Specific volume is expressed in ft^3/lb, gal/lb, or $ml/gram$.

Spectrophotometer   An instrument used to measure and quantify colors, and used as an aid in the formulation of colorants to match a given sample under all types of illumination. The instrument produces a curve representing the amounts of light energy the specimen will absorb over the visible spectrum range. Matching this curve assures that the developed compound will match the control color under all lighting conditions.

Spectroscopy   A branch of analytical chemistry devoted to identification of elements and elucidation of atomic and molecular structure by measurement of the radiant energy absorbed or emitted by a substance in any wavelength of the electromagnetic spectrum in response to excitation by an external source. According to the wavelength involved, spectroscopy is usually identified as: gamma, X-ray, ultraviolet, visible, infrared, microwave, and radiofrequency.

Spectrum   The radiant energy fingerprint emitted by a substance as a characteristic and diagnostic band of wavelengths, by which it can be unequivocably identified.

Spherulite   A round aggregate of radiating crystals with a fibrous appearance present in most crystalline polymers. They originate from a nucleus such as a catalyst residue, a chance fluctuation in density, a contaminant particle, etc.

Sphygmomanometer   The familiar instrument for measuring arterial blood pressure, consisting of: a rubberized cuff, a bulb to create pressure, and a gauge that indicates the blood pressure values.

SPI   Abbreviation for *Society of the Plastics Industry*.

Spinneret   An extrusion machine fitted with a die containing multiple tiny openings, through which a plastic melt or solution is forced to produce fine fibers and filaments. Most synthetic yarns are fabricated in this fashion, including dacron, nylon, acrylic, and polyurethane.

Spinning   The process of forming synthetic fibers by extrusion of a plastic melt or solution. There are three main processes: (1) melt spinning, in which the polymer compound is heated to melt temperature; (2) dry spinning, where the extrudate is subjected to a hot atmosphere that removes the solvent by flash evaporation; and (3) wet spinning, where the jet or spinneret is immersed in a nonsolvent fluid, which either diffuses the solvent or chemically reacts with the fiber composition. The spinning operation is often followed by stretching to orient the polymer molecules, conferring a high degree of mechanical properties to the fibers.

Spirometer, Diagnostic   A Class II device used in pulmonary function testing to measure the volume of gas moving in and out of the lungs.

Spirometer, Monitoring   A Class II device used to continuously measure tidal volume (volume of gas inhaled during each respiration cycle) or minute volume (tidal volume multiplied by the rate of respiration for 1 minute) for evaluation of ventilatory status.

Spontaneous Combustion   The process of increasing the temperature of a material to a point where it ignites without drawing heat from its surroundings.

Spontaneous Ignition   A substance proceeding without constraint by internal impulse or outside energy (flame, sparks, hot or glowing bodies) to kindle or set fire. Due to quick oxidation or combustion due to chemical, electrical, bacterial, or physical processes (vibration, pressure, friction).

Spray Coating   The application of a plastic coating to a substrate by means of a spray gun.

Spray Drying   The method by which a polymerized emulsion is sprayed onto a heated cylinder or conical bottomed container, and from which the dried resin is mechanically removed by scraping or by a pneumatic blast.

Spread Coating   A process for coating fabrics, sheets, films, and the like with fluid resins, such as solutions, plastisols, etc. The substrate is supported on a carrier, and the fluid material is applied by means of a blade that regulates the thickness of the coating. The deposit is then fused to the substrate by heat, evaporation, chemical reaction, etc.

Sprue   In injection or transfer molding, the main feeding channel that connects the mold filling orifice with the runners leading to each cavity.

Stabilization   The act of reducing or eliminating unwanted degradative effects on polymers. Achieved by physical incorporation of the agent(s), or by copolymerization.

Stabilizer   Any substance that tends to keep a compound, mixture, or solution from changing its form or chemical nature. Stabilizers retard, preserve, and inhibit unwanted chemical reactions. The most important stabilizers are those that protect plastics from the effects of heat, evidenced by a change in color, lowering of physical properties, and exudation of components. Other stabilizers perform specialized functions such as: an emulsion stabilizer serves to keep emulsions, suspensions, and the like from separating. A viscosity stabilizer is used to retard viscosity increases on aging. An antioxidant is used primarily to protect rubber and plastics from deterioration by oxidation. An ultraviolet stabilizer functions primarily by absorbing UV light, thus protecting the polymer from light degradation.

Stain   Any compound, or mixture of dyes, used to color bacteria, tissue, cells, etc., to facilitate microscopic examination.

Standard   (1) Anything taken as an objective basis of comparison. (2) Anything taken by general consent as the basis of comparison. Standards attempt to create a common language, and frequently encompass four descriptive areas:

- The recommended practice is a type of standard that describes an accepted procedure for doing something. Example: AAMI recommended practice on sterilization and sterility assurance.
- A testing method is an agreed upon way of measuring something.
- A standard classification describes categories of objects or concepts. Example: white-cell differential test in which white cells are categorized in a standardized fashion based on cellular morphology.
- A specification, which is perhaps the most common of all standards, sets limits on the characteristics of a product or material. Specifications can be of two types: design and performance.

See also ASTM CONSENSUS STANDARDS.

Standards, International Organizations   To date the only ''standard'' has been established by ASTM, while the other organizations have provided ''guidelines.'' These guidelines have tended to follow ASTM fairly closely. The following is a current list of organizations:

ASTM:	American Society for Testing and Materials 1916 Race Street Philadelphia, PA
TRIPARTITE:	Tripartite biocompatibility guidance for medical devices. Developed by medical device authorities of the U.S.(FDA), United Kingdom, and Canada, April 24, 1987.
BSI:	British Standards Institute 2 Park Street London, England W1A 2BS

AFNOR: French Normalization Committee
                    S90−700 December 1986
ISO: International Organization for Standardization
                    ISO/TC 150: Focuses on biocompatibility and hemocompatibility.
                    ISO/TC 194: Focuses on biological evaluations of medical/dental materials and devices.

Static Eliminators   Mechanical devices for removing electrostatic charges from plastic articles by creating an ionized atmosphere in close proximity to the surface, which neutralizes the static charges.

Statistically Significant   When the difference between a predicted and an observed value is so large that it is improbable that it could be attributed solely to change.

Stenosis   The pathological narrowing of a channel, duct, or passage in the body.

Stent, Ureteral   A Class II implantable device. It is a catheter (stent) inserted into the ureter to provide ureteral rigidity and allow the unimpeded passage of urine. The device may have distal protrusions or hooked ends to keep the device in place during treatment of ureteral injuries and obstructions.

Step-Growth Polymerization   One of the fundamental types of polymerization, the others being chain-growth polymerization and ring-opening polymerization.

Stereoblock Polymer   A polymer with molecules arranged in blocks or long sections of identical stereospecific structure, interspersed with sections of another type of structure.

Stereochemistry   A subdiscipline of organic chemistry that studies the three-dimensional spatial configuration of polymers. One aspect deals with stereoisomers, compounds with identical chemical constitution, but different arrangement of atoms in space. Stereoisomers fall into (1) optical isomers and (2) geometric (cis-trans) isomers. Another aspect of stereochemistry deals with the synthesis and control of the molecular configuration of polymers by the use of stereospecific catalysts.

Stereograft Polymer   A polymer consisting of chains of an atactic polymer grafted to chains of an isotactic polymer. For example, atactic polystyrene can be grafted to isotactic polystyrene under the proper conditions.

Stereoregular Polymerization   A polymerization method that produces a significantly stereoregular polymer structure. Many vinyl polymers are STEREOSPECIFIC.

Stereoregular Polymers   Polymers with chain configurations consisting of small, regularly oriented units. See also ISOTACTIC and SYNDIOTACTIC.

Stereospecific   Implies a specific or definite order of molecular arrangement in space. This ordered regularity permits close packing of the chains, and leads to high crystallinity, in contrast to branched or random arrangement, which prevents close molecular proximity.

Stereospecific Polymers   Polymers whose molecular chains are arranged in a specific or definite order. There are five types of stereospecificity: cis, trans, isotactic, syndiotactic, and tritactic structures. These structures are most commonly produced in polyolefins, by means of Ziegler-Natta catalysts derived from a transition metal halide and a metal alkyl.

Steric Hindrance   A characteristic of molecular structure in which the molecules have a spatial configuration of their atoms such that a given reaction with another molecule is prevented or retarded.

Sterilization   Complete destruction of all bacteria and other infectious organisms from a medical device. The methods may involve (1) wet or dry heat, (2) chemicals, such as ethylene oxide or formaldehyde, (3) ionizing irradiation, such as gamma or electron beam.

Sterilization, Comparative Methods   A comparison between Ethylene Oxide (EtO) and Gamma sterilization methods is shown below:

EtO	GAMMA RADIATION
Surface sterilant	Volume sterilant
Depends on moisture	Depends on dosage (time)
Some organisms are resistant	Kills all organisms
Needs biological indicators	No indicators
Toxic compounds may form	Optical color changes
Deaeration time required	Immediate use

Steroid   One of a group of polycyclic compounds closely related biochemically to terpenes. They include cholesterol, hormones, precursors of certain vitamins, bile acids, certain drugs, and poisons. Steroids are classed as lipids because of their solubility in organic solvents and insolubility in water.

Stethoscope   A Class I device. The familiar instrument for listening to the heart, arteries, and other sounds within the body, consisting of two ear pieces connected via tubes to a cup or disc-shaped device that is applied to the skin.

Stiffness   The inherent ability of a material to resist elastic displacement under stress, such as bending. As opposed to hardness, which is resistance to indentation.

Stimulator   A device that applies electrical current to a nerve to treat certain chronic conditions.

Stimulator, Cranial Electrotherapy   A Class III device intended to provide electrical stimulation to a patient's head to treat insomnia, depression, or anxiety.

Stimulator, Diaphragmatic/Phrenic Nerve   A Class III implantable device that provides electrical stimulation to the phrenic nerve and produces normal breathing during hypoventilation (a state in which an abnormally low amount of air enters the lungs), caused by brain stem disease, high cervical spinal cord injury, or chronic lung disease. The stimulator consists of an implanted receiver with electrodes placed around the phrenic nerve and an external transmitter for stimulating pulses across the skin to the implanted receiver.

Stimulator, Diaphragmatic/Subcortical Nerve   A Class III implantable device that applies electrical current to subsurface areas of the brain to treat severe intractable pain. The stimulator consists of an implantable receiver with electrodes placed within the brain, and an external transmitter for the stimulating pulses across the skin to the implanted receiver.

Stimulator, Neuromuscular   A Class II implantable device that provides electrical stimulation to the peroneal or femoral nerve causing muscle contraction, thus improving the gait in a paralyzed leg. The stimulator consists of an implanted receiver with electrodes placed around the nerve, and an external transmitter for the stimulating pulses across the skin. The external transmitter is activated by a switch in the heel of the patient's shoe.

Stimulator, Spinal Cord   A Class III implantable device used to help in emptying the bladders of paraplegics with complete transsection of the spinal cord, who are unable to empty their bladders by reflex means or by intermittent use of catheters. The device consists of an implanted receiver with electrodes placed on the conus medullaris, and an external transmitter for stimulating pulses across the skin to the implanted receiver.

Stochastic Process   A process characterized by the occurrence of certain probabilities of events, which make up the process. For example, the copolymerization of many resins can be mathematically analyzed by considering the probabilities of certain events occurring at specific times.

Stoichiometry   The branch of chemistry that deals with the quantities of substances that enter and are produced during chemical reactions. For example, when methane unites with oxygen in complete combustion, 16 grams of methane require 64 grams of oxygen (reactants). At the same time, 44 grams of carbon dioxide and 36 grams of water are formed (reaction products). The mathematical calculations of what and how much is needed and produced during chemical reactions is the major concern of stoichiometry.

Stoke   The e.g.s. unit of kinematic viscosity. It is calculated by dividing the absolute viscosity of a fluid by its density. A CENTISTOKE is one hundredth of a stoke.

Stoma   An opening. A term used to describe an artificial surgical opening in a body part, e.g., a COLOSTOMY, an opening into the colon made through the abdominal wall.

Strain   In tensile testing, the ratio of the elongation to the original length of the test specimen, i.e., the change in length per unit of original length. The term also applies in a broader sense to a dimensionless number that characterizes the change in dimensions of an object during deformation or flow.

Strain Energy   The pure elastic energy stored in a strained body, resulting from the work done in deforming the body. A pure elastic material will recover instantaneously upon removal of the deforming stress.

Strain Gauges   Metallic grid elements that can be adhered to plastic surfaces to measure the deformation occurring immediately below each gauge. The deformation causes a change in electrical resistance proportional to the amount of deformation, which difference is measured with a sensitive galvanometer.

Strain Softening   The reduction in the slope of the stress-strain curve when a polymer has been stressed beyond its yield point.

Strength, Dry   The physical strength of an adhesive joint determined immediately after drying under specified conditions.

Strength, Wet   The physical strength of an adhesive joint determined immediately after removal from a liquid in which it has been immersed under specified conditions of time, temperature, and pressure.

Stress   The force producing or tending to produce deformation in a unit area of a substance. Engineering stress is the ratio applied to the original cross section. The "true" stress is the applied load per instantaneous cross-sectional area. Most of the stress values given for polymers in the literature represent engineering stress.

Stress Concentration   The magnification of the level of an applied stress in the region of a notch, void, inclusion, or discontinuity.

Stress Corrosion   The preferential attack of areas under stress in a corrosive environment, when the environment alone would not have caused corrosion.

Stress Crack   External cracks in a polymer caused by tensile stresses well below its short-term mechanical strength. When the development of such cracks is accelerated by the environment to which the polymer is exposed, the phenomenon is then referred to as Environmental Stress Cracking.

Stress Crazing   A form of environmental stress cracking that occurs when glassy polymers are exposed to certain organic solvents, and is evidenced by the formation of surface cracks shortly after solvent evaporation.

Stress Relaxation   Due to the viscoelastic nature of polymers, the amount of stress necessary to produce a given amount of deformation gradually decreases each time the stress is applied. This decay of stress at a constant strain is called stress relaxation.

Stress Rupture   The sudden, complete failure of a plastic specimen held under a definite load for a given period of time at a specific temperature. Loads may be applied by tensile, bending, flexural, biaxial, or hydrostatic methods.

Stress Whitening   The local appearance of white regions in a polymer while it is being stressed, due to crystallization with corresponding changes in the refractive index in the stressed regions, due to microcrazes.

Stress Wrinkles   Distortions in the face of a laminate caused by uneven web tensions, slowness of adhesive setting, selective adsorption of adherends, reactions of the adherends with the adhesive, or residual stresses.

Stress-Strain Diagram   The curve plotting the calculated applied stress on a test specimen in tension versus the corresponding strain. The test is conventionally carried out at a constant rate of elongation, on test specimens that had been preconditioned at a specified temperature and humidity for a given period of time.

Stretch Forming   A plastic sheet forming technique in which the heated thermoplastic sheet is stretched over a mold, and subsequently cooled. Also called *drape forming, thermoforming* and *vacuum forming*.

Stretching   See ORIENTATION.

Striae   Surface or internal thread-like inhomogeneities in transparent plastic.

Striation   In blow molding, a rippling of thick parisons caused by a local orientation effect in the melt imparted by the spider legs.

Stringiness   The property of an adhesive that results in the formation of filaments or threads when adhesive transfer substrates are forcibly separated.

Strippable Coatings   (Sacrificial Coatings). Temporary coatings applied to finished articles to protect them from abrasion, corrosion, or deterioration during shipping and storage. Prior to use, the coatings are designed to be removed easily, without damage to the substrate.

Structural Adhesive   A bonding agent used for transferring required loads between substrates exposed to service environments typical for the intended use.

Structural Foam Molding   A process of molding thermoplastic articles with a cellular core and an integral solid skin in a single operation. The resin containing a blowing agent is rapidly forced into a mold, with the charge being only about one half of the mold volume. As the foam expands, the cells in contact with the cold mold surface collapse to form a solid skin.

Styrene   (Vinyl Benzene). A colorless liquid, easily polymerized by exposure to light, heat, or a peroxide catalyst. It is the monomer from which polystyrene is produced.

Styrene Butadiene Rubbers (SBR, Buna-S, GRS)   A group of synthetic rubbers comprising about 3 parts of butadiene copolymerized with 1 part of styrene. Prepared as latices, in which form they are sometimes used. The latices are coagulated to produce crumb-like particles resembling natural crepe rubber.

Styrene-Acrylonitrile Copolymers (SAN)   Copolymers of 70% styrene and 30% acrylonitrile, with higher rigidity, tensile strength, chemical and impact resistance than straight polystyrene. They may be blended with butadiene, either as a terpolymer, or by grafting onto the butadiene, to form Acrylonitrile Butadiene Styrene (ABS) resins.

Styrene-Butadiene-Styrene Thermoplastics   A family of rubber elastomers that behave like thermoplastics during processing. They are linear block copolymers produced by lithium-catalyzed solution polymerization, with a segmented structure comprising amorphous polybutadiene centers surrounded by crystalline polystyrene ends. The materials are available as fully compounded pellets ready for processing by conventional thermoforming processes such as extrusion, blow molding and injection molding.

Styrene-Ethylene/Butylene-Styrene Block Copolymers   A hydrogenated version of styrene-butadiene-styrene copolymers, in which the

213

polybutadiene portion has been saturated, resulting in a much improved oxidation and chemical resistance.

Subacute Toxicity   How poisonous a substance is to an animal or person after repeated small doses under long exposure.

Sublimation   The direct conversion of a substance from solid to vapor without appearing in the intermediate (liquid) state. An example is carbon dioxide.

Substance   Any chemical element or compound that is homogenous, and is characterized by a unique and identical constitution.

Substrate   (1) Any solid surface on which a coating or layer of a different material is deposited. (2) A material upon the surface of which an adhesive-containing substance is spread for any purpose such as bonding or coating. (3) A substance on which an enzyme is active.

Suffixes   Medical suffixes are formed from nouns, adjectives, or verbs. Examples:

SUFFIX	MEANING	EXAMPLES
algia	Pain	Myalgia— muscle pain
		Neuralgia—nerve pain
esthesia	Feeling	Hyperesthesia—high sensitivity to touch
		Paraesthesia—abnormal sensation
gen	Origin	Hematogenous—derived from blood
genesis		Neurogenic—derived from nerves
opia	Vision	Hemiopia—vision in one-half field
path	Disease	Myopathy—muscle disease
plegia	Paralysis	Hemiplegia—unilateral paralysis
scope	Viewing	Microscope
		Endoscope—viewing internal cavities
trophy	Nourishment	Atrophy—wasting
	Development	Hypertrophy—tissue volume increase

Sulfide Staining   A discoloration of a plastic caused by the reaction of stabilizers (such as lead, cadmium, antimony, copper, etc.), with a sulfide to which the plastic article is exposed. The color is due to the formation of chromophoric metallic sulfides.

Sulfonate-Carboxylate Copolymers   See POLYSULFONATE COPOLYMERS.

Sulfonation   The formation of sulfonic acid, a compound containing the radical: ($-SO_2OH$). Common sulfonating agents are: concentrated sulfuric acid, sulfur trioxide, pyrosulfates, chlorosulfonic acid, etc. Sulfonating polyurethane elastomers renders the surfaces more hydrophilic, and thus more hemocompatible.

Sunlight Resistance   See LIGHT RESISTANCE.

Supermolecular Structure   Morphological polymeric structures observable at a level above that of individual polymer molecules. They include: (1) crystal structure, (2) crystallite formation, (3) multilayer crystallinity, (4) spherulitic and fibrillar morphologies, and (5) segmentation.

Supernatant   A liquid or fluid forming a distinct layer on the surface of another liquid.

Superoxide   A compound characterized by the presence in its structure of the superoxide ion. In these compounds each oxygen has an oxidation number of $-1/2$ instead of -2, as a normal oxide.

Supersaturation   The unstable condition in which a solvent contains more dissolved solute than is present in a saturated solution of the same components at similar temperature. These solutions precipitate readily upon mere addition of solute crystals, agitation, or shaking.

Surface   The area of contact between two different phases or states of matter. Three general categories of phases are recognized: (1) powders and air (solid-gas); (2) liquids and air (liquid-gas); and (3) insoluble powders and liquid (solid-liquid). Surfaces are the sites for physicochemical activity between the phases, responsible for such phenomena as adsorption, reactivity, biocompatibility, catalysis, etc.

Surface Area   The total area of exposed surface of a powder, foam, or textured material. Since biological and chemical activity is greatest at the surface, i.e., the boundary between the surface and its environment, the larger the surface area of a given mass of substance, the more reactive it becomes.

Surface Chemistry   The observation and measurement of forces acting at the surfaces of gases, liquids, and solids, or at the interfaces between them. This includes the surface tension of liquids (vapor pressure, solubility); emulsions (liquid/liquid interfaces); fine powders (adsorption, catalysis); semipermeable membranes (breathability); microporous materials (water vapor transport); and biological phenomena such as osmosis, cellular function, and metabolic mechanisms.

Surface Conductance   The direct current conductance between two electrodes in contact with a specimen of solid insulating material when the current is passing only through a thin film of moisture on the surface of the specimen.

Surface Preparation   A physical or chemical preparation, or both, of a substrate to render it suitable for adhesion or coating.

Surface Resistance   The surface resistance between two electrodes in contact with a material is the ratio of the voltage applied to the electrodes to that portion of the current between them that flows through the surface layers.

Surface Resistivity   The ratio of the potential gradient parallel to the current along the surface of a material to the current per unit width of the surface. Surface resistivity is equal to the surface resistance between opposite sides of a square of any size when the current flow is uniform.

Surface Tension   The attractive forces exerted by the molecules of a liquid below the surface upon those at the surface/air interface, resulting from the high molecular concentration of a liquid compared to the low molecular concentration of a gas. An inward force is created, which tends to restrain the liquid from flowing. Polar liquids have high surface tension (water = 73 dynes/cm); nonpolar liquids have lower values (benzene = 20 dynes/cm, ethyl alcohol = 22.3 dynes/cm) and thus flow more readily than water. Mercury, with the highest surface tension (480 dynes/cm) does not flow at all, but disintegrates into small droplets.

Surfactant   A widely used contraction of *Surface Active Agent*, a substance that generally reduces the surface tension of a liquid in which it is dissolved. If it were not for surface tension, all liquids would be freely miscible in each other. Surfactants allow the formation of stable mixtures between normally immiscible fluids, solids, and gases. Surfactants are classified as:

NAME	REDUCE INTERFACIAL TENSION BETWEEN
Wetting Agent	Liquid/solid
Dispersant	Liquid/solid
Emulsifier	Liquid/liquid
Defoamer	Liquid/gas

Surgery   The branch of medicine that deals with external diseases (skin excepted) and all other diseases and accidents amenable to operative, interventional, or manual treatment. Surgical methods are used in general surgery, and also in some independent disciplines, shown below:

BRANCH OF SURGERY	INVOLVING
Anesthesiology	Anesthetic methods
Gynecology	Female genital tract
Neurosurgery	Surgical treatment of the nervous system
Obstetrics	Managing pregnancies and childbirth
Ophthalmology	Eye diseases
Orthopedics	Bones and joints
Otolaryngology	Ear, nose, and throat
Plastic surgery	Reconstructive surgery
Thoracic surgery	Diseases of the chest organs
Urology	Diseases of the urinary organs

Surgical Treatment   Surgical treatment is usually causal—an attempt is made to remove the cause of the disease, and is designated according to the following nomenclature:

NAME	INVOLVING
Anastomosis	Communication between blood vessels
Ectomy	Removal of whole organ
Extirpation	Complete removal of tumor
Incision	Opening tissue with knife
Plastic Surgery	Restore shape and function
Resection	Removal of part of organ
Transplantation	Grafting an organ from one patient to another or from one place on the body to another.

Suspension   A system in which very small particles of solid, semi-solid or liquid are uniformly dispersed in a liquid or gaseous medium. If the particles are small enough to pass through a filter membrane, the system is called a colloidal suspension. See also DISPERSION and EMULSION.

Suspension Polymerization   (Pearl, Bead, Granular Polymerization). A polymerization process in which the monomer or mixture of monomers is dispersed by mechanical agitation in a second liquid phase, usually water, in which both the monomer and the polymer are essentially insoluble. The monomer droplets, containing initiators and catalysts, are polymerized while maintained in suspension by continuous mixing. The resulting polymers may be in the form of pearls, beads, spheres, or granules. Used primarily for PVC, PVAc, PMMA, PTFE, and polystyrene.

Sustained Release Dosage   A term that indicates that a drug has been manufactured so that predetermined portions of each tablet are released over a prolonged period of time.

Suture   Strands of material used for ligating or tying blood vessels and tissues together until healing takes place. The present worldwide market for sutures is approximately $950 million. Sutures are divided into two classifications: absorbable and nonabsorbable.

Suture, Absorbable   A sterile, flexible strand prepared from collagen or synthetic polymer, and capable of being resorbed by living mammalian tissue.

Suture, Nonabsorbable   A flexible strand of material that is suitably resistant to the action of living mammalian tissue.

Swelling Ratio   In extrusion, the ratio of extrudate diameter to the extrusion die diameter. In general, the swelling ratio is about 1.5 to 3 for most polymers.

Symmetry   Arrangement of the constituents of a molecule in a definite and continuously repeated space pattern or coordinate system. It is described in terms of three parameters: (1) center of symmetry, (2) plane of symmetry, and (3) axis of symmetry.

Syndiotactic   Pertaining to a type of polymer molecule in which groups of atoms that are not part of the primary backbone structure alternate regularly on opposite sides of the chain. See also STEREOSPECIFIC.

Syndiotactic Polypropylene   Polypropylene in which the asymmetric carbon atoms have opposite configurations on each alternate asymmetric center. See also SYNDIOTACTIC.

Syndrome   (1) The constellation of symptoms that describes a particular disease state. (2) A characteristic set of symptoms that occur together, and are given a name to indicate that particular combination, e.g., Reye's syndrome, Adams-Stokes syndrome, Cushing's syndrome.

Syneresis   The spontaneous contraction of a gel upon standing, with the concomitant exudation of liquid. The separation of plasma from a blood clot is an example.

Synergism   (1) A chemical phenomenon in which the effect of two active components of a mixture is more than just additive. (2) Relating to the total effect of two or more discrete agents acting at the same time being greater than the sum of the individual effects. (3) The opposite of antagonism.

Syntactic Foams   Composites containing tiny hollow spheres of glass, phenolic, or epoxy resins. The spheres are premixed with the reactive resin, curing agents, additives, etc., to form a fluid mass that can be cast into molds and cured with heat to form the finished article.

Synthesis   Artificial creation of a substance that either duplicates a natural product, or is a unique material not found in nature, produced by means of chemical reactions, or (for elements) by a nuclear change. Syntheses are among the most important activities practiced in the fields of polymer chemistry and organic chemistry.

Synthetic Polymer   A polymer produced by polymerization of its monomer or monomers in a chemical reaction fully conducted in a laboratory. Contrasts with a polymer produced in nature by biosynthesis, giving rise to a natural polymer such as collagen elastin or cellulose. Several natural polymers have been chemically modified for subsequent use, and these are referred to as semi-synthetic.

Systemic   Relating to the organism as a whole—to the physiologic machine working as an integrated unit.

Systole   The phase of the cardiac cycle during which the myocardium is contracting, and ejecting blood into the arteries. Atrial systole is the contraction of the atria, forcing blood into the ventricles, contributing approximately 20% of ventricular filling. Ventricular systole is the contraction of the ventricles, forcing blood into the aorta and pulmonary arteries, performed with atrioventricular and semilunar valves.

T

Tack   The stickiness of an adhesive, measurable as the force required to separate a substrate from it by viscous or plastic flow of the adhesive.

Tack, Dry   The property of certain adhesives to adhere with themselves on contact at an intermediate step in the evaporation of volatile constituents, even though they seem dry to the touch.

Tack Range   The period of time in which an adhesive is expected to remain in a sticky condition after application to a substrate, under specified conditions of temperature and humidity.

Tackifier   A substance added to synthetic resins or elastomeric adhesives to improve the initial and extended TACK RANGE of the deposited adhesive film.

Tacticity   The regularity or symmetry in the molecular arrangement or structure of a polymer molecule. In contrast to random positioning of substituent groups along the polymer backbone, or random position with respect to one another of successive atoms in the backbone chain of a polymer molecule. Also see STEREOSPECIFIC.

Tamponade Accumulation of blood or pericardial fluid within the pericardial cavity, to the point that the heart is prevented from fully relaxing in diastole, ventricular filling during systole is inhibited, and cardiac output is thus compromised.

Tare (1) The weight of a container, wrapper, or liner, which is deducted in determining the net weight of a material. (2) A weight used in analytical work to offset the weight of a container.

Tautomerism A type of isomerism in which migration of a hydrogen atom results in two or more structures, called tautomers. For example, acetoacetic acid acts both as an unsaturated alcohol and a ketone, with the tautomers called enol and keto.

TDI Abbreviation for *toluene diisocyanate* (also known as *tolylene diisocyanate*), an 80–20 mixture of 2,4- and 2,6-toluene diisocyanate monomers. See TOLUENE-2,4 -2,6 DIISOCYANATE.

TDI Index The TDI content of a polyurethane formulation. A 105 index means there is a 5% excess of isocyanate groups over all other reactants.

Techelic Polymer A polymer with deliberately introduced end groups of a specified type. Techelic polymers are prepared by reacting, and subsequently end-capping, a living polymer with a desired agent. Example: carboxy or hydroxy-terminated polybutadiene is formed by reaction of the living polymer with carbon dioxide or ethylene oxide respectively. Many macroglycols are end-capped with ethylene oxide to allow subsequent reactivity with isocyanates.

Technology The systematic application of fundamental scientific phenomena and principles in a device, process, or concept that performs a useful function, and has commercial value. See also HIGH TECHNOLOGY.

Telomer A low molecular weight addition polymer, in which the growth of the molecule is terminated by a radical-supplying chain transfer agent. The term is also used synonymously with *oligomer*, meaning simply a polymer with very few (2 to 10) repeating units.

Telomerization A polymerization performed in the presence of large amounts of an active chain transfer agent (the telogen) so that only polymers of low molecular weight are produced (the telomers).

Temper To increase the hardness and strength of a metal or alloy by quenching or heat treatment.

Temperature, Curing The temperature to which an adhesive, coating, composite, etc., is subjected to effect specific changes in physicochemical characteristics.

Temperature, Drying The temperature-time relationship to which an adhesive or coating is subjected to dry the spread surface.

Tenacity A textile term denoting the strength of a filament of given size. Expressed as the grams of breaking force per denier of yarn or filament, when pulled at a rate of 12 inches per minute.

Tensile Impact Test   A test similar to the Izod test, except that the specimen is clamped in a fixture attached to the swinging pendulum, and is ruptured by tensile stresses as it strikes an anvil.

Tensile Modulus   See MODULUS OF ELASTICITY.

Tensile Product   The product of tensile strength and elongation at break, divided by 10,000. Also the product of tensile strength and gauge length plus deformation at break. (The latter definition being only an approximation to actual rupture stress).

Tenter Frame   (1) A machine for stretching thermoplastics performed by tenter pins which run the materials through heating chambers. (2) A machine that treats and dries a fabric while maintaining the fabric uniformly stretched by tenter pins running on two parallel endless chains.

Tentering   The process of uniaxial stretching of films and sheets while heating, when the stretching is performed by holding the material on a TENTER FRAME. In the plastics industry the term is frequently used in connection with ORIENTATION.

Tera   Prefix signifying 10^{12} units (symbol T).

Teratogen   An agent that causes growth abnormalities in embryos, genetic modifications in cells, etc. Certain chemicals and ionizing radiation are known to cause this effect.

Ternary   Descriptive of a chemical compound having three constituent elements or groups.

Terpolymer   The product of simultaneous polymerization of the different monomers, or the grafting of one monomer to the copolymer of two different monomers. Example: Acrylonitrile Butadiene Styrene (ABS) resin.

Test Measurement   A single quantitative value obtained from a material test.

Test Method   A definitive standardized procedure for the identification, measurement, and evaluation of characteristic properties of a material or product.

Test Result   A value obtained by applying a TEST METHOD.

Test of Significance   A statistical procedure to ascertain whether a particular effect could be attributed to chance.

Test Specimen   A suitably prepared sample for evaluating any or all the chemical, physical, mechanical, or metallurgical properties of a material.

Testicular Prosthesis   A Class III implantable device that consists of a solid or gel-filled silicone rubber prosthesis implanted within the scrotum to resemble a testicle.

Testing, Chemical   Identification of an unknown substance by means of reagents, chromatography, spectroscopy, and other chemical analytical procedures.

Testing, Physical   Application of any procedure used to determine the mechanophysical properties of a material. There are four major categories: (1) direct measurements, e.g., tensile strength; (2) those that subject the material to actual service conditions, e.g., exposure to sun; (3) accelerated tests, requiring simulated conditions on an exaggerated scale; and (4) non-destructive testing, e.g., by X-ray or radiography.

Testing, Physiological   Determination of the toxicity or biocompatibility of a substance or product by administering it to laboratory animals orally, by skin application, by injection, or by surgical implant.

Tetrafluoroethylene $F_2C:CF_2$. (TFE, perfluoroethylene). A colorless gray gas derived by passing chlorodifluoromethane through a heated tube. Used as the monomer for the synthesis of polytetrafluoroethylene resins.

Tetrahydrofuran (THF)   A colorless solvent obtained from the catalytic hydrogenation of furan. A powerful solvent for many synthetic resins. THF has been polymerized to polytetramethylene ether glycol (PTMEG), the most widely used macroglycol for the synthesis of medical-grade polyurethane elastomers.

Tetramer   A polymer synthesized by uniting four different simple molecules.

Textile   Originally a woven fabric, but now applied to staple fibers, filaments, yarns, nonwovens, and fabrics.

Texture   The structural quality of a solid that results from the shape, arrangement and proportions of its surface. The texture of a biomaterial influences the degree of tissue adhesion to it, as well as the intensity of the foreign body reaction around it.

TFE   Abbreviation for *Tetrafluoroethylene*.

T_g A symbol for the temperature of GLASS TRANSITION.

TGA   Abbreviation for *Thermogravimetric Analysis*.

Therapeutic Dosage   The quantity of a drug calculated to improve the condition for which it is being prescribed.

Therapeutic Index   The relationship between the desired and undesired effects of a drug is commonly expressed as the therapeutic index, defined as the ratio between a drug's median toxic dose and its median effective dose, TD50/ED50. Thus a drug with a therapeutic index of 15 would be expected to have a greater margin of safety in its use than a drug with a therapeutic index of 5. For drugs with indexes as low as 2, extreme caution must be exercised.

Therapeutic Indices   Examples of therapeutic indices for some drug substances are shown below.

DRUG SUBSTANCES WITH THERAPEUTIC INDICES

LESS THAN 5	BETWEEN 5 AND 10	GREATER THAN 10
Amitriptylene	Barbiturates	Acetaminophen
Chordiazepoxide	Diazepam	Bromide
Diphenhydramine	Digoxin	Choral hydrate
Ethchorvynol	Imipramine	Glutethimine

LESS THAN 5	BETWEEN 5 AND 10	GREATER THAN 10
Lidocaine	Meperidine	Meprobamate
Methadone	Paraldehyde	Nortriptyline
Procainamide	Primodone	Pentazocine
Quinidine	Thioridazine	Propoxyphene

Thermal Analysis   One of a number of analytical techniques for determining the temperature dependence of certain polymer properties. Comprises: (1) THERMOGRAVIMETRIC ANALYSIS (TGA); (2) DIFFERENTIAL THERMAL ANALYSIS (DTA); (3) Differential Scanning Calorimetry (DSC); (4) THERMAL VOLATILIZATION ANALYSIS (TVA); (5) Dynamic Mechanical Spectroscopy; (6) TORSIONAL BRAID ANALYSIS; and (7) THERMAL OPTICAL ANALYSIS (TOA).

Thermal Black   See CARBON BLACK.

Thermal Conductivity   The rate at which heat is transferred by conduction through a unit cross-sectional area of a material when a temperature gradient exists perpendicular to the area.

Thermal Decomposition   Decomposition resulting entirely from the action of heat. It occurs at a temperature at which some components of the material are separating or reacting together, with a modification of the macro/microstructure, and a general lowering of the physicomechanical properties.

Thermal Diffusivity   A measure of the rate at which a temperature disturbance travels through the mass of a substance. It is expressed by the relationship k/dC_p, where k is the coefficient of thermal conductivity, d is the density, and C_p is the specific heat at constant pressure.

Thermal Impulse Sealing   See IMPULSE SEALING.

Thermal Optical Analysis (TOA)   Any of a group of techniques based on the measurement of transmitted light intensity variation in a specimen subjected to a constant temperature increase. The techniques are particularly useful to the detection of the melting, glass transition, and crystallization points of polymers.

Thermal Polymerization   A polymerization process performed solely by heat, in the absence of a catalyst. Resins such as polystyrene, polymethylmethacrylate, and aromatic polyurethanes can be thermally polymerized.

Thermal Sealing   (Heat Sealing). The method of bonding two or more layers of thermoplastics by pressing them between heated dies or tools that are maintained at a relative high temperature.

Thermal Stability   See HEAT STABILITY.

Thermal Stress Cracking (TSC)   Surface crazing and cracking of some thermoplastic resins resulting from overexposure to elevated temperatures.

Thermal Volatilization Analysis (TVA)   An analytical method for the determination of volatile thermal degradation products of a polymer. By using a series of detectors and cold traps for condensing volatiles at different temperatures, mixtures of products can be analyzed in terms of fractions evolved with high sensitivity.

Thermally Foamed Plastic   A cellular plastic article produced by applying heat to effect gaseous decomposition, or volatilization of a blowing agent.

Thermochemistry   A branch of chemistry comprising the measurement and interpretation of heat changes that accompany changes of state and chemical reactions. It is closely related to chemical thermodynamics.

Thermocompression Bonding   The joining of two thermoplastic materials without an intermediate material by the application of pressure and heat, in the absence of an electrical current.

Thermocouple   A pair of dissimilar metal wires welded at one end, which when heated at the welded junction generate a small electrical current through a circuit connected to the opposite ends of the wires. The current strength is proportional to temperature, and can be measured with a millivoltmeter calibrated in degrees of temperature. A system comprised of a thermocouple and a detecting instrument is called a PYROMETER, a widely used instrument in the plastics industry.

Thermodilution   A method for obtaining cardiac output, where a bolus of 10 ml of cold saline is injected into the right atrium. After mixing, a temperature curve is obtained from a thermistor in the pulmonary artery, from which an algorithm allows the calculation of cardiac output values. This method can be used for many repeated measurements, since there is no buildup of foreign substances in the body.

Thermodilution Probe   A Class II device that monitors cardiac output by means of thermodilution techniques. The device is commonly attached to a catheter that may have one or multiple probes.

Thermoelasticity   Rubber-like elasticity exhibited by a normally rigid plastic resulting from an increase in temperature. Retention of desired shape may be achieved by cooling in place after THERMOFORMING.

Thermoforming   The process for forming thermoplastic sheet into a desired three-dimensional shape by clamping the sheet in a frame, softening by heat, then applying differential pressure to force the sheet to conform to the shape of a mold positioned below the frame. When the pressure differential is obtained entirely by vacuum, the process is called VACUUM FORMING. When air pressure is employed to partially preform the sheet prior to the application of vacuum, the process is called air assisted vacuum forming.

Thermogram   A curve plotting weight loss of a specimen against temperature. See also THERMOGRAVIMETRIC ANALYSIS.

Thermographic Transfer   A modification of the hot stamping process wherein the design to be delivered is first printed on a film, from which it is transferred to the plastic part by means of heat and pressure.

Thermography   A diagnostic device that uses the temperature in various body parts to determine the presence of abnormal conditions in those areas.

Thermogravimetric Analysis (TGA)   A technique where the weight of a specimen is continually recorded while being heated in a thermobalance. Data may be recorded either isothermally (static TGA), or at a constant heating rate (dynamic TGA). Widely used in degradation kinetic studies, volatilization during cure, or weight loss due to component evaporation.

Thermomechanical Analysis (TMA)   A technique for analyzing the deformation of a small sample of film, sheet, fiber, disc, etc., as a function of temperature. Deformation is accomplished by nonoscillating penetration, expansion, bending, shear flow, or torsion loads. The results are displayed as a thermomechanical fingerprint.

Thermomechanical Spectrum   A plot of the variation in mechanical properties of a polymer versus temperature. Usually the plots are of storage or loss moduli or of tangent of the loss angle (tan δ).

Thermoplastic   Resins or compounds which in their final state as finished articles are capable of being repeatedly softened by an increase in temperature, and are subsequently hardened to their original physical properties by a corresponding decrease in temperature.

Thermoplastic Elastomer   An elastomer that displays the typical high elasticity, tensile strength, and toughness of vulcanized rubber, but which does not need to be cross-linked through covalent bonds. The rubbery polymer chains are thought to be tied by physical cross-links, such as hydrogen bonds, Van der Waals forces and other short-distance molecular interactions. These physical cross-links are thermoreversible, so the materials may be processed by all known thermoforming techniques, with the ''cross-links'' reformed upon cooling.

Thermoplastic Elastomers, Classification   TPE's are identified according to the multifactorial classification shown below:

CHEMICAL COMPOSITION

HARD PHASE	SOFT PHASE	POLYMER TYPE	NATURE OF HARD PHASE
Polystyrene	Polybutadiene	Triblock (SBS)	Amorphous
Polystyrene	Polyisoprene	Triblock (SIS)	Amorphous
Polystyrene	EB copol*	Triblock	Amorphous
Polyester	Amorph polyester	Multiblock	Crystalline
Polyurethane	Macroglycol	Segmented	Crystalline
Polyamide	Polyether	Multiblock	Crystalline
Polypropylene	EPDM	Graft/blend	Crystalline

* EB copolymer refers to poly(ethylene-co-butene-1).

Thermoplastic Polyurethane (TPU)   Trade names of Medical-Grade TPU's: Biomer, Mitraflex, Pellethane, ChronoFlex, Tecoflex. A linear, or slightly cross-linked polyurethane that displays all the properties of vulcanized rubber, but without needing to be cross-linked. TPU's vary from soft elastomeric materials, to hard elastoplastics.

Thermoplastic Polyurethane Elastomers (TPUE)   A type of linear, segmented elastomers, in which crystalline hard blocks are covalently interspersed among amorphous soft segments. When the hard blocks are composed only of urethane linkages, the materials are true thermoplastics. However, when the hard blocks are also rich in substituted urea linkages, the amount of hydrogen bonding is very high, thus rendering the material nonthermoplastic. This phenomenon is known as pseudocross-linking. The polymers are formed by the reaction between isocyanates, macroglycols, and chain extenders.

Thermoreversible Cross-Link   A physical cross-link that is destroyed during heating, but which reforms after cooling. Present in thermoplastic elastomers, thereby enabling them to be thermoprocessed, but which exhibit the high physical properties of vulcanized elastomers.

Thermosetting Plastics   (Thermosets). Resins or compounds which in their final state as finished articles are substantially infusible and insoluble. Thermosets are often liquids at some stage in their manufacture or processing, which are cured by heat, catalysts, and other means. After full cure, thermosets cannot be resoftened by heat or solvents.

Thermotropic   A polymer that exhibits a transition from a glassy crystalline state to a liquid crystalline state at a characteristic temperature, without being diluted by an organic solvent.

Theta Solvent   A solvent that performs in an ideal manner (activity coefficient = 1) in dilute solution measurements of molecular weight.

Theta Temperature   (Flory Temperature). With respect to molecular interactions in dilute polymer solutions, the temperature at which the second virial coefficient disappears.

THF   Abbreviation for *Tetrahydrofuran*.

Thickening Agent   Any of a variety of hydrophilic substances used to increase the viscosity of aqueous mixtures and organic solutions, and as stabilizers due to their emulsifying properties. They are classified into four broad categories: (1) Natural Agents, i.e., starches, gums, casein, gelatin, and phycocolloids; (2) Semisynthetic polymers, i.e., cellulose derivatives; (3) Synthetic resins, i.e., vinyl alcohol, polyvinyl pyrrolidone, etc.; and (4) Inorganic powders, i.e., bentonite, magnesium oxide, silicates, and colloidal silica.

Thickness   (1) The distance between the upper and lower surfaces of a sheet, film, wall, etc.

Thin Layer Chromatography   A chromatographic technique where the stationary phases are characteristically spread as a thin layer on an inert carrier, such as paper or plastic, to enhance separation. See also CHROMATOGRAPHY.

Thinner   A fluid substance incapable of dissolving a resin, but which can partly substitute for a true solvent, and at the same time reduce the viscosity of a coating, adhesive, etc. See also DILUENT.

Thio   A prefix in chemical nomenclature to indicate the presence of sulfur in a compound, usually as a substitute for oxygen.

Thiol   Any of a group of organic compounds resembling alcohols, but having the oxygen of the hydroxyl group replaced by sulfur.

Thixotropic Agents   The ability of certain substances in solution to cause gelation or thickening upon standing. See also THICKENING AGENTS.

Thixotropic Fluids   See THIXOTROPY.

Thixotropy   A flow characteristic evidenced by a decrease in viscosity of a fluid when it is stirred or is subjected to increasing shear. When the stirring or shearing is discontinued, the apparent viscosity of the fluid is gradually restored to the original value. Changes in both directions are dependent on time as well as shear. See also RHEOLOGY, DILATANCY.

Thoracentesis   Withdrawal of a fluid from the pleural cavity to relieve hydrostatic pressure on the lungs.

Thoracic Cavity   The space within the chest, enclosed by the ribs, spine, sternum, clavicles, and scapulae. Contains the lungs, heart, and the great vessels. The walls of the cavity and the lungs are lined with the pleura; in the center of the thoracic cavity, the pleura folds end establishes the confines of the MEDIASTINUM.

Thoracotomy   An operation in which the chest wall is opened surgically, and the pleural space entered. The usual procedure for myocardial lead placement, artificial heart implant, etc.

Thorax   The chest. The upper portion of the trunk, beginning superiorly with the neck, separated from the abdomen by the diaphragm.

Threshold   The point where a physiological or toxicological effect begins to be produced by the smallest degree of stimulation or challenge.

Threshold Limit Value (TLV)   A set of standards established by the American Conference of Governmental Industrial Hygienists for concentrations of airborne substances to which nearly all persons can be exposed day after day, without adverse effects. They are time-weighed averages based on conditions that are believed representative of the environment to which workers may be exposed repeatedly without adverse effects. The TLV values are revised annually, and provide the basis for OSHA Safety Regulations. Some of the most important are:

(1) *TLV-TWA* — The allowable Time-Weighed Average concentration for a normal 8-hour workday of a 40-hour work week.

(2) *TLV-STEL* — The Short-Term-Exposure Limit, or maximum concentration for a continuous 15-minute exposure period (maximum of four such periods per day, with at least 60 min. between exposure periods and provided that daily TLV-TWA is not exceeded).

(3) *TLV-C* — The Ceiling exposure limit — the concentration that should not be exceeded even instantaneously.

(4) *TLV-Skin* — A ''skin'' notation is sometimes used with TLV. It indicates that the stated substance may be absorbed by the skin, mucous membranes, and eyes — either airborne or by direct contact.

Thrombin   A proteolytic enzyme that catalyzes conversion of fibrinogen to fibrin, and is thus an essential part of the clotting cascade. It circulates as an inactive precursor, prothrombin. When bleeding occurs, it is activated to thrombin, which in turn activates the formation of fibrin.

Thrombocytes   (Platelets). The smallest of the formed blood elements, averaging 1.5 μm in diameter and from 0.5 to 1 μm in thickness. Normally about 250×10^3 mm^3 are present in the circulation. Microscopically they appear as flat discs, remaining viable in man for 9 to 12 days. The interior of the platelets contains two storage granules called, respectively, dense and α granules; interactions between platelets and foreign surfaces (collagen, synthetic polymers) cause the release of granular material. Degranulation causes the following:

 − Recruitment of additional platelets, initiating mural thrombus
 − Activation of the intrinsic coagulation sequence

Platelets are products of megakaryocytes, which are extremely large cells of the granulocytic system formed in bone marrow. The normal blood concentration of platelets is between 150,000 and 300,000 per cubic mm.

Thrombosis   The manifestation of those functions in blood normally responsible for the arrest of bleeding. The principal mechanisms that have evolved in blood are platelet adhesion, platelet aggregation, and fibrin formation (coagulation).

Time, Assembly   The time interval between the spreading of an adhesive on the substrate(s), and the application of heat, pressure, or both, to the assembly.

Time, Curing   The period of time during which an assembly is subjected to heat, pressure, or both, to cure the adhesive, coating, ink, or composite.

Time, Drying   The period of time during which an adhesive, coating, or ink on a substrate is allowed to dry, with or without the application of heat and/or pressure.

Time-Resolved Spectroscopy (TRS)   An infrared spectroscopic technique for the acquisition of high resolution spectra in a short time. It is used to study deformation and relaxation in organic fibers and matrices where changes in frequency and intensity can be related to molecular stress, chain orientation, and conformational analysis.

Tincture   An alcoholic or aqueous alcoholic solution of a drug or chemical substance. The tincture of most drugs is a 10% solution. Tinctures are more dilute than fluid extracts, and less volatile than spirits.

Tissue   A collection of similar cells and the surrounding intercellular substances. Tissues are divided into four general types: (1) Epithelial Tissue, (2) Connective Tissue, including blood, bone, and cartilage, (3) Muscle Tissue, and (4) Nerve Tissue.

Tissue, Connective   The mechanical framework of the body, formed of fibrous proteins and ground substance. Connective tissues are composed of: areolar, adipose, white, fibrous, elastic, mucous, lymphoid, cartilage, and bone.

Blood and lymph are connective tissues where the ground substance is a liquid.

Tissue, Epithelial The cellular, avascular layer covering all the free surfaces—cutaneous, mucous, and serous—including the glands and other derivative structures.

Tissue, Muscle One of three varieties (skeletal, cardiac, and smooth) tissues, characterized by the ability to contract upon stimulation.

Tissue, Nerve A highly differentiated tissue composed of nerve cells, dendrites, and the supporting neuroglia.

Tissue Capsule In newly developing granulation tissue, fibroblasts hypertrophy and actively synthesize collagen. With further healing there is an increase in extracellular material, a decrease in leukocytes, macrophages, and blood vessels. The end result is a scar that surrounds the implanted prosthesis composed of collagen, fibroblasts, and blood vessels, referred to as a "tissue capsule." A tissue capsule is part of a FOREIGN BODY REACTION.

Tissue Culture The process where small amounts of cells or living tissue are isolated from an organism and grown aseptically in a defined or semi-defined culture nutrient medium. The term covers both cell culture (in which cells are propagated as cell suspensions or as an attached monolayer) and organ culture (in which a piece of tissue or organ is grown, retaining tissue architecture, cell interaction, physiological functions, and histological-biochemical differentiation).

Titanium Dioxide TiO_2. A white powder available in two crystalline forms, the anatase and rutile types. The rutile form has the higher refractive index (2.75 vs. 2.55 for the anatase form) and thus has the greater opacifying power. Both are widely used as opacifying pigments, used alone when whites are desired, or in conjunction with other pigments when tints are desired. They are inert, light-fast, and are resistant to heat and migration.

Titration Any of a number of methods for the volumetric determination of concentration of dissolved substances. Performed by adding a standard solution of known volume and concentration until the reaction is completed, usually by an indicator color change. Both aqueous and organic-solvent based solutions may be used in this determination.

Tolerance (1) The guaranteed maximum deviation from the specified value of a component characteristic at standard or stated environmental conditions. (2) The upper and lower limit between which a dimension must be held. (3) The precision and accuracy criteria for balances, weights, and other measuring instruments.

Toluene-2,4 -2,6 Diisocyanate $CH_3C_6H_3(NCO)_2$. An 80/20 mixture of isocyanate isomers used in the production of polyurethane foams, elastomers, coatings, and adhesives. Elastomers made from this monomer exhibit low modulus of elasticity and good recovery properties. Flexible foams synthesized from this monomer are quite resilient, and can be made reticulated.

Toner An organic pigment that does not contain inorganic pigments or base. In other words, full-strength organic pigments. Important toners are: Pigment Green 7, Pigment Blue 15, Pigment Yellow 12, and Pigment Blue 19. See also PIGMENTS.

Topical   A medical term meaning "applied directly to the surface of the skin."

Topical Anesthetic   An anesthetic agent directly applied to the area where pain relief is needed.

Topochemical Reaction   Any chemical reaction that is not expressible in stoichiometric relationships. Such reactions are characteristic of collagen cross-linking, or with cellulose. They can take place only at certain sites on the molecule where reactive groups are available.

Torr   A pressure unit used chiefly in vacuum technology. It is the pressure required to support 1 millimeter of mercury at $0^{\circ}C$.

Torsion   Stress caused by any twisting force.

Torsional Braid Analysis   A method of performing torsional tests on small amounts of materials that cannot support their own weight, i.e., liquid thermosetting resins. A glass braid is impregnated with a solution of the test material, and after solvent evaporation, the torsional modulus is measured by oscillating the braid as it is being heated at a programmed rate.

Torsional Test   Tests for determining the stiffness properties of plastics, based on measuring the torque required to twist the specimen to a predetermined degree of arc.

Tortuosity Factor   The distance a molecule must travel to pass through a film divided by the thickness of the film.

Toughness   A loose term implying a lack of brittleness, having high elongation accompanied by high tensile strength. One proposed definition for toughness is the energy required to break a material, equal to the area under the stress-strain curve.

Toxemia   The condition caused by poisonous substrates in the blood.

Toxic   Poisonous. Relating to or caused by a toxin. Substance capable of causing injury by contact or systemic action to plants, animals, or humans. Among the recognized groups of toxic agents are: aldehydes, anilines, alkaloids, allyl compounds, barbiturates, chlorinated hydrocarbons, corrosive materials, organic phosphate esters, and radioactive compounds.

Toxicity   The degree of being poisonous. Capacity of a poisonous compound to produce deleterious effects in organisms, such as alteration of behavioral patterns, biological productivity or death. "Acute" toxicity refers to exposure of short durations; "chronic" toxicity refers to exposure of long duration, or repeated exposures. Toxicity is objectively evaluated on the basis of test dosages made on experimental animals under controlled conditions. Most important of these are the LD_{50}, (Lethal Dose, 50%), and the LC_{50} (Lethal Concentration, 50%).

Toxicology   The science of poisons. The systematic study of substances that exert deleterious effects on living organisms, as well as their chemistry in relation to mode of action, antidotes, and pathophysiological effects. The subject is subdivided into (1) clinical, (2) environmental, (3) forensic, and (4) occupational.

TPU Abbreviation for *Thermoplastic Polyurethane*, a material usually supplied as pellets ready for thermoforming operations.

Tracheal Tube A Class II device inserted into the trachea via the nose or mouth and used to maintain an open airway.

Tracking A phenomenon wherein a high voltage source current creates a leakage or fault across the surface of an insulating material by slowly forming a carbonized path.

Trade Name The official name under which a company does business.

Trade Secret Confidential information (formula, process, device, or compilation of data) that gives the owner an advantage over competitors.

Trademark A word, symbol, or insignia designating one or more proprietary products, which has been officially registered with the government trademark agency. The accepted designation is a superior capital R enclosed in a circle.

Trans A prefix denoting an isomer in which certain atoms or groups are located on opposite sides of a plane.

Transabdominal Amnioscope (Fetoscope). A Class III device designed to permit direct visual examination of the fetus by means of a telescopic system through an abdominal incision. The device is used to ascertain fetal abnormalities, to obtain fetal blood samples, or to obtain fetal biopsies. The device is composed of: trocar and cannula; instruments associated with an amnioscope; a light source; cables; and components.

Transalkylation A type of disproportionation reaction by which toluene is hydrogenated to benzene and mixed xylene isomers, while avoiding the formation of methane resulting from the conventional hydroalkylation process.

Transcutaneous Electrical Nerve Stimulator (TENS) A Class II device used for pain relief by applying an electrical current to electrodes fixed on the skin. The applied electric current is thought to prevent pain signals travelling in the nerves from reaching the brain.

Transducer A Class II device used to measure pressure by converting mechanical inputs to electrical signals.

Transducer, Catheter Tip Pressure A Class II device incorporated into the distal end of a catheter. When placed in the bloodstream its mechanical or electrical properties change in relation to changes in blood pressure. These changes are in turn transmitted to accessory equipment for analysis.

Transducer, Extravascular Blood Pressure A Class II device used to measure blood pressure by changes in mechanical or electrical properties of the device. The proximal end of the transducer is connected to a pressure monitor that produces analog or digital electrical signals paralleling changes in blood pressure.

Transducer, Heart Sound   A Class II device consisting of an external transducer that exhibits changes in mechanical or electrical properties in relation to cardiac sounds.

Transducer, Pressure   A Class II device used to measure the pressure between a device and soft tissue by converting pressure inputs to analog electrical signals.

Transducer, Ultrasonic   A Class II device applied to the skin to transmit and receive ultrasonic energy. Used in conjunction with an echocardiograph, as an aid in imaging cardiovascular structures. The device includes phased arrays and two-dimensional scanning transducers.

Transducer, Vessel Occlusion   A Class II device used to supply an electrical signal corresponding to sounds produced in a partially occluded vessel. The device may include motion, sound, and ultrasonic transducers.

Transfer Mold   A chamber, pot, or cylinder in which a resin is softened by heat and pressure, in preparation for injection into a final mold.

Transfer Molding   A molding process used with thermosetting resins and vulcanizable elastomers where the molding material is preheated in a chamber, pot or cylinder. The hot material is injected into the curing mold by means of a plunger. Following a curing cycle, the mold is opened, and the finished part is ejected.

Transfer Molding Pressure   The pressure applied to the cross-sectional area of the material chamber, pot, or cylinder, expressed in lbs/in^2.

Transferase   An enzyme whose activity causes the relocation (transfer) of a radical from one molecule to another. Examples: transaminases, transacetylases, and transmethylases, which cause the transfer of amino, acetyl, and methyl groups respectively.

Transfusion   Any fluid introduced into a vein, but generally refers to blood given as replacement for blood loss due to hemorrhage, surgery, injury, or to increase an inadequate blood supply due to a blood disease.

Transition Section   In an extruder the section of the screw that contains material in both the solid and molten states.

Transition Temperature   The temperature at which a polymer reversibly changes from a viscous or rubbery condition to a hard and relatively brittle one.

Transplant   The surgical transfer of tissue or an organ from one body area to another, or from one person to another, to replace a missing, diseased, or nonfunctioning body part.

Transplantation, Nomenclature   The nomenclature of transplantation has been redefined in the past several years as follows:

TYPE	OLDER TERM	RELATIONSHIP
Autograft	Autologous	Donor and recipient are same individual
Allograft	Homologous	Two individuals from the same species
Xenograft	Heterologous	Individuals from two different species

231

Trauma   Any injury produced by external force. An external blow can cause a wound (cut), perforation (hole), laceration (slash), contusion (bruise), dislocation (bone displacement), or fracture (bone breakage).

Tribasic   Pertaining to acids or salts that have three displaceable hydrogen atoms per molecule. Substances having one displaceable hydrogen are called MONOBASIC, and those with two are called DIBASIC.

Trichlorofluoromethane   A blowing agent for foamed plastics, particularly polystyrene.

Trimer   A molecule formed by the union of three molecules of a monomer. See also POLYMER.

s-**Trioxane**   (Metaformaldehyde). The stable trimer of formaldehyde; a colorless crystalline solid, which may be further polymerized to form Acetal Resins.

Trioxane Copolymers   See ACETAL RESINS.

Triple Bond   A highly unsaturated linkage between the two carbon atoms of acetylenic compounds (alkynes).

Triple Point   The temperature and pressure at which the solid, liquid, and vapor of a substance coexist in equilibrium. The triple point of water is $+0.072°C$ at 4.6 mm Hg; it is of special significance since it is the fixed point for the absolute scale of temperature.

Tritactic Polymers   Isotactic or syndiotactic polymers that are also of the cis- or trans- form because the molecules are unsaturated and have double bonds.

Trocar   A Class I device consisting of a sharp-pointed instrument used in conjunction with a cannula for piercing a vessel or chamber to facilitate insertion of the cannula. In neurology, a trocar is a needle used to puncture an artery prior to catheterization for cerebral angiograms.

Tubal Occlusion Device (TOD)   A Class III device designed to close the fallopian tube with a mechanical structure such as band, or clip on the outside of the tube, or a plug or valve on the inside, to prevent pregnancy.

Tube Feeding   Procedure performed on patients unable to take nourishment by eating or drinking normally. A nasogastric tube is inserted into the stomach or duodenum, through which liquids or blended foods can be given at prescribed intervals.

Tumbling Agitators   Cylindrical or cone-shaped vessels rotating about a horizontal or inclined axis, with internal ribs that lift the material and then tumble back into the charge. Used primarily for compounding solids, such as adding color concentrates to molding resins.

Tumor   (Neoplasm). An uncontrolled growth of cells that serve no useful purpose. Tumors may be benign or malignant. Benign tumors have well-defined borders, growing like a bladder, then gradually expanding. A malignant tumor infiltrates the surrounding tissue and the tumor grows in between normal cells, extending to other parts by (1) infiltration (via blood vessels and lymph) and (2) by implantation (dissemination of daughter tumors). The tissue from which dissemination has occurred is known as the primary tumor; secondary tumors are daughter tumors or metastases, which have originated from the primary tumor. Depending on their origin tumors are classified as:

NAME	ORIGIN	EXAMPLE
Oma	Tumor in general	Fibroma; lipoma
Angioma	Vascular tumor	Hemangioma, lymphoma
Carcinoma	Epithelial tumor	Adenosarcoma
Sarcoma	Connective tissue	Osteosarcoma, lymphosarcoma
Glioma	Glial cells	

TWA   Time-Weighed Average for a normal workday in relation to THRESHOLD LIMIT VALUE.

Two-Dimensional Chromatography   A variation of paper chromatography, used for the separation of complex mixtures of polypeptides. The mixture is first chromatographed in one direction, the paper dried, and the mixture is chromatographed with a different solvent at right angles to the first. In this fashion, a two-dimensional map is obtained.

U

UF   Abbreviation for *Urea-Formaldehyde*. See AMINOPLASTS.

Ultimate Elongation   Alternative name for *Elongation at Break*. Term used to describe the maximum stretch a material will withstand when subjected to an applied load during a tension, or bending test.

Ultimate Tensile Strength   Alternative name for tensile strength. Term used to describe the maximum unit stress a material will withstand when subjected to an applied load during compression, tension, or shear test.

Ultraaccelerator   An accelerator for the sulfur-based cross-linking of rubber, which is particularly reactive, and thus promotes very rapid cure. Two types are most frequently used: (1) dithiocarbamates and (2) thiuram disulphides.

Ultracentrifuge   A centrifuge capable of rotating at speeds of 20,000 to 60,000 RPM, thereby creating forces up to several hundred thousand times greater than gravity. Weight average and molecular weight distributions of high polymers may be studied by sedimentation rates obtained during ultracentrifugation.

Ultrafiltration   (Membrane Filtration). A fast version of dialysis in which pressure is used to filter molecules through a membrane. The range of particle size separation of ultrafiltration is between 10^{-3} and 10 microns. This range includes substances such as albumin, vitamin B_{12}, and glucose. Applications of ultrafiltration include hemodialyzers, blood fractionation, cell harvesting, membrane bioreactors, tissue culture, and enzyme and protein separation.

Ultramarine Blue Pigments   Pigments comprising complexes of double silicates of sodium and aluminum in combination with sodium polysulfide. They produce bright colors, resistant to temperature, which are light-fast.

Ultramicroscope   An improvement over traditional instruments, this microscope is capable of resolving suspended particulate matter in the 5 millimicron range. The ultramicroscope detects suspended particles because of the light-scattering effects of the particles as they move in the suspension.

Ultramicrotomy   Microtomy technique in which extremely thin slices are produced, often necessary for assessment of biological cells and segmented polymers under transmission electron microscopy.

Ultrasonic Cleaning   A method used for cleaning plastic parts for implantation. Based on the principle that high frequency vibrations in the cleaning medium will extricate contaminants from the smallest crevices, normally inaccessible by brushing or similar mechanical rubbing.

Ultrasonic Degradation   A type of mechanochemical degradation induced in a polymer exposed to ultrasonic radiation. Cavitation (rapid collapse of low-pressure regions) occurs, resulting in regions of high localized shear, which in turn are capable of lowering the molecular weight of polymers by chain scission.

Ultrasonic Frequencies   Frequencies above the limit of human audibility, approximately 18,000 hertz.

Ultrasonic Insertion   A method of incorporating metallic inserts into plastic articles by means of ultrasonic energy and some light pressure. In this technique, ultrasonic vibrations are applied to the metal part as it is being inserted, which causes the polymer to flow around threads, knurls, or under-cuts on the insert, mechanically locking the insert in place.

Ultrasonic Welding   Welding method utilizing ultrasonic frequencies to heat the polymer articles due to vibrational friction at the interfaces. The process is best utilized with rigid plastics, since the energy is rapidly dissipated in soft, elastomeric materials.

Ultrasonics   The study of effects of sound vibrations beyond the limits of audible frequencies.

Ultrasonography   A diagnostic technique that utilizes the reflection and transmission of ultrasonic waves to determine abnormality or disease of internal body structures.

Ultrasound, Imaging   Imaging with ultrasonic techniques is a valuable supplement to radiological examinations. The reason is that many different soft-tissue structures, such as muscle, connective tissue, nerve tissue, blood, and to some extent fat, can be imaged by ultrasonic techniques although their mass attenuation coefficients and densities do not differ sufficiently to produce X-ray contrast. Ultrasonic diagnosis differs from conventional radiological diagnosis in that normally no shadow images are obtained. In the majority of cases, sectional images that appear similar to radar images are obtained through parts of the body.

Ultrasound and Muscle Stimulator   A Class II device used in applying therapeutic deep heat and muscle stimulation by means of ultrasonic energy at frequencies beyond 20,000 cycles per second, and passes electrical currents through the affected body area to relax muscles. May also be used for the relief of muscle spasm pain, and joint contractures.

Ultraviolet   Radiation in the region of the electromagnetic spectrum including wavelengths from 10 to 400 nm where it merges with the lower limit of visual perception. Ultraviolet is the most popular radiant energy source for radiation curing.

Ultraviolet Absorber   A type of UV stabilizer, soluble in the polymer matrix, so they do not bloom. These compounds are stable to ultraviolet light themselves, are transparent, have low volatility and good thermal stability, and are capable of dissipating ultraviolet energy as heat by internal rearrangement. The main types are: (1) benzophenones, (2) benzotriazoles, and (3) derivatives of salicylic acid.

Ultraviolet Curing   Ultrafast method of polymerization via actinic radiation. Molecules known as photoinitiators set off a free-radical reaction, cross-linking the monomers and/or oligomers in seconds, or fractions of a second. Most industrial UV-producing lamps range from 200–400 nm, with power in the 4 to 6 electron volt range. UV below 200 nm is highly penetrating, and is seldom used.

Ultraviolet Screen   A type of ultraviolet stabilizer that is insoluble in the polymer matrix, and which is colored, thereby rendering transparent polymers opaque. Carbon black is the most effective ultraviolet screen known, followed by zinc oxide and rutile titanium dioxide.

Ultraviolet Spectrophotometry   An analysis similar to Infrared Spectrophotometry, except that the spectrum is obtained with ultraviolet light. It is less sensitive than IR for polymer analysis, but is quite effective for detecting leachable antioxidants, stabilizers, plasticizers, and other UV-absorbing species.

Ultraviolet Stabilizers   (UV Absorbers). A chemical agent that absorbs or screens out radiation beyond the violet end of the visible spectrum. UV stabilizers are of three types: (1) Agents that screen the polymer by absorbing UV radiation and then dissipating the energy as heat. They require high concentration to be effective and are ineffectual when the polymers are highly pigmented. Example: 2-hydroxy-4-n-octoxy benzophenone. (2) Stabilizers that act by quenching molecules activated by UV radiation, and also function as antioxidants. These agents are typically nickel-based coordination complexes, and can be used effectively in pigmented systems. Example: [2,2′-Thiobis(4-t-octylphenolato)]-n-butylamine nickel II. (3) Hindered Amine Light Stabilizers (HALS), which interrupt the radical chain degradation mechanism, and are effective in very low concentrations. Example: Dimethyl succinate polymer with 4-hydroxy-2,2,6,6-tetramethyl-1-piperidine ethanol.

Undercure   Inadequate cross-linking in a thermosetting resin, resulting in substandard physical properties. May be due to insufficient temperature or time during the curing cycle.

Undercut   An indentation, protuberance, or surface texturing in a mold that tends to impede withdrawal of a molded part at the end of the cycle. Slight undercuts are sometimes deliberately formed in one half of the mold to cause the article to remain in the desired mold half until ejected.

Uniaxial Load   A condition whereby a material is stressed in only one direction.

Uniaxial Orientation   A method of orientation in which the orienting stress is applied only in one direction.

Unicellular Plastic   A term sometimes used for *Closed Cell Foamed Plastic*.

Unidirectional Laminate   A reinforced plastic laminate in which the fibers are substantially oriented in the same direction.

Unit Elongation   In tensile testing, the ratio of the elongation to the original length of the specimen. That is, the change in length per unit of original length.

Unit Operation   In chemical engineering terminology, a physical change used in the industrial production of various chemicals and related industries. Filtration evaporation, distillation, drying, fluid flow, and heat transfer are examples.

Unit Process   A process characterized by a particular kind of chemical reaction, such as oxidation, hydrolysis, esterification, and nitration.

Uns   Abbreviation for *Unsymmetrical*. A prefix denoting the structure of organic compounds in which substituents are arranged unsymmetrically around the carbon skeleton, or to a functional group.

Unsaturation   The state at which not all available valence bonds along the alkyl chain are satisfied. In such compounds, the extra bonds form double or triple bonds (chiefly with carbon).

Urea Plastics   See AMINO RESINS.

Urea-Formaldehyde Plastics   See AMINO RESINS.

Uremia   The presence of an abnormally high level of urea in the blood and other nitrogenous waste substances in the blood, caused by poorly functioning or nonfunctioning kidneys.

Ureteral Cather   (Fiberoptic). A Class II device consisting of a fiberoptic bundle that emits light throughout its length and is inserted into the ureter to visualize the path.

Ureteral Stone Dislodger   A Class II device consisting of a bougie or catheter with an expandable wire basket and a flexible stone dislodger near the distal tip. Used to remove stones from the lower ureters when inserted through a cystoscope.

Urethane Foam   A cellular plastic where the chemical reaction causes foaming simultaneously with the polymer-forming reaction. As in the case of polyurethane resins, the polymeric constituent of urethane foams is made by reacting a polyol with an isocyanate. When water is added as a compounding ingredient, the isocyanate-water reaction produces carbon dioxide gas, which expands the mixture. Three basic processes are used for making urethane foams: (1) the prepolymer technique, (2) the semi-prepolymer technique, and (3) the one-shot method.

Urethane Linkage   (urethan, carbamate, linkage). The linkage (HNCOO−), typical of urethane polymers. Strangely, urethane is not used directly in the production of polyurethane plastics or foams. Typically, the urethane linkage is obtained by the reaction of an isocyanate group with a hydroxyl moiety. The relative rate of isocyanate reaction with the hydroxyl moiety is: Primary Hydroxyl = 1.000; Secondary Hydroxyl = 0.300; and Tertiary Hydroxyl = 0.005.

Urethane Plastics   See POLYURETHANES, URETHANE LINKAGE, TPU.

Urethome   A Class II device that is inserted into the urethra and is used to cut urethral strictures under direct visual observation, and thus enlarge the urethral diameter. It consists of a metal instrument equipped with a dorsal-fin cutting blade that can be elevated from its sheath.

Urinary Continence Device   (Electrical). A Class III device that consists of a receiver implanted in the abdomen, electrodes for pulsed-stimulation implanted either in the bladder wall or in the pelvic floor, and an extracorporeal battery-powered transmitter.

Urinary Incontinence   Inability to retain or control urine.

Urine Culture   A laboratory technique used to determine the presence and type of harmful microorganisms in the urinary tract, so appropriate treatment may be instituted.

Urological Catheter   A family of Class II devices which include: radiopaque urological catheter; ureteral catheter; urethral catheter; coude catheter; ballon retention catheter; upper urinary tract catheter; double lumen female urethrographic catheter; male urethrographic catheter; and urological catheter accessories.

Urological Catheter, Suprapubic   A Class II device consisting of a flexible tube that is inserted percutaneously through the abdominal wall into the urinary bladder with the aid of a trocar and cannula. Used to pass fluids to and from the urinary tract. Accessories include: catheter and tube, malecot catheter, punch, drainage tube, and suprapubic cannula and trocar.

Urology   The branch of medical science that embraces the study, diagnosis and treatment of the genitourinary tract.

USP   Abbreviation for *United States Pharmacopeia*. Founded in 1820 by physicians concerned with the proper identification and uniformity of medicines. The approach was to standardize articles believed safe and effective, through the provision of formulations by which they could be consistently compounded. Preparations were given definitive names so as to avoid confusion. In the late 1800s, the formula for compounding gave way to the standardization of end-product characterization, utilizing the analytical procedures of chemistry, physics, and microbiology.

USP Standards Standards designed to "identify or characterize an acceptable product that would reasonably be expected to produce the desired result or therapeutic effect in humans." Unlike many other bodies, the standards-setting process in the USP is not based on consensus. Rather, the USP Convention utilizes a "republic-type" system in which scientific decisions are voted on by experts elected by individuals representing the various organizations in the pharmaceutical, medical, and other health related fields. Because of its widespread acceptance—USP quality became the "official" compendium of medicine and pharmacy—USP quality was expected, and became the rule; a "not USP" product was an exception. The first federal food and drug act simply incorporated this theory and provided that a drug sold under a name recognized in the pharmacopeia shall be deemed adulterated unless it met the standards of strength, quality, and purity contained in the pharmacopeia.

V **Vacuum Casting** A method used for casting fluid thermosetting resins to avoid entrapment of gas bubbles. The mold is placed under vacuum, filled with resin, then the vacuum is released.

Vacuum Deposition The process of coating a substrate by evaporating a metal under high vacuum and condensing it on the surface of the substrate to be coated, which is usually a polymer or another metal. See also VACUUM METALLIZING.

Vacuum Distillation Distillation at a pressure less than atmospheric, but not so low that it would be considered molecular distillation. Since lowering pressure also lowers the boiling point, this process is useful for distilling high-boiling and heat-sensitive materials, such as vitamins, antibiotics, fatty acids, etc.

Vacuum Forming A method of forming plastic sheets or films into three-dimensional shapes, in which the plastic sheet is clamped in a frame suspended above a mold, heated, drawn into contact with the mold by vacuum, and cooled in that position.

Vacuum Metallizing A protective and decorative process used to make plastic objects resemble shiny metals. Aluminum is frequently used for this purpose, with a top coat of lacquer applied to the metal coating.

Vaginal Pessary   A Class II device consisting of a removable structure placed in the vaginal cavity to support the pelvic organs. Used to treat such conditions as: uterine prolapse (fallen uterus); uterine retroposition (backward displacement of the uterus); and gynecological hernias.

Vaginal Stent   (Vaginal Dilator). A Class II device designed to completely fill the vaginal cavity, in order to enlarge the vagina following reconstructive surgery.

Valence   A integral number that represents the combining power of one element with another. Measured by the number of hydrogen one atom can hold in combination if negative, or can displace in a reaction if positive. By balancing these integral valence numbers in a given compound, the relative proportions of the elements present can be accounted for. In inorganic compounds it is necessary to assign either a positive or negative value to each valence number, so that valence-balancing will give a zero algebraic sum. Negative numbers are called polar valence numbers (-1 and -2), and positive numbers are called nonpolar. Chlorine may have five valences (-1, $+1$, $+1$, $+5$, and $+7$). In organic chemistry however, only nonpolar valence numbers are used.

Valence Electrons   Electrons that are gained, lost, or shared in a chemical reaction.

Validation   Establishing documented evidence that provides a high degree of assurance that a specific process will consistently produce a product meeting its predetermined specifications and quality attributes.

Validation Change Control   A formal monitoring system by which qualified representatives of appropriate disciplines review proposed or actual changes that might affect validated status and cause corrective action to be taken that will ensure that the system retains its validated state of control.

Validation Committee   Representatives from various disciplines within the company who are responsible for reviewing and approving validation protocols and final results. Typically, these individuals are from quality control, quality assurance, regulatory affairs, manufacturing, research and development, and engineering departments.

Validation Protocol   A written procedure stating how the validation study will be conducted, including parameters, product attributes, product equipment, and decision points on what constitutes acceptable test results. The protocol also identifies individuals responsible for various tasks.

Validation Report   A documentation package summarizing the results of a validation study, including protocol, quality control, quality assurance, and a validation committee review/approval sign-off form.

van der Waals Forces   Weak attractive forces acting between molecules of a substance after all of the primary valences within covalent molecules are saturated. Weaker than hydrogen bonds, and much weaker than interatomic valences. Also called *Secondary Valence Forces* or *Intermolecular Forces*.

Vapor   An air dispersion of molecules of a solid or liquid substance, such as water vapor and benzene vapors. Vapors of organic liquids are also called fumes. Gas is most frequently used for a substance that remains gaseous at room temperature.

Vapor Barrier   A continuous layer, sheet, film, or material through which water will not pass readily, if at all.

Vapor Pressure   The pressure characteristic at any given temperature of a vapor in equilibrium with its liquid or solid form, expressed in mm Hg.

Vapor Transmission   See WATER VAPOR TRANSMISSION.

Vaporizer, Anesthetic   A Class II device used to atomize (vaporize) liquid anesthetic, and deliver a controlled amount of the vapor to the patient.

Varnish   An organic protective coating, which does not contain a colorant, and which undergoes a chemical reaction during "curing" or "hardening."

Vascular   Pertaining to blood vessels. As compared to circulatory system, a more comprehensive term that includes the heart.

Vascular Grafts, Markets   In the U.S., approximately 90,000 surgical procedures are performed annually to repair occlusions or aneurysms of the aorta and/or other major arteries. These cases involve the implantation of a vascular graft to replace or repair the diseased artery.

Vascular Grafts, Performance Characteristics   Vascular surgeons choose a vascular graft based on graft performance in the following areas:

- Handling: ease of suturing and conformability to artery
- Healing: ease of tissue ingrowth into the graft
- Porosity: leakage of blood through graft at implantation
- Strength: no deterioration or dilation over time

Historically, knitted grafts have been shown to offer excellent handling and healing but have high porosity and low strength compared to wovens, which offer low porosity and excellent strength, but poor handling and healing.

Vascular Grafts, Small Bore   A Class III device of less than 6 mm in diameter, used to replace sections of small arteries. While both woven and knitted dacron, and blown PTFE have been used, these devices have not performed as adequately as the alternatives for endarterectomy and autogenous vein grafting.

Vasoconstrictor   An agent or drug that causes blood vessels to constrict or narrow.

Vasodilator   An agent or drug that causes blood vessels to dilate or expand.

Vectorcardiograph   A Class II device used to process and interpret the electrical signal transmitted through ECG electrodes, and to produce a visual display of the magnitude and direction of the cardiac electrical signals.

Ventilator, Emergency   A Class II device, it is a demand valve or inhalator used to provide emergency respiratory support through a facemask or catheter inserted into the airway.

Ventilators   When artificial respiration must be maintained for a long time, a ventilator is used. Ventilators operate in different modes: controlled breathing, where ventilators take over all the breathing work; and assisted breathing, where the patient's own spontaneous attempt to breathe causes the ventilator to cycle during inspiration.

Ventricular Assist Devices   A Class III device that mechanically helps the right or left ventricle in maintaining proper circulatory blood flow. These devices may be either totally or partially implanted in the body.

Vertical Extruder   An extruder arranged so the barrel is vertical, and thus the extrudate flows downward.

Vicat Softening Point   The temperature at which a flat-ended needle of fixed cross section (1 sq mm) will penetrate a thermoplastic specimen to a depth of 1 mm, under a specified load using a uniform temperature rise. Used for thermoplastics that have no definite melting point.

Vinyl   The unsaturated group $CH_2:CH-$, which is the basis for all vinyl plastics.

Vinyl Acetate   A colorless liquid obtained from the reaction of acetylene and acetic acid in the presence of catalysts, usually mercuric oxide. It is the monomer used in the synthesis of polyvinyl acetate, and a comonomer and intermediate for many members of the vinyl family of plastics.

Vinyl Alcohol   (ethanol). A theoretical material, since it only exists in the form of its esters and the polymer POLYVINYL ALCOHOL, which actually is not derived directly from the ''vinyl alcohol.''

Vinyl Benzene   See STYRENE.

Vinyl Chloride $CH_2 = CHCl$ (chloroethylene, monochloroethylene). A colorless gas at room temperature, liquefying at $-13.9°C$, in which form it is usually handled. It is the monomer for the synthesis of POLYVINYL CHLORIDE.

Vinyl Cyanamide   See ACRYLONITRILE.

Vinyl Ethers   See VINYL ETHYL ETHER, VINYL ISOBUTYL ETHER, and VINYL METHYL ETHER.

Vinyl Ethyl Ether   (EVE, ethyl vinyl ether). A colorless liquid, which can be easily polymerized either in the liquid or gaseous state, used as a comonomer and intermediate.

Vinyl Fluoride   (fluoroethylene). A colorless gas, used as the monomer for the synthesis of POLYVINYL FLUORIDE.

Vinyl Foams   Cellular materials that can be manufactured by (1) chemical blowing, (2) frothing, and (3) leaching of soluble ingredients. Vinyl foams are extensively utilized in packaging.

Vinyl Formic Acid   See ACRYLIC ACID.

Vinyl Isobutyl Ether   A colorless, flammable liquid used in the production of polymers and copolymers used in surface coatings, adhesives and lacquers, modifiers for alkyd resins and polystyrene, and a plasticizer used in conjunction with cellulose nitrate.

Vinyl Methyl Ether   A colorless gas polymerizable to POLYVINYL METHYL ETHER.

N-Vinyl Pyrrolidone   A monomer derived from acetylene and formaldehyde, used to synthesize POLYVINYL PYRROLIDONE, and as a comonomer in hydrogels.

Vinyl Resins   Term referring to vinyl chloride plastics, as well as:

polyvinyl acetal	polyvinyl acetate	polyvinyl alcohol
polyvinyl butyral	polyvinyl carbazole	polyvinyl dichloride
polyvinyl formal	polyvinyl chloride	polyvinyl pyrrolidone
polyvinyl isobutyl ether		

NOTE: While polystyrene, polymethyl methacrylate, and copolymers are also "vinyl" resins, their commercial importance has earned them a separate classification.

Vinylation   The process of forming a vinyl derivative by reaction of alcohols, amines, or phenols with acetylene. These derivatives are used as polymerization intermediates.

N-Vinylcarbazole   A monomer derived from acetylene and carbazole, used in the production of POLYVINYL CARBAZOLE.

Vinylethylene   See BUTADIENE.

Vinylidene Chloride   A colorless, volatile liquid used as the monomer for the synthesis of POLYVINYLIDENE CHLORIDE, and as a comonomer with vinyl chloride (Saran) and other monomers such as acrylonitrile.

Vinylidene Fluoride   A colorless gas, which polymerizes readily in the presence of free-radical initiators to produce POLYVINYLIDENE FLUORIDE, and is also copolymerized with other olefins to make fluorocarbon elastomers.

Virgin Plastic   Any plastic compound or resin that has not been subjected to use or processing other than that required for its original manufacture.

Virology   The study of viruses and of diseases caused by viral agents.

Virus   An infectious agent composed almost entirely of protein and nucleic acids. Viruses only reproduce within living cells, since they lack metabolism, are unable to synthesize macromolecules, to grow or die. Therefore they are parasites, relying on a living host cell. They account for many diseases, including mumps, measles, scarlet fever, smallpox, influenza, and are implicated in cancer, in those instances when viral DNA becomes irreversibly bound to the host DNA.

Viscoelasticity   The time-dependent property of certain polymers to respond to stress as if they were a combination of purely elastic solids and viscous liquids. This property, exhibited to some extent by all polymers, predicts that while plastics have solid-like characteristics, such as elasticity, strength, tear resistance, abrasion resistance, etc., they also have liquid-like characteristics such as flow, which are dependent on (1) time, (2) temperature, and (3) rate and amount of loading.

Viscometer   (Viscosimeter). An instrument used to measure the viscosity and flow characteristics of fluids. A commonly used type (Brookfield Viscometer) measures the force required to rotate a disc or hollow cup immersed in the test fluid at a predetermined speed. Instruments used for measuring flow properties of highly viscous fluids or molten polymers are called plastometers and rheometers, respectively.

Viscosity   A measure of the internal friction resulting when one layer of a fluid is forced to move in relationship to another layer. The units of measure are (1) POISE: shear stress in dynes/cm^2 divided by the rate of shear in seconds, and (2) STOKE: viscosity in poises divided by the fluid density. The following table of approximate viscosities in centipoises provides a useful perspective:

Water . . . . 1 cp
Glycerine . . . . 1000 cp
Corn syrup . . . . 10,000 cp
Molasses . . . . 100,000 cp

Viscosity Coefficient   The shearing stress tangentially applied that will induce a unit velocity flow gradient in a material. In the metric system, the viscosity coefficient is expressed in poises, units being dyne-sec/cm^2.

Viscosity Depressant   A substance capable of significantly lowering the viscosity of fluids when added in small amounts.

Viscous   A term implying a material that is thick and sluggish in flow, rather than thin and free-flowing.

Viscous Elasticity   A degree of elasticity in which the time necessary to completely recover initial dimensions is longer than a stated time by 5%.

Viscous Flow   A type of fluid movement in which all particles flow in a straight line, parallel to the axis of a straight pipe or channel, with little or no mixing or turbulence.

Vitamin   Any of a number of complex organic compounds, present in natural products, which are essential in small proportions in the diet. Some are fat-soluble (A,D,E,K); others are water-soluble (B complex, C).

Vitamins   A vitamin is an organic compound needed in small quantities for operation of normal bodily metabolism that cannot be synthesized in the cells of the body. From a clinical standpoint the agents that are considered to be vitamins are those organic compounds that occur in the diet and, when lacking, can cause specific metabolic deficits. The recommended daily requirements (RDR) of the vitamins are summarized below.

VITAMIN	DAILY REQUIREMENT
A	3.1 mg
Thiamine	1.3 mg
Riboflavin	1.8 mg
Niacin	18 mg
Ascorbic acid	80 mg

Vitamins

VITAMIN	DAILY REQUIREMENT
D (children; during pregnancy)	11 μg
E	Unknown
K	None
Folic Acid	Unknown
B_{12}	Unknown
Inositol	Unknown
Pyridoxine	Unknown
Panthotenic acid	Unknown
Biotin	Unknown
Para-aminobenzoic acid	Unknown

Void (1) An unfilled space in a cellular plastic substantially larger than the average diameter of individual cells. (2) An empty space in any material or medium.

Volatile Capable of being evaporated as a vapor at room or slightly elevated temperatures.

Volatile Content The percent of volatiles evaporated as a vapor from a plastic, coating, adhesive, etc.

Volatile Loss The loss in weight of a substance caused by evaporation of a constituent.

Voltage Breakdown See DIELECTRIC STRENGTH.

Volume Resistance The ratio of the direct voltage applied to two electrodes that are in contact with or embedded in a specimen, to that portion of the current between them that is distributed through the volume of the specimen.

Volume Resistivity The ratio of the potential gradient parallel to the current in a material, to the current density.

Vulcanization A coined term, derived from Vulcan, the god of fire and sulfur. Refers to the sulfur-based cross-linking reaction that occurs in rubber during cure. After cure, the rubber elastomer has decreased plastic flow, reduced surface tack, increased elasticity, greater tensile strength, better abrasion resistance, and significantly reduced solubility. Currently many thermoplastic materials, polyethylene, polyurethanes, etc., are being "vulcanized" (cross-linked without sulfur), thereby increasing resistance to deformation, flow, and chemical attack.

Vulcanize To subject an uncured rubber to vulcanization or heat cure.

W

Warp   Those threads in a woven fabric that are parallel to the selvedge, placed lengthwise in the loom. Opposite of WEFT.

Water Absorption   The amount of water absorbed by a plastic specimen when immersed in water for a stipulated period of time. All plastics will absorb moisture to some extent, varying from almost zero in the case of PTFE, to complete solubility for some types of PVA, polyethylene oxide, PVP, etc. Water absorption may cause swelling, dissolving, leaching, plasticizing, and/or hydrolyzing events. These events, in turn, may result in discoloration, embrittlement, loss of mechanical and electrical properties, lowered resistance to heat and weathering, and stress cracking, although the amount of water absorbed by any particular polymer is not predictive of the extent of harmful results.

Water Permeability   (of Some Polymers). The amount of water permeating through a given area of a plastic film. The test polymer is maintained at a constant temperature, with the water touching the underside of the test film. The data is typically expressed in "Barrers," which have the units: $cc(STP)/cm^2/mm/second/cm\,Hg \times 10^{-10}$. Typical values of some polymers are shown in the table below:

POLYMER	TRADE NAME	PERMEABILITY
Polychlorofluoroethylene	Kel-F	3–360
Polyvinylidine chloride	Saran	15–1000
Polyethylene	–	120–2000
Polytetrafluoroethylene	Teflon	350–400
Butyl rubber	–	400–2000
Chlorinated polyethylene	Hypalon	12,000
Polychloroprene	Neoprene	18,000
Silicone rubber	Silastic	85,000–110,000
Polyurethane	Mitraflex	95,000–175,000

Water Vapor Transmission (WVT)   The amount of water vapor diffusing through a given area of a plastic sheet, film, or membrane in a given time. The test plastic is maintained at a constant temperature, when its faces are exposed to certain different relative humidities. The results are expressed in grams of water, per square meter, per day. WVT of different polymers is frequently compared to the amount of water vapor normally perspired by humans, which is about 500 $g/cm^2/day$. Synonymous with *MVT* (*Moisture Vapor Transmission*).

Water-Soluble Resins   Polymers that are capable of being dissolved in water either by their polar/ionic character (polyvinyl pyrrolidone, polyacrylamide, polyvinyl alcohol, etc.), or by chemical modification (carboxymethyl cellulose, ethyl cellulose, etc.).

Weatherometer   An instrument utilized to test by ability of polymers to withstand exposure to weather. Performed by subjecting the test specimens to simulated accelerated weathering conditions, e.g., a potent UV source and water spray.

Web (1) Any continuous sheet in process in a machine. In extrusion coating, the molten web is the sheet that is extruded by the die, and the substrate web is the material being coated. (2) Any continuous length of sheet material handled in roll form, as contrasted with the same material cut into sheets.

Web Coating See EXTRUSION COATING, SPREAD COATING.

Webbing Filaments or threads that may form when adhesive transfer surfaces are forcibly separated.

Weft The transverse threads or fibers in a woven fabric. Those fibers running perpendicular to the length of the loom. See also WARP.

Weight-Average Molecular Weight (M_w). The first moment of a plot of the weight of polymer in each molecular weight range against molecular weight. The value can be estimated by light scattering or sedimentation equilibrium measurements. See also MOLECULAR WEIGHT, MOLECULAR WEIGHT DISTRIBUTION.

Welding Permanent joining of two or more pieces of plastic by fusion at adjoining or nearby areas, with or without the addition of plastic from another source.

Wet Flexural Strength The flexural strength measured after boiling the specimen in water for a certain period of time.

Wetting The tendency of a liquid to spread over another surface. Perfect wetting occurs if the surface tension of the spreading liquid is much higher than the surface tension of the substrate; in this case the wetting angle is zero. Conversely, in poor wetting, the wetting angle is 180 degrees, as seen when liquid mercury droplets fall on a glass surface.

Wetting Agents Compounds that cause a liquid to penetrate more easily, or to spread over the surface of another material.

White Blood Cell (Lymphocyte). A constituent of blood, formed in the bone marrow and the lymph glands. They protect against body infection, participate in rejection reactions, and constitute some of the cells that adhere to the surfaces of biomaterials implanted in circulating blood.

Working Life (Pot Life). The period during which a reactive compound, after mixing with catalyst, coreactants, or other compounding ingredients, remains at a viscosity suitable for further use.

Worst Case A set of conditions encompassing upper and lower processing limits and circumstances, including those within standard operating procedures, which pose the greatest chance of process failure when compared to ideal conditions. Such conditions do not necessarily induce product or process failure.

Wound Any disruption in the anatomy or physiology of tissue. Wounds are caused either surgically or accidentally, e.g., burns or trauma. Wounds vary in severity from a minor skin scratch to complicated trauma.

Wound Culture   A laboratory procedure to determine whether a wound is infected, and to identify the microorganism(s) that cause the infection.

WVT   Abbreviation for *Water Vapor Transmission.*

WVTR   Abbreviation for *Water Vapor Transmission Rate.*

Xenogeneic   In transplantation biology, denoting individuals or tissues from individuals of different species and hence of disparate cell type.

Xenograft   A graft of tissue transplanted between animals of different species; the older term was *Heterograft.*

Xenon Arc Light Aging   A test for evaluating the light stability of polymers. The test utilizes a xenon gas discharge lamp, which emits radiation duplicating the spectrum of natural sunlight better than most artificial sources.

XPS Derivatization   An analytical technique in which surface organic groups such as carbonyl, hydroxyl, and carboxy are treated with selective organic reagents, prior to XPS analysis.

X-radiation   (Roentgen Rays, X-rays). Electromagnetic radiation of short wavelength (0.06 to 120 Å), emitted as a result of electron transitions in the inner orbits of heavy atoms bombarded by cathode rays in a vacuum tube. Its properties are: (1) Penetration of solids of moderate density, such as human tissue; retarded by bone, barium sulfate, bismuth, lead, and other dense materials. (2) Ionization of gases. (3) Ability to damage or destroy diseased tissue.

X-ray Microscopy   The technique of examining X-rays by means of a microscope. In a variation called Point Projection Microscopy, an enlarged image is obtained from X-rays emitted from a pinhole source. This technique is useful for the characterization of foamed plastics, laminates, fibers, and multifilaments.

X-ray Photoelectron Spectroscopy (XPS, ESCA)   A variation of Electron Spectroscopy where X-ray photons (electrons ejected from an atom under X-ray bombardment) produce primary photoelectrons. By measuring the kinetic energy of photoelectrons ejected, a fingerprint characteristic of individual atoms (above hydrogen) is obtained. This is truly a surface probe, since XPS measures a maximum depth of 40–50 Å of the surface.

Yarn   A geometric collection of fibers laid or twisted together, ready for the production of textiles, which are spun or woven from these yarns. The number of filaments may vary from one (monofilament), to several hundred (multifilament), but is usually in the range of 15–100.

Yield Value   In viscosity measurements, yield value is (1) the force that must be applied to a fluid layer before any observable movement is produced; (2) the stress at which a marked increase in deformation occurs, without an increase in load.

Young's Modulus   The ratio of tensile stress to tensile strain below the proportional limit. See also MODULUS OF ELASTICITY.

Zahn Viscosity Cup   A small hand-held U-shaped cup, with an orifice of any of five sizes. The cup is completely immersed into the test fluid, and quickly withdrawn. The time in seconds from the moment the top of the cup emerges from the fluid until the stream from the orifice first breaks is a measure of viscosity.

Z-Calender   A calender with four rolls arranged in a geometric cross section resembling the letter Z.

Zeta Potential   (Electrokinetic Potential). The potential across the interface of all solids and liquids. Specifically, the potential across the diffuse layer of ions surrounding a charged colloidal particle, which is largely responsible for colloidal stability.

Ziegler Catalysts   A large family of catalysts made by reacting a compound of a transition metal chosen from groups IV through VIII of the periodic table with an alkyl, hydride, or other compound of a metal from groups I through III. Typically, titanium chloride is added to aluminum alkyl in a hydrocarbon solvent to form a dispersion or precipitate of the catalyst complex. Originally developed by Karl Ziegler for the polymerization of ethylene, G. Natta subsequently showed that similar catalysts are useful in the synthesis of stereoregular polyolefins.

Zone Electrophoresis   ELECTROPHORESIS in which a protein is held in a rigid, narrow hydrophobic matrix across which an electric field is applied. After the protein components are separated electrophoretically and stained, the concentrations may be calculated since optical density is proportional to the amount of the protein component.

Zymogen   (Proenzyme). The inactive precursor of an enzyme, from which the active enzyme is derived by cleavage of peptide fragment(s). Many monomeric enzymes are first produced as zymogens.

APPENDIX I

POLYMERS IN MEDICAL APPLICATIONS

POLYMER	APPLICATION
Acrylics	Hemostatic agents; bone replacement; corneas; facial prosthesis
Cellulose	Dialysis membranes
Cellulose acetate	Nerve regeneration; packaging material; dialysis membranes
Copolymer silicone— polyurethane (Avcothane®)	Left ventricular assist devices; intra-aortic balloon devices
Epichlorohydrin rubber (Hydrin®)	Flexible mold; impression material; dental applications
Fluorocarbons	Blood vessels; reconstructive surgery
Gelatin/resorcinol formaldehyde	Tissue adhesives
Polyacrylic acid	Dental cement
Polyacrylonitrile (PAN)	Dialysis membranes
Polyalkylsulfone	Membrane oxygenators
Polyamide (Nylon 6)	Sutures
Polyamides	Syringes; blood transfusion sets; vascular implants
Polycarbonate (Lexan®)	General use oxygenator valve occluders; cranioplasty
Polycarbonates	Syringes; containers
Polycyanoacrylates	Tissue adhesives
Polydihydroxypropyl methacrylate	Antithrombogenic surfaces; tubing; plastic surgery; drug release; contact lenses
Polyethylene	Tubing; syringes; heart valves; knee joints

POLYMER	APPLICATION
Polyethylene (high molecular weight)	Orthopedic; acetabular cup
Polyethylene terephthalate	Woven vascular prostheses; heart valve suture rings
Polyformaldehyde (Delrin®)	Heart valve occluders; general structural polymer
Polyglycolic acid	Resorbable sutures
Polyhydroxyethyl-methacrylate	Antithrombogenic surfaces; tubing; plastic surgery; drug release; contact lenses
Polymethylmethacrylate	Neurosurgery; cranioplasty; orthopedics; grout for artificial joints; ophthalmolgy lenses; contact lenses; dental
Polyphenoxy	Oxygenator membranes
Polypropylene	Syringes; catheters; oxygenators; dialysis; heart valves; occluders; sutures; bones and joints
Polysulfide rubber (mercaptan)	Dental impressions
Polytetrafluoroethylene (Teflon TFE®)	Orthopedics; coating stem prostheses; coating tips; neurosurgery; aneurism clips
Polytetrafluoroethylene-hexafluoropropylene copolymer (Teflon FEP®)	Orthopedics
Polyurethanes	Plastic surgery; biodegradable sutures; artificial hearts; catheters
Polyurethanes (segmented)	Catheters; tubing; artificial heart ventricles; pumps
Polyvinyl chloride	Surgical tubing; blood collection and administration; blood vessels sets; blood bags; bubble oxygenators; oxygenator and dialysis tubing; catheters
Resin: diglycidyl ether of bisphenol A (DGEBA)	Packaging pacemakers; central restorations
Silicones	Tubing; catheters; lubricants; tissue substitutes; heart and related components
Silicone-polycarbonate copolymer	Oxygenator membranes

APPENDIX II

DRUG-RELATED DEVICES CLASSIFICATION

FDA CLASSIFICATION	DEVICE NAME	21 CFR SECTION	CLASS
1. ANESTHESIOLOGY			
	Bourdon gauge flowmeter	868.2300	II
	Thrope tube flowmeter (uncomp)	868.2320	II
	Thrope tube flowmeter (comp)	868.2340	II
	Anesthesia conduction catheter	868.5120	II
	Anesthesia conduction filter	868.5130	II
	Anesthesia conduction needle, gas machines, or analgesia	868.5150	II
	Laryngotracheal topical anesthesia applicator	868.5170	II
	Anesthesia breathing circuit	868.5240	II
	Nasal oxygen cannula	868.5340	I
	Nasal oxygen catheter	868.5350	I
	Nonrebreathing mask	868.5570	II
	Oxygen mask	868.5580	II
	Scavenging mask	868.5590	II
	Venturi mask	868.5590	II
	Medical nonventilatory nebulizer (atomizer)	868.5640	I
	Portable liquid O_2 unit	868.5655	II
	Nonpowered oxygen tent	868.5700	II
	Electric-powered O_2 tent	868.5710	II
	Anesthetic vaporizer	868.5880	II
	Manual emergency ventilator	868.5915	II
	Powered emergency ventilator	868.5925	II

FDA CLASSIFICATION	DEVICE NAME	21 CFR SECTION	CLASS
2. CARDIOVASCULAR			
	Continuous-flush catheter	870.1210	II
	Percutaneous catheter	870.1250	II
	Prog. diagnostic computer	870.1425	II
	Single-function, preprogrammed diagnostic computer	870.1435	II
	Withdrawal-infusion pump	870.1800	II
	CPB catheter, cannula, tubing	870.4210	II
	CPB fitting, stopcock, adaptor	870.4290	II
	CPB oxygenator	870.4350	II
	CPB blood reservoir	870.4400	II
3. DENTAL			
	Dental injection needle	872.4730	II
	Cartridge syringe	872.6770	II
	Perio/endodontic irr. syringe	872.6800	I
	Manual toothbrush	872.6855	I
	Powered toothbrush	872.6865	II
4. EAR, NOSE, AND THROAT			
	Nasopharyngeal catheter	874.4175	I
	ENT drug administration set	874.5220	I
5. GASTROENTEROLOGY/ UROLOGY			
	Biliary catheter and accessories	876.5010	II
	Urological catheter and acc.	876.5130	II
	Enema kit	876.5210	I
	Colonic irrigation system	876.5220	II,III
	Peritoneal dialysis system	876.5630	II
	GI tube and accessories	876.5980	II
6. GENERAL AND PLASTIC SURGERY			
	Inflatable breast prosthesis	878.3530	II
	Gauze, sponge, wound dressing	878.4060	I
	Intro/drainage catheter and acc.	878.4200	II
	Surgical drape and accessories	878.4370	II
7. GENERAL HOSPITAL AND PERSONAL USE			
	Intravenous container	880.5025	II
	Intravascular catheter	880.5200	II
	Intravasc. administ. set	880.5440	II

FDA CLASSIFICATION	DEVICE NAME	21 CFR SECTION	CLASS
	Hypodermic single-lumen needle	880.5570	II
	Infusion pump	880.5725	II
	Piston syringe	880.5860	II
	Irrigating syringe	880.6960	I
8. OBSTETRICAL/ GYNECOLOGICAL			
	Uterotubal CO_2 insufflator	884.1300	II
	OB/GYN vaginal applicator	884.4520	I
	Obstetric anesthesia set	884.5100	II
	Contraceptive diaphragm	884.5350	II
	Therapeutic vaginal douche	884.5900	II
	Vaginal insufflator	884.5920	II
9. OPHTHALMIC			
	Vitreous aspiration/cutting inst.	886.4150	III
	Ocular surg. irrigation device	886.4360	I
	Eye pad	886.4650	I
	Ophthalmic sponge	886.4790	II
10. ORTHOPEDIC			
	PMMA cement with antibiotic	888.3027	III
11. PHYSICAL MEDICINE			
	Ultrasonic diathermy	890.5300	II,III
	Iontophoresis device	890.5525	II,III

APPENDIX III

CRITICAL DEVICE (Class III) LISTING

FDA CLASSIFICATION	DEVICE NAME	21 CFR SECTION
PART 868 – ANESTHESIOLOGY DEVICES		
	Indwelling blood oxygen analyzer	868.1200
	Breathing frequency monitor	868.2375
	Emergency airway needle	868.5090
	Gas machine for anesthesia	868.5160(a)
	Anesthesia breathing circuit	868.5240
	Electroanesthesia apparatus	868.5400
	Portable oxygen generator	868.5440
	Hyperbaric chamber	868.5470
	Membrane lung for chronic support	868.5610
	Esophageal obturator	868.5650
	Bronchial tube	868.5720
	Tracheal tube	868.5730
	Tracheal/bronchial diff vent.tube	868.5740
	Inflatable tracheal tube cuff	868.5750
	Tracheostomy tube and tube cuff	868.5800
	Airway connector	868.5810
	Autotransfusion apparatus	868.5830
	Continuous ventilator	868.5895
	Noncontinuous ventilator (IPPB)	868.5905
	Manual emergency ventilator	868.5915
	Powered emergency ventilator	868.5935
PART 870 – CARDIOVASCULAR DEVICES		
	Arrhythmia detector and alarm	870.1025
	Catheter guide wire	870.1330

Appendix III

FDA CLASSIFICATION	DEVICE NAME	21 CFR SECTION
	Trace microsphere	870.1360
	External programmable pacemaker pulse generator	870.1750
	Withdrawal infusion pump	870.1800
	Vascular clip	870.3520
	Vena cava clip	870.3260
	Arterial embolization device	870.3300
	Cardiovascular intravascular filter	870.3375
	Vascular grafts <6 mm DIA	870.3540
	Vascular grafts >6 mm DIA	870.3460
	Intracardiac patch or pledget	870.3470
	Intra-aortic ballon and control system	870.3535
	Ventricular bypass (assist) device	870.3545
	External pacemaker pulse generator	870.3600
	Implantable pacemaker pulse generator	870.3610
	Pacemaker, lead adaptor	870.3620
	Pacemaker polymeric mesh bag	870.3650
	Pacemaker charger	870.3670
	Cardiovascular permanent or temporary pacemaker electrode	870.3680
	Pacemaker programmers	870.3700
	Pacemaker repair or replacement material	870.3710
	Annuloplasty ring	870.3800
	Carotid sinus nerve stimulator	870.3850
	Replacement heart valve	870.3925
	CPB pulsatile flow generator	870.4320
	CPB bypass oxygenator	870.4350
	Nonroller-type CPB blood pump	870.4360
	Roller-type CPB blood pump	870.4370
	External cardiac compressor	870.5200
	External counter-pulsating device	870.5225
	DC-defibrillator (including paddles)	870.5300
	External transcutaneous cardiac pacemaker (noninvasive)	870.5550
	Percutaneous transluminal coronary angioplasty (PTCA) ballon dilation cath.	–
	Automatic implanted cardioverter defibrillator system	–

FDA CLASSIFICATION	DEVICE NAME	21 CFR SECTION
PART 872 – DENTAL DEVICES		
	Endosseous implant	872.3640
PART 874 – EAR, NOSE, AND THROAT DEVICES		
	ENT synthetic polymer material	874.3620
	Mandibular implant facial prosthesis	874.3695
	Laryngeal prosthesis (Taub design)	874.3730
	Endolymphatic shunt	874.3820
	Endolymphatic shunt tube with valve	874.3850
	Tympanostomy tube with semipermeable membrane	874.3930
	ENT natural polymer-collagen material	–
PART 876 – GASTROENTEROLOGY-UROLOGY DEVICES		
	Penile inflatable implant	876.3350
	Implanted electrical urinary continence device	876.5270
	A-V shunt cannula	876.5540
	Peritoneal dialysis system and acc.	876.5630
	Hemodialysis system and acc.	876.5820
	Sorbent hemoperfusion system	876.6870
	Isolated kidney perfusion and transport system and acc.	876.6880
	Peritoneo-venous shunt	876.5955
	Urethral sphincter prosthesis	–
	Urethral replacement	–
PART 878 – GENERAL AND PLASTIC SURGERY DEVICES		
	Absorbable surgical sutures	–
	Nonabsorbable surgical sutures	–
	PTFE (Teflon) injectable	–
	Surgical mesh	878.3300
	PTFE with carbon fibers composite implant material	878.3500
	Silicone gel-filled breast prosthesis	878.3540
	Implanted mammary prosthesis of composite saline/gel-filled design	–
	Esophageal prosthesis	878.3610

FDA CLASSIFICATION	DEVICE NAME	21 CFR SECTION
	Tracheal prosthesis	878.3720
	Implantable clip	878.4300
	Implantable staple	878.4750
	Maxillofacial prosthesis	–

PART 880 – GENERAL HOSPITAL AND PERSONAL USE DEVICES

	Infant radiant warmer	880.5130
	Neonatal incubator	880.5400
	Neonatal transport incubator	880.5410
	Infusion pump	880.5725
	Implanted infusion pump	–

PART 882 – NEUROLOGICAL DEVICES

	Methyl methacrylate for aneurysmorrhaphy	882.5030
	Intravascular occluding catheter	882.5150
	Aneurysm clip	882.5200
	Implanted malleable clip	882.5225
	Burr hole cover	882.5250
	Methyl methacrylate for cranioplasty	882.5300
	Preformed alterable cranioplasty plate	882.5320
	Preformed nonalterable cranioplasty plate	882.5330
	Cranioplasty plate fastener	882.5360
	Central nervous system fluid shunt and components	882.5550
	Implanted cerebral stimulator	882.5820
	Implanted diaphragmatic/phrenic nerve stimulator	882.5830
	Implanted intracerebral/subcortical stimulator for pain relief	882.5870
	Implanted spinal cord stimulator for bladder evacuation	882.5850
	Implanted neuromuscular stimulator	882.5860
	Implanted peripheral nerve stimulator for pain relief	882.5870
	Implanted spinal cord stimulator for pain relief	882.5880
	Epidural spinal electrode	882.5890
	Preformed craniosynostosis strip	882.5900
	Dura substitute	882.5910

FDA CLASSIFICATION	DEVICE NAME	21 CFR SECTION
	Artificial embolization device	882.5950
	Lyophilized human (cadaver) dura mater	—
	Stabilized epidural spinal electrode	—
	Implanted intracranial pressure monitor	—
	Totally implanted spinal cord stimulator for pain relief	—

PART 884 – OBSTETRICAL AND GYNECOLOGICAL DEVICES

	Contraceptive intrauterine device (IUD) and introducer	884.5360
	Contraceptive tubal occlusion device (TOD) and introducer	884.5380

PART 886 – OPHTHALMIC DEVICES

	Absorbable implant (scleral bucking method)	886.3300
	Keratoprosthesis	886.3400
	Intraocular lens	886.3600
	Eye valve implant	886.3920